THE PERICARDIUM

Developments in Cardiovascular Medicine

232. A. Bayés de Luna, F. Furlanello, B.J. Maron and D.P. Zipes (eds.):
      Arrhythmias and Sudden Death in Athletes. 2000   ISBN: 0-7923-6337-X
233. J-C. Tardif and M.G. Bourassa (eds): *Antioxidants and Cardiovascular Disease*.
      2000.   ISBN: 0-7923-7829-6
234. J. Candell-Riera, J. Castell-Conesa, S. Aguadé Bruiz (eds): *Myocardium at
      Risk and Viable Myocardium Evaluation by SPET*. 2000.ISBN: 0-7923-6724-3
235. M.H. Ellestad and E. Amsterdam (eds): *Exercise Testing: New Concepts for the
      New Century*. 2001.   ISBN: 0-7923-7378-2
236. Douglas L. Mann (ed.): *The Role of Inflammatory Mediators in the Failing
      Heart*. 2001   ISBN: 0-7923-7381-2
237. Donald M. Bers (ed.): *Excitation-Contraction Coupling and Cardiac
      Contractile Force, Second Edition*. 2001   ISBN: 0-7923-7157-7
238. Brian D. Hoit, Richard A. Walsh (eds.): *Cardiovascular Physiology in the
      Genetically Engineered Mouse, Second Edition*. 2001 ISBN 0-7923-7536-X
239. Pieter A. Doevendans, A.A.M. Wilde (eds.): *Cardiovascular Genetics for Clinicians*
      2001   ISBN 1-4020-0097-9
240. Stephen M. Factor, Maria A.Lamberti-Abadi, Jacobo Abadi (eds.): *Handbook of
      Pathology and Pathophysiology of Cardiovascular Disease*. 2001
                                                         ISBN 0-7923-7542-4
241. Liong Bing Liem, Eugene Downar (eds): *Progress in Catheter Ablation*. 2001
                                                         ISBN 1-4020-0147-9
242. Pieter A. Doevendans, Stefan Kääb (eds): *Cardiovascular Genomics: New
      Pathophysiological Concepts*. 2002   ISBN 1-4020-7022-5
243. Daan Kromhout, Alessandro Menotti, Henry Blackburn (eds.): *Prevention
      of Coronary Heart Disease: Diet, Lifestyle and Risk Factors in the Seven
      Countries Study*. 2002   ISBN 1-4020-7123-X
244. Antonio Pacifico (ed.), Philip D. Henry, Gust H. Bardy, Martin Borggrefe,
      Francis E. Marchlinski, Andrea Natale, Bruce L. Wilkoff (assoc. eds):
      Implantable Defibrillator Therapy: A Clinical Guide. 2002
                                                         ISBN 1-4020-7143-4
245. Hein J.J. Wellens, Anton P.M. Gorgels, Pieter A. Doevendans (eds.):
      *The ECG in Acute Myocardial Infarction and Unstable Angina: Diagnosis and Risk
      Stratification*. 2002   ISBN 1-4020-7214-7
246. Jack Rychik, Gil Wernovsky (eds.): *Hypoplastic Left Heart Syndrome*. 2003
                                                         ISBN 1-4020-7319-4
247. Thomas H. Marwick: *Stress Echocardiography*. Its Role in the Diagnosis and
      Evaluation of Coronary Artery Disease 2nd Edition. 2003
                                                         ISBN 1-4020-7369-0
248. Akira Matsumori: *Cardiomyopathies and Heart Failure: Biomolecular, Infectious
      and Immune Mechanisms*. 2003   ISBN 1-4020-7438-7

249. Ralph Shabetai: *The Pericardium* 2003   ISBN 1-4020-7639-8

Previous volumes are still available

THE PERICARDIUM

Ralph Shabetai, M.D., F.R.C.P. (Edin), F.A.C.P., F.A.C.C.
Professor of Medicine, University of California, San Diego, CA

Kluwer Academic Publishers
Boston/Dordrecht/London

Distributors for North, Central and South America:
Kluwer Academic Publishers
101 Philip Drive
Assinippi Park
Norwell, Massachusetts 02061 USA
Telephone (781) 871-6600
Fax (781) 681-9045
E-Mail: kluwer@wkap.com

Distributors for all other countries:
Kluwer Academic Publishers Group
Post Office Box 322
3300 AH Dordrecht, THE NETHERLANDS
Telephone 31 786 576 000
Fax 31 786 576 254
E-Mail: services@wkap.nl

 Electronic Services < http://www.wkap.nl>

Library of Congress Cataloging-in-Publication Data

A C.I.P. Catalogue record for this book is available
from the Library of Congress.

The Pericardium by Ralph Shabetai
ISBN 1-4020-7639-8

Permission for books published in Europe: permissions@wkap.nl
Permissions for books published in the United States of America: permissions@wkap.com

Printed on acid-free paper.

Printed in the United States of America.

The Publisher offers discounts on this book for course use and bulk purchases.
For further information, send email to <Melissa Ramondetta@wkap.com>.

Dedication

I dedicate this book to the memory of my beloved daughter Karen.

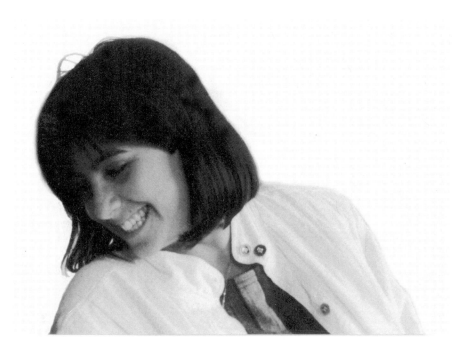

Contents

Preface

Many noteworthy advances in our knowledge of the pericardium, its functions and diseases and their relation to heart failure have been made since the first edition of this book appeared in 1981; and no other book that covers in detail the physiology and pathophysiology has since been published. The first edition was favourably received, and I have frequently been asked to write a new edition. My own knowledge in the years that have passed since then, and my clinical and research experience in the field of the subject have both increased. For all these reasons, I decided that the second edition was overdue. The long time that has elapsed between editions necessitated rewriting, rather than simply revising, most of the text. For the same reason, many of the figures are new. Most of the references I have cited appeared in the literature after 1981, but I have retained a number of earlier ones, either because they are classics or, in my opinion, have not yet been bettered. It is my hope that the new edition will be a useful resource for clinicians called upon to manage patients with pericardial disease and for physiologists when the pericardium is relevant to their investigations. I make no apology for the in-depth treatment of the pericardial physiology and pathophysiology throughout the book, for they are the foundation on which diagnosis, hemodynamic and imaging studies, and management must rest. It is often instructive, as well as fascinating, to trace the origin of ideas underlying current concepts of pericardial physiology, pathophysiology and diseases. I have therefore included some brief sections on historical background in the hope that they will make the volume more enjoyable.

Ralph Shabetai
La Jolla, CA, 2003

Acknowledgments

I am happy to express my gratitude to the late Noble O. Fowler M.D. who, in 1961, encouraged me to begin investigating the pericardium and its diseases. He continued to stimulate this research during the time we were both at the University of Cincinnati, and subsequently after I had moved, first to the University of Kentucky, and then to the University of California, San Diego. In San Diego, James Covell M.D. provided the needed laboratory space and was ever ready with insights and practical help with the experiments. Many of the cardiology faculty members and fellows there contributed to my research, and then branched out into their own pericardial research while they remained in San Diego and after they had left to assume more senior positions elsewhere. In this capacity, I must especially acknowledge Martin M. LeWinter M.D., Brian D Hoit M.D., and Gregory Freeman M.D. My thanks are also owing to the many physicians worldwide who consulted me about difficult or particularly interesting cases or new research ideas.

A deep debt of gratitude that I will never be able to adequately repay is owing to my dear wife, Estelle, for her incomparable editorial assistance and thoughtful evaluation of every chapter, without which I could never have completed the work. She willingly gave up much of her time, and made it as much her objective as my own to see the work completed. I thank V. Bhargava Ph.D. for scanning and his skill in enhancing the figures, and Melissa Romandetta, my editor at Kluwer Academic, for her encouragement and much helpful advice.

Chapter 1

ANATOMY

The entire heart is covered with a certain membranous involucrum, to which it is joined at no point. This involucrum is much more ample than the heart and is moistened by an aqueous humour. (Realdus Columbus, De Re Anatomica, 1599)

The pericardium is something of an enigma. Like the vermiform appendix, we can very well do without it, yet when it becomes diseased it can, because of its strategic position, place a stranglehold around the heart and thus threaten life itself.

The pericardium has another peculiarity: while seldom the primary seat of a systemic disease, it may be involved in almost every such disease. In some instances pericardial involvement overshadows all other features of the systemic disease, whereas in others, pericardial involvement may escape detection, unless specifically sought out. Pericardial disease is a successful mimic; for example, pericardial pain may simulate that of a thoracic catastrophe such as acute myocardial infarction, pulmonary embolus, or dissecting hematoma of the aorta. The pericardial friction rub may be a patient's most dramatic physical sign, but it may simulate a cardiac murmur. Pulsus paradoxus seldom fails to excite the interest of physicians, but may be mistaken for pulsus alternans or arrhythmia, especially when the examiner is not suspecting cardiac tamponade. Finally, the electrocardiographic abnormalities may be alarmingly like those of ischemic heart disease.

This chapter deals with the structure of the pericardium. In a discussion of the structure of an organ, one should perhaps avoid too teleological an argument. Although Galen stated "nature has made nothing without reason," to concede that the pericardium has specific functions does not prove that it was designed to carry out these functions. Rather, as is so often the case in nature, the functions may come about by chance, and the pericardium may exert its influence on the heart and circulation simply because of its structure and location - a stiff membrane that closely envelops the heart, the origins of the great arteries and the terminations of the great veins. Possession of a protective membrane is not unique to the heart, since all important organs of the body are enveloped in an invaginated membrane that contains a small volume of fluid between its layers. The heart is not different in this regard, but in regard to its vulnerability to serious effects from a relatively small effusion or modest fibrosis.

1.   GROSS ANATOMY

A pericardium is found in vertebrates ranging from the lower forms to humans, and it has been studied in a wide variety of animals. It is commonly stated that the human pericardium is up to three millimetres thick. Measurements from autopsy, computer assisted tomograms, magnetic resonance images and trans-oesophageal echocardiograms agree fairly closely. A recent study, however, using high resolution computerized tomography in 100 patients found that the thinnest portion of the pericardium measured 1.2 using 10 mm. slices and 0.7 using 1 mm. slices (*Bull, Edwards, Dixon, 1998*) (see also Chapter 6). A study using magnetic resonance imaging visualized an average pericardial length of 60 mm. The average thickness was 1.7 mm (range 1.5 - 2 mm.) (*White 1995*).

1.1   Layers of the pericardium

The mammalian pericardium comprises a serous membrane, composed of a single layer of mesothelial cells and a fibrous outer layer. The inner layer is intimately applied to the surface of the heart and epicardial fat, where it constitutes the visceral pericardium. It is reflected back so that it lines the inner aspect of the fibrous pericardium, together with which it forms the parietal pericardium.

1.2   Sinuses of the pericardium

A short tube-like extension encloses the origins of the aorta and pulmonary artery and is known as the arterial mesocardium. The pulmonary veins and venae cavae likewise are invested by the venous mesocardium. The oblique sinus lies behind the left atrium and within the sweep of an inverted U formed by the venous mesocardium and the transverse sinus, another serosal tunnel which lies posterior to the arterial mesocardium and anterior to the atria and superior vena cava. The transverse sinus is thus a passage between the anterior and posterior mesocardia (Figure. 1). The anatomy of the pericardial sinuses and recesses has been described in a beautiful study of human cadavers *(Choe, Im, Park 1987)*. They can be visualized on computer-assisted electron beam tomography *(Groell, Schaffler, Rienmueller 1999)* (see Chapter 6) and by trans-oesophageal echocardiography. Thin-section helical computerized tomography shows that near water density behind the pulmonary artery and its main right branch is a normal finding *(Kubota, Sato, Ohgushi 1996)*. It represents pericardial fluid in the recesses of the oblique and transverse sinuses.

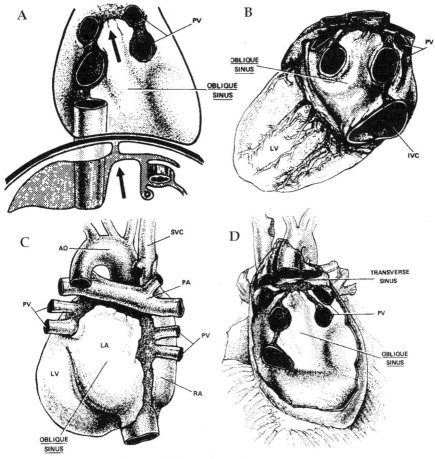

Figure 1E and legend on next page

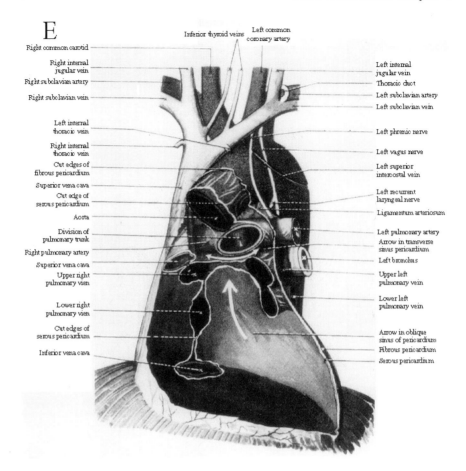

Figure 1. *Anatomy of the Pericardial Sinuses. Anatomy of the pericardial sinuses, (A) The posterior aspect of the heart viewed from the front to show the oblique sinus, which ends as a blind pouch at the level of the superior pulmonary veins (PV). (B) Posterior oblique view of the heart to show the relation of the oblique sinus to the left atrium and pulmonary veins. (C) The oblique sinus viewed from behind. LA, left atrium: PV, pulmonary veins; LV, left ventricle; AO, aorta; PA, pulmonary artery; SVC, superior vena cava; RA, right atrium. (D) Relation of the transverse sinus to the oblique sinus. The transverse sinus is a blind pouch bounded in front by the aorta and the main pulmonary artery. The postero-lateral boundaries are the atria with their appendages and the superior vena cava. (A and C from Grants JBC: Method of Anatomy, (ed. 10), 1980; B and D Modified by permission from Grants JBC: An Atlas of Anatomy, (ed 7), 1978, The Williams & Wilkins Company.) (E) Relations of the pericardium. (From Romanes GJ: Cunningham's Text Book of Anatomy (ed 10), London, Oxford University Press, 1964. Reprinted with permission.)*

The oblique sinus is important in applied anatomy because its presence means that, strictly speaking, the left atrium is not entirely an intrapericardial chamber, its posterior wall being separated from the pericardial space by the oblique sinus. This feature is thought to permit left atrial enlargement and explain *p mitrale* in constrictive pericarditis. Similarly, when an ultrasound sweep of a pericardial effusion is performed, the echo-free space often disappears as the beam is swept from the posterior wall of the left ventricle to behind the left atrium. On the other hand, a large enough pericardial effusion may enter the oblique sinus and cause the effusion to be visualized behind both the left ventricle and the left atrium.

1.3   Distribution and quantity of pericardial fluid

Normally, a small quantity of pericardial fluid is present between the two serosal layers of the pericardium. Necropsy studies have suggested that as much as 50 ml of pericardial fluid may be found in normal subjects. In dogs, the volume of pericardial fluid was measured as 0.29 ml/kg (*Santamore, Constantinescu, Bogen 1990*). Extrapolated to humans, a 75 kg subject would have approximately 30 ml of pericardial fluid This fluid prevents apposition of the visceral and parietal surfaces of the pericardium. Over the flatter surfaces of the heart, only a thin film of fluid separates the layers, whereas over the grooves that separate the cardiac chambers from each other and in the sinuses, fluid volume is more substantial. Thus only a potential space is present over much of the surface of the heart. This feature, discussed in Chapter 2, has important implications for measuring pericardial pressure and estimating the restraining effect of the pericardium on cardiac volume.

1.4   Attachments of the pericardium

The fibrous pericardium is thick and forms a flask-like sac, the neck of which is closed by its attachment to the roots of the great vessels. The thickness and strength of the fibrosa tend to vary inversely with the thickness and strength of the underlying chamber wall. The presence of strong ligaments explains why pericardial compliance *in vivo* is less than *in vitro*. The pericardium is attached anteriorly by the superior pericardiosternal ligament to the manubrium sterni and to the xiphoid process by the inferior pericardiosternal ligament, posteriorly to the vertebral column, and inferiorly to the central tendon of the diaphragm. These attachments are firm and of considerable mechanical importance. The ligament of the left superior vena cava is a triangular fold of visceral pericardium that lies between the pulmonary artery and the subjacent pulmonary veins. The fibrous pericardium blends with the adventitia of the great arteries, the cervical fascia and the central tendon of the diaphragm. It is more loosely attached to the oesophagus and descending aorta posteriorly and to the left leaf of the diaphragm inferiorly. The superior and inferior pericardiosternal ligaments are slack. The fibrous pericardium contacts the chest wall behind the fifth to the seventh costal cartilages, an area referred to as the triangle of safety, because it provides safe access for instrumentation of the pericardium (see Chapter 5).

1.5   Species differences

There are interesting and physiologically important differences in the pericardia of different species (*Elias and Boyd, 1960*). The mediastinum of dogs is extremely flimsy and the fibrous pericardium considerably less substantial than in humans; dogs also have no venous mesocardium, no triangle of safety or oblique sinus (*Spodick, 1959*). These differences should be kept in mind when the results of studies of pericardial function performed on dogs are applied to humans, and when picking an animal model for pericardial research. The fibrous pericardium is well developed in humans and pigs, and attachment to the diaphragm is extensive; the horse has strong attachments to the sternum and in herbivore in general the fibrous layer tends to be thick.

The lower gill-breathing vertebrates lack a thoracic cavity with rhythmically fluctuating pressure and gas-filled lungs surrounding the pericardium. Instead, the pericardium is located within, and is firmly attached to a single body cavity, in which respiratory variations in pressure and dimensions are considerably less than in mammals and, therefore, respiratory variations on hemodynamics are diminished. In the elasmobranch, the pericardium is composed of dense fibrous tissue firmly attached to the cartilaginous skeleton, except in its caudal surface. The only part of the elasmobranch pericardium that resembles the mammalian is thus the caudal surface (septum) that separates the heart from the peritoneal cavity. Other distinguishing features are the large ratio of pericardial to cardiac volume, failure of the pericardial cavity to collapse after the heart is removed and, most intriguing of all, the presence of a canal that allows one way transfer of fluid from the pericardial to the peritoneal cavity (*Shabetai, Abel, Graham 1985*). The function of this canal is discussed in Chapter 2. The pericardium of the African lungfish surrounds the heart like a rigid box, thereby providing an excellent model for the study of the effects of the pericardium on hemodynamics (*Johansen, Lenfant, Hanson 1968*).

1.6   Pericardial weight

We owe much of our knowledge of the gross structure of the pericardium to Dr. Joseph P. Holt who did significant original work on this subject (*Holt,*

Rhode, Kines 1960) and published comprehensive reviews (*Holt 1970*). In one review, he showed that just as heart weight in normal adult mammals is a function of body weight, so too is the thickness of the pericardium. The pericardium of the horse is about 15 times thicker than that of the rabbit. Hort and Braun *(1962)* published a graph of the weight in mg/cm^2 of parietal pericardium from rabbits, dogs, swine, cattle, horses, and humans. They assumed the specific gravity of the pericardium to be essentially the same in all mammals and therefore the weight of the pericardium was taken as proportional to the wall thickness (Figure 2). Humans fall somewhat above the line of best fit, suggesting that, regarding this particular attribute at least, we are superior to the lower animals.

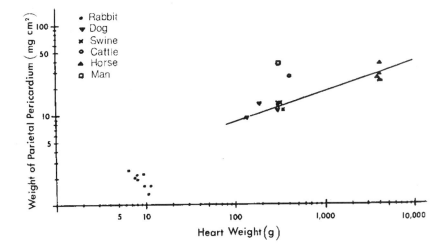

Figure 2. Heart Weight versus Pericardial Weight. Relation between heart weight and an average square centimeter of the parietal pericardium in rabbits, dogs, swine, cattle, horses and humans. (From Hort and Braun, quoted by Holt). Assuming the specific gravity of the pericardium is approximately the same in all mammals, the weight of 1 cm^2 is proportional to the wall thickness. Note that the thickness of the pericardium increases with the size of the heart. *(From Holt JP. The normal pericardium. Am J Cardiol 1970; 26:455-465. Reprinted with permission.)*

1.7   Pericardial fluid and the lymphatic system

Surprisingly little is known about the formation and removal of pericardial fluid. This regrettable deficiency is due in part to the paucity of comprehensive studies, especially in human subjects, and in part to the difficulties in distinguishing between the dynamics of normal pericardial fluid and those of an abnormal effusion. Confusion may be lessened by distinction between cardiac lymph and pericardial fluid. The details of lymphatic drainage of the pericardium, whether the same as, or different from ventricular lymphatic drainage, and whether principally to the right lymphatic duct, or to the thoracic duct, is still disputed. Even the fundamental question of whether pericardial fluid is an ultrafiltrate of plasma or merely excess fluid weeping from the epicardium, much as fluid weeps from the cirrhotic liver to form ascites, is unsettled. For sheep, it has been estimated by experiments that mediastinal lymphatic pathways remove a volume equivalent to the pericardial volume every 5.4 to 7.2 hours (*Boulanger, Yuan, Flessner 1999*).

The haemodynamic substrate should also be considered; for instance, the force of systole may influence the rate of lymph drainage and the central venous pressure, and thus the pressure in the right lymphatic and thoracic ducts. Therefore, the heartbeat modulates the rate of fluid removal from the heart and pericardium. The effects of lymphatic blockage are discussed in Chapter 3.

1.7.1   Active constituents of pericardial fluid

The number of biologically active substances and their significance is too large to permit comprehensive treatment here. Many of these are associated with specific diseases and will be discussed in that context in subsequent chapters. Normal pericardial fluid is clear in appearance. Much of the more recent data originate from studies of pericardial fluid obtained during thoracotomy. Investigators are endeavouring to establish databases. The recent development of techniques to sample pericardial fluid through a catheter in the absence of a pericardial effusion may contribute a new source of material, although it is very unlikely that any of the techniques would be routinely employed in normal subjects. Prostoglandin, cyclo-oxygenase, synthetase (*Herman, Claeys, Moncada 1978*) and 6 keto-PGE1$_{alpha}$ have been identified in rabbit pericardial fluid.

Both atrial naturetic peptide (ANP) and brain naturetic peptide (BNP) are present in pericardial fluid. Pericardial concentration of both peptides is higher than in plasma, suggesting that, at least in part, the source is not ultrafiltration of plasma but directly from the myocardial interstitium. Ventricular dysfunction is associated with greatly increased pericardial BNP, but only slightly elevated ANP (*Tanaka, Hasegawa, Fujita 1998*). It is possible that ANP and BNP exert paracrine and autocrine influences, since it is known that when isolated myocytes are exposed to these peptides, functional changes are observed. Furthermore, both ANP and BNP increase the production of $_c$GMP. They also inhibit DNA synthesis in cardiac fibroblasts and thus may modify cardiac remodeling in heart failure. In the bloodstream, they are diuretic, naturetic and vasodilators; thus their role in heart failure is complex and awaits clarification. The concentration of ANP in normal dogs exceeds that of plasma (*Szokodi, Horkay, Kiss 1997*).

Endothelin-1 in pericardial fluid may also exert autocrine or paracrine influence on cardiac function. Endothelin-1 is found in high concentration in the pericardial fluid of patients undergoing cardiac surgery (*Rubanyi and Polokoff 1994*). Furthermore, cultured rat pericardial mesothelial cells produce endothelin-1 and possess endothelin ET_B receptors. Endothelins increase intracellular concentration of calcium in pericardial mesothelial cells.

These findings support the opinion that pericardial endothelin functions in an autocrine or paracrine fashion, in this case, on signal transduction (*Kuwahara and Kuwahara, 1998*).

Methods of collection, storage and measurement influence determinations of complement in pericardial fluid. Kinney et al. *(1979)* determined normal ranges of pericardial fluid content of C3, C4, and CH50 were 35 to 127 mg/l, 6.3 to 23 mg/l and 1.9 to 9.1 units respectively. The comparative values for serum are C3, 70 to 176 mg/l; C4, 16 to 45 mg/l; and 25 to 30 units for CH50. The normal ranges are narrow, allowing for easy recognition of abnormal values. (See also Chapters 3 and 9.)

1.7.2   Anatomy of the pericardial and cardiac lymphatics

The classic descriptions are those of Patek (1939) and Kampmeier (1929), which include the embryology. The arrangement of lymphatic vessels is complex. The dog has an extensive subpericardial plexus with drainage vessels divided into five orders that accompany the blood vessels and empty into a single vessel and lymph node. There is also a myocardial plexus, uniform in density from endocardium to epicardium which drains into the subpericardial plexus. Controversy exists regarding whether or not the cardiac valve cusps are supplied by lymphatics (*Symbas, Schlant, Gravanis 1969)* and, if so, whether they play a role in thickening of the valves by disease processes.

Miller et al. (1961) and Leeds et al. (1977) demonstrated that, in dogs, the earlier view (*Courtice and Simmonds 1954*), that lymph from the pericardium drains almost exclusively to the right lymphatic duct, was in error, but drains via multiple pathways into both the right lymphatic duct and the thoracic duct. The complexity of this system may play an important role in the prevention or amelioration of the effects of lymphatics by neoplasm or inflammation. Uhley et al. (1969) found a fourfold increase in lymph flow after complete ligation of the coronary sinus, but (and of greater interest) cardiac lymph flow did not increase in congestive heart failure, although apparently it does during hypoxia (*Drinker, Warren, Maurer 1940*). In a more recent study, Miller, whose major research interest over the past several decades has been the cardiac lymphatic system, studied the pericardial lymphatics in 35 human cadavers with more recent associates, and gave a detailed account of regional lymph drainage (*Eliskova, Eliska, Miller 1995*). The lymphatics that drain the thoracic surface of the diaphragm and the postero-inferior pericardium have been described in detail after a study of 68 cadavers (*Shimada, Fujii, Sato 1995*) (only the abstract is in English).

It is commonly held that pericardial fluid and cardiac lymph drain by the same route. Uhley et al. *(1969)* used micropulverized barium sulphate to demonstrate radiographically that both the pericardium and myocardium drained to the pretracheal and thence to the cardiac lymph nodes, with some additional drainage from the pericardium to retrosternal nodes. Thanikachalam et al. (1978), using radio-opaque contrast injected either into the myocardium or into pericardial space, found that drainage of the former was via the pretracheal node to the cardiac node, whereas the pericardium drained predominantly to the retrosternal nodes. In this study, ligation of a coronary artery did not cause lymph flow to increase, but rather produced peri-infarctional stasis.

Hollenberg and Dougherty (1969) used the absorption of radioactive albumin injected into the pericardial sac of nine patients with pericardial effusion of various aetiologies to model the resorptive function of the pericardium. They reasoned that the effusions were created by increased capillary permeability in response to tissue injury, and argued that proteins do not pass back again across the capillary membrane to enter the blood directly, but rather are removed exclusively by the lymphatics. Thus the rate of removal of albumin from a pericardial effusion may be used as a measure of pericardial lymph flow. These investigators observed losses of albumin from the pericardial cavity amounting to 1.86 ± 0.57 g/day. The albumin disappeared from the pericardial cavity in exponential fashion and accumulated in corresponding concentrations in the blood. Serial precordial scans demonstrated decreasing radioactivity over the pericardium, but no activity in the pleura, indicating drainage directly into the lymphatics without transit through the pleura. This finding is not in accord with the results obtained by Gibson and Segal *(1978)*, or by Pegram and Bishop (1975), in experimental animals in which pericardial fluid was shown to drain into the lymphatic system, in part via the pleural cavity.

1.7.3 Membrane function

Pegram and Bishop (1975) postulated that the small rigidly confined pericardial space would make the heart highly prone to cardiac tamponade, unless the membrane characteristics of the pericardium and the lymphatic drainage system combined to favour removal over accumulation of pericardial fluid. To ascertain the permeability qualities of the pericardium, they measured three phenomological coefficients. These coefficients, the hydraulic coefficient (volume flow per unit of hydrostatic pressure), the reflection coefficient (ratio of the osmotic flow produced by the concentration of a test molecule to that produced by a known pressure head), and the permeability coefficient (a velocity term measured at zero volume flow, indicating the ability of substances to diffuse across a membrane) were calculated using dog and rabbit pericardium.

The investigators found large hydraulic conductances, suggesting that, with increasing pericardial fluid pressure, bulk transfer across the parietal pericardium into the pleural space takes place. This would constitute a highly favorable arrangement because, normally, pericardial pressure is only about one mmHg higher than pleural pressure, so little or no bulk transfer would occur. When pericardial pressure rises to dangerous levels, however, a large pressure gradient favouring bulk transfer of fluid from the pericardium to the pleura is developed.

1.7.4 How pericardial fluid is formed

A considerable body of evidence suggests that pericardial fluid is an ultrafiltrate of plasma. One of the better studies supporting this view (*Gibson and Segal, 1978*) found sodium and chloride concentrations were those predicted for an ultrafiltrate of plasma. Small differences in greyhounds were resolved by *in vitro* dialysis of plasma against pericardial fluid. Calcium and magnesium were present in concentrations compatible with ultrafiltration of plasma. Protein concentrations were one quarter to one third of those in plasma whereas albumin concentration was higher, reflecting its lower molecular weight and ease of transport. The osmolarity of pericardial fluid was slightly less than that of plasma, as would be anticipated for an ultrafiltrate. A particularly interesting finding in this and other studies is that potassium was present in the pericardial fluid in concentrations appreciably higher than those of plasma. This difference, which could be abolished by *in vitro* dialysis, was ascribed to "lability of the intracellular potassium during contraction." Fundamental studies of the formation and flow of cardiac lymph and pericardial fluid were published six decades ago from Drinker's famous laboratory (*Maurer, Warren, Drinker 1940; Drinker, Warren,*

Maurer 1940). The first of these was a meticulous analysis of pericardial fluid obtained from an interesting array of animals, including 34 dogs, 1 rat, 2 cats, 2 hens, 2 ducks, 7 rabbits, and 2 humans. They used the chloride levels to demonstrate that the pericardium obeys the Donnan law of membrane equilibrium, a conclusion consistent with pericardial fluid formation by filtration from the plasma. To clarify fluid dynamics, they injected horse serum and acacia intravenously and subsequently detected their presence in pericardial fluid, thereby providing further support for filtration. Soliman et al. (1966), from their studies of the physiochemical properties of pericardial fluid obtained from healthy adult camels, again confirmed that pericardial fluid is an ultrafiltrate of plasma, a view also accepted by Holt. Drinker's view was that plasma is filtered by the epicardial blood capillaries, passing through, not only their epithelial walls, but also through the epicardial endothelium. He stated, "...pericardial fluid contains the blood proteins in lower concentration than the (cardiac) lymph, owing to a double filtration; the concentration in the cardiac lymph representing the approximate concentration in the tissue fluid of the heart, and the pericardial fluid representing that of the tissue fluid, reduced slightly by a second filtration through the epicardium." Tysall and Segal (1979) used the isolated perfused rat heart to show that the rate of formation of fluid on the surface of the heart varies with the hydrostatic pressure. To that extent, their study supported the formation of pericardial fluid from myocardial interstitial fluid. The ionic content of the pericardial fluid, however, remained identical to that of the perfusate at all hydrostatic pressures, an observation more in keeping with the formation of pericardial fluid by filtration.

Miller et al., based on their extensive experimental work, adopted the opposing view that pericardial fluid is not filtered from the plasma, but is an overflow of myocardial interstitial fluid (*Miller, Ellis, Katz 1964; Miller, Pick, Johnson, 1971*). Subsequently, Miller published a scholarly but very readable book on the cardiac lymphatics, in which he detailed the surprisingly long history of the subject and reviewed all the work published on it up to that time (*Miller, 1982*).

1.7.5   Cardiac lymph flow and lymphatics

1.7.5.1   Dynamics of lymph flow

The classic descriptions are those of Patek (1939) and Kampmeier (1929). They proposed that lymphatic flow is promoted by systolic shortening of the long axis of the heart, driving lymph from the myocardial to the subepicardial lymphatic plexus, and that flow is maintained in diastole by the pressure of the heart at maximal volume against the pericardium, driving lymph from the subepicardial plexus to the main lymphatic trunks.

1.8 Pericardial volume

The total volume within the pericardium is the volume within the heart and intrapericardial portions of the great vessels together with that of the pericardial fluid. The curve relating pericardial pressure to volume is extremely steep (Figure 3) because pericardial tissue is very stiff, and the reserve volume of the pericardium is relatively small (*Fineberg 1936*).

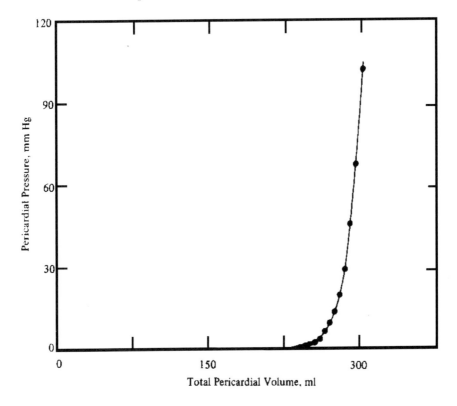

Figure 3. *Pericardial Pressure-Volume Curve. Total pericardial pressure-volume curve from a dead dog. The heart was first drained of blood and the great vessels were ligated. The pericardial space was cannulated, and fluid was slowly injected. The heart was then removed and its volume determined. The volume of the heart was added to the volume of the fluid injected to obtain the pressure-total volume curve.* (From Holt 1970. Reprinted with permission.)

The reserve volume is the amount that pericardial volume exceeds that of its contents in euvolemic subjects. This reserve explains the flat initial portion of the curve and allows for physiologic changes in cardiac volume, such as those associated with straining or changes in posture to take place without significant impact on pericardial and, therefore, transmural cardiac pressures. The importance of the steep portion of the curve is that it limits acute cardiac distension. As is discussed in Chapter 2, this same feature explains why a small but hyperacute increase in pericardial fluid volume causes severe cardiac tamponade and, conversely, why subsequent removal of only a small portion of the fluid is followed by dramatic relief.

1.9   Pericardium as bioprosthetic material

1.9.1   Model of the pericardium

Biological material should be characterized by its stress-strain relation rather than by simple pressure-volume data. Stress (force per unit area) is more relevant than pressure because it takes into consideration the dimensions and thickness of the tissue as well as the pressure exerted on it. Strain is a change in dimension from a previous state and thus is normalised to zero. Figure 4, taken from the classic work of Rabkin and Ping (1975), using canine pericardium, demonstrates its stiff nature. These authors modelled pericardium as two sets of springs connected in parallel to represent the collagen and elastic fibers (Figure 4). The collagen fibers were set initially at less than their unstretched length to take into account their wavy appearance microscopically. The springs were considered stabilised by the extension of collagen into the surrounding mediastinal structures. The initial, shallow portion of the curve is inscribed as the wavy collagen fibers gradually straighten out. The steep portion commences when the fibers are fully straightened. In this model, acute volume overload stretches the springs, which then compress the heart to limit over-distension.

A small, low-pressure effusion compresses only the lighter elastin fibers, whereas, in cardiac tamponade, the heavier collagen springs are compressed. In constrictive pericarditis, according to this model, the springs are tightly applied to the pericardium, limiting ventricular diastolic volume. The early diastolic dip of ventricular diastolic pressure is analogous to the creation of suction by sudden expansion of the springs from their compressed systolic state. When the break point of several pericardial strips is measured, variation up to an order of magnitude is found. Furthermore, when pericardial volume is increased by 8 percent, the resulting increase in pericardial pressure ranges over a considerable span (Figure 5). The model is also consistent with the hemodynamics of pericardial effusion and cardiac tamponade (Figure 6). Low-pressure effusion compresses only the elastic springs and pericardial pressure rises little. Tamponade compresses the stiffer collagen springs and pericardial pressure rises much more (Figure 6, right panel).

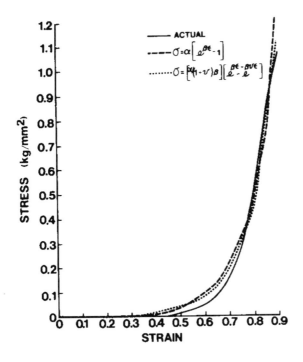

Figure 4. *Stress-strain Curve of Canine Pericardium.* (From Rabkin and Ping, 1975. Reprinted with permission.)

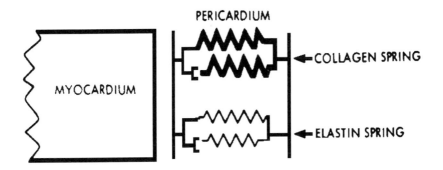

Figure 5. *Rabkin's Model of the Pericardium. The heart is the open square, the parietal pericardium is the two sets of springs connected by dashspots, and the pericardial cavity is the space between pericardium and myocardium.* (From Rabkin and Ping, 1975. Reprinted with permission.)

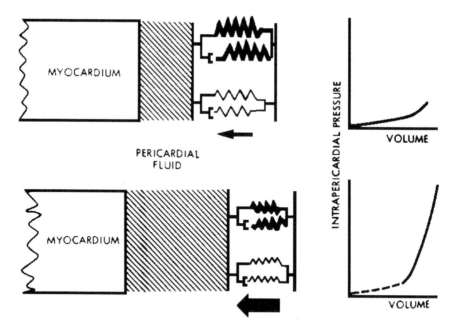

Figure 6. **Top:** *Model of pericardial effusion under slightly increased pressure, sufficient to compress the elastic springs.* **Bottom:** *Model of cardiac tamponade, which compresses the heavier collagen springs.* (From Rabkin and Ping, 1975. Reprinted with permission.)

Canine pericardium is anisotropic; furthermore, its biomechanical properties vary regionally, depending not only on its thickness, but also on the direction of the major collagen fibers. Biaxial testing is therefore more appropriate than uniaxial as a determinant of the suitability of pericardium for patching or incorporation in a bioprosthetic valve (*Sacks, Chuong, More 1994*). The region over the heart from which the pericardium is taken is likewise critical to its suitability for specific applications. While regional differences in biomechanical behaviour are not sufficient to identify a specific area for manufacturing bioprostheses, histological testing suggests that pericardium over the right ventricle is preferred (*Braile, Soars, Souza 1988*). The mechanical properties of chemically treated bovine pericardium have been reviewed in a more recent publication (*Sacks and Chuong, 1998*).

1.9.2   Pericardium as a bio-prosthesis

The parietal pericardium is composed largely of Types 1 and 3 collagen with some elastin fibers. These collagen types are also the predominant ones in natural cardiac valve leaflets. Pericardium, usually bovine, has therefore been used where a strong material that is not highly thrombogenic is required as a patch to cover natural defects, or those created intentionally by surgeons in the course of operative treatment of congenital heart disease.

Pericardium treated with gluteraldehyde has been used in a number of bioprosthetic heart valves. These valves have a better hemodynamic profile than mechanical valves or other more commonly used bioprosthetic valves, but are more prone to deterioration (*Duran, 1991*), a feature associated with gluteraldehyde treatment. Commercially prepared pericardium calcifies more slowly than pericardium preserved only by gluteraldehyde (*Quintero, Lohre, Hernandez* 1998). While bovine pericardium has much to commend it as a material from which to fashion bioprosthetic valves, its final place remains to be established (*Duran, 1991*). The wavy appearance of collagen bundles has been noted earlier in connection with the biomechanics of pericardial tissue. (*Ferrans, Hilbert, Jones 1991*). Crimping is relevant to the function of valve leaflets, because it allows them to alter their geometry in response to stress. It is thought to exert this effect by even distribution of the forces occurring in the leaflets when they open and close, and thus may prevent tears. Once crimping is fully straightened out, the collagen is virtually inextensible (mobility is critical for normal function).

The valve in pericardial extra-cardiac conduits, used for complex congenital heart disease with discontinuity between the pulmonary ventricle and the pulmonary artery, develops increasingly severe regurgitation for the first three to five years, but diminishes thereafter. Stenosis, however, is progressive for the duration of the graft (*Ando, Imai, Takanashi 1997*). Heterologous pericardium has been used to close the pericardium when closure could not be accomplished by sutures alone, but may cause reactions and therefore remains controversial (*Mills, 1986*). Glisson's capsule, alone or in combination with bovine pericardium, may be used to construct bioprostheses (*Kagramanov, Kokshenev, Dobrova 1998).*

2.   HISTOLOGY

Histological examination of the pericardium provides structural evidence supporting models based on pairs of light and heavy springs. The mesothelial cells are attached to the fibrous pericardium by delicate connective tissue rich in elastic fibers (*Holt, 1970*). Superficial, middle and deep layers of collagen fibers interlaced with elastic fibers can be distinguished within the fibrous layer. In humans, the collagen fibers are straight at birth, become increasingly wavy until young adulthood, and progressively straighten again with advancing age, suggesting that the pericardium is less compliant in the elderly (Figure 7). The contribution made by increased pericardial stiffness to altered left ventricular diastolic properties in the elderly has not been elucidated, but a first step would be to measure biaxial biomechanical properties of human pericardium across a spectrum of age.

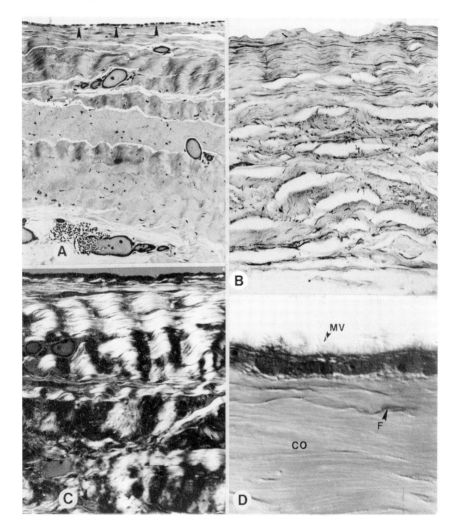

Figure 7. *Histology of Parietal Pericardium. (**A**) Sections through the entire thickness of parietal pericardium show the mesothelial cell layer (arrow heads); several layers of collagen fibres; small thin wall vessels, and a few scattered connective tissue cells. (**B**) Similar section stained by elastica-von Gieson method to demonstrate small elastic fibres (shown in black) throughout the thickness of the pericardium. (**C**) Polarized light macrograph of an area similar to (**A**) showing wavy collagen fibres. (**D**) High magnification of mesothelial cells showing microvilli (MV) and dense collagen fibres (CO). Note elongated fibroblast-like cell (F) between collagen fibers.* (Figures supplied through the courtesy of Dr. Victor Ferrans, from Ishihara, Ferrans, Jones 1980).

2.1   Electron microscopy

The pericardium is composed primarily of dense connective tissue lined on either side by mesothelial cells (Figure 8). Numerous microvilli protrude from the epicardial and parietal aspects, and they play a role in the distribution of pericardial fluid, and the gliding of the two mesothelial surfaces during the cardiac cycle. Cells of the enoplasmic reticulum may be involved in the production of components of pericardial fluid. Tight junctions are present, but the cells do not form a syncytium.

A comprehensive account of the ultrastructure of the pericardium (*Ishihara, Ferrans, Jones 1980*) included Figure 7 and Figures 9 to 11, reproduced below, from their work, and given to me by the authors. These figures will surprise readers who suppose the pericardium is inert. Figure 8 was given to me by Drs. Borg and Caulfield, who have studied the mechanical properties and ultrastructure of the pericardium and their interrelationship. The serosal layer is completely covered by mesothelial cells containing numerous microvilli. In some areas the microvilli completely cover the cell surface. In others they are concentrated in the central portion or around the periphery of the cells. Single cilia, larger than the microvilli, are present in smaller numbers. The microvilli provide the pericardium with specialized friction-bearing surfaces and greatly increase the surface area available for fluid transport. The cilia are capable of sweeping motions mediated through the side arms on their microtubles. The microvilli and cilia permit the pericardium to accommodate to changes in the size and shape of the heart occurring in the cardiac cycle. Large areas of overlap and interdigitation between adjacent cells facilitate stretching of the mesothelium in diastole, but stability of cell shape is assured by a cytoskeleton of fine filamentous bundles.

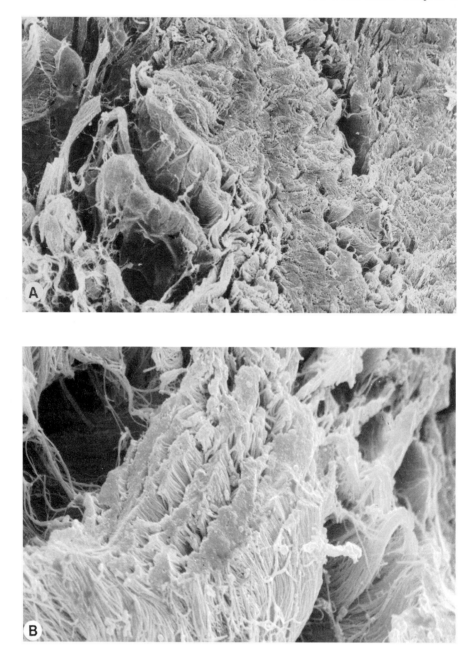

Figure 8. *Electron microscopic scans of pericardium (A) dense collagen fibres (x1000) (B) Parallel arrangement of the fibres (x6000).* (Figures supplied through the courtesy of Thomas K Borg, and JB Caulfield, University of South Carolina.)

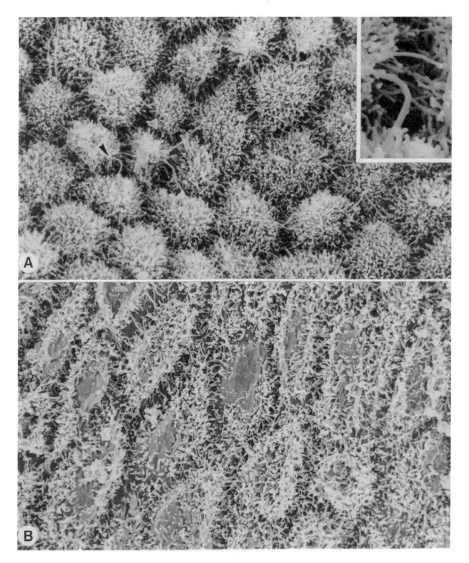

Figure 9. *Scanning electron micrographs of human parietal pericardium. (A) View of area in which the serosal surfaces of the mesothelial cells are completely covered by microvilli. Cilia (arrow head), which are thicker and longer than microvilli, are also distinguishable. Inset shows higher magnification of a cilium indicated by arrowhead. (B) View of area in which microvilli tend to form rings near peripheral portions of the cells, leaving smooth central portions.* (Figures supplied through the courtesy of Dr. Victor Ferrans, from Ishihara, Ferrans, Jones, 1980)

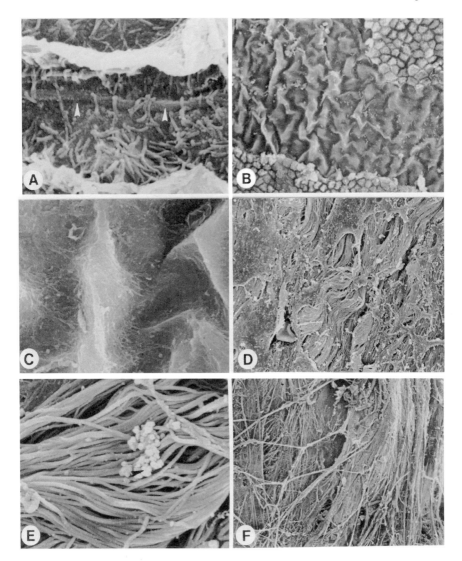

Figure 10. *Scanning electron micrograph of human pericardium (A) Intercellular junction appears as a slightly elevated ridge (arrow heads) (B) Area of partial denudation of mesothelial cell layer. Some mesothelial cells remain (bottom and upper right). Surface of the denuded area has a wavy configuration that reflects arrangement of underlying collagen. (C) High magnification view of area similar to that shown in B. The surface is relatively smooth; it is composed of basal lamina material and collagen fibrils are not evident. (D) Area of surface from which the mesothelial cells have been completely denuded and the basolamina has been partly removed, exposing underlying bundles of collagen fibrils. (E) High magnification view of centre of area shown in (D). Collagen fibres are seen as discrete units, together with some cellular debris. (F) Low magnification view showing large coarse collagen bundles in the pericardial surface that faces the sternum.* (Figures supplied through the courtesy of Dr. Victor Ferrans, from Ishihara, Ferrans, Jones 1980.)

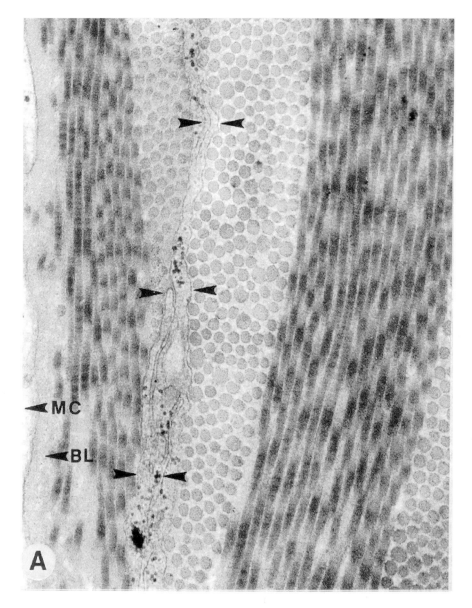

Figure 11. Transmission electron micrographs of pericardial connective tissue. (A) Section through submesothelial area showing the basal surface of a mesothelial cell (MC), the basolamina (BL), several layers of variously oriented collagen fibrils and part of the cytoplasm (arrow heads) of a greatly elongated fibroblast-like cell. (B) Demonstration of elastic fibres. The elastin cores are darkly stained, (upper right). Other elastic fibres (centre and bottom) contain abundant microfibrils and small elastin cores. (C) Nuclear region of elongated fibroblast-like cell in pericardial tunica fibrosa. A small elastic fibre (arrow head) is shown in upper right. (Figures supplied through the courtesy of Dr. Victor Ferrans, from Ishihara, Ferrans, Jones 1980).

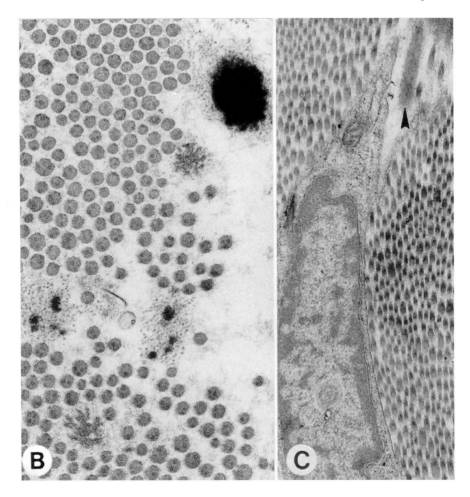

See figure legend on previous page

2.2   Nerve supply

The pericardium is innervated by the vagus, the left recurrent laryngeal nerve and the oesophageal plexus. Sympathetic innervation is also abundant from the stellate and first dorsal ganglia, and from the aortic, cardiac and diaphragmatic plexuses.

The phrenic nerves run along the pericardium to the diaphragm, a relationship important in surgical anatomy, because care must be exercised when performing cardiac or pericardial operations to avoid injury with consequent paralysis of a hemidiaphragm. The phrenic nerve may also be injured by local hypothermia during cardiac surgery. Intrathoracic neoplasm may involve the phrenic or recurrent laryngeal nerve with resulting diaphragmatic or vocal cord paralysis. Phrenic innervation of both the pericardium and diaphragm and the contiguity of the two structures account for diaphragmatic pain in acute pericarditis.

2.2.1   Pain perception

The pain of acute pericarditis may be pleuritic or simulate that of myocardial ischemia. Patients are usually aware of fluid (or gas) injected into the pericardium and often are somewhat aware of its temperature. Balloon pericardiotomy and instillation of a substance like tetracycline for chemotherapy are both painful procedures.

2.2.2   Historical perspective

Early in the twentieth century, sensory perception by the pericardium was recorded in a patient in whom part of the chest wall had been excised to treat suppuration (*Alexander, Macleod, Barker 1929*). The observations were made during pericardiostomy under local anaesthesia and for 16 days postoperatively. Pain could not be elicited from the lateral and posterior regions of the parietal pericardium. Temperature and vibration were not perceived. Pressure against the anterior chest wall from within the pericardial sac caused severe sub-sternal pain. Pinching and pricking the parietal pericardium also induced sub-sternal pain, but the epicardium was insensitive to these stimuli. Pain could not be evoked from the lateral and posterior regions of the parietal pericardium. Temperature and vibration were not perceived.

The venerable William Harvey reported the case of a young nobleman who had a large defect of the anterior chest wall that was the result of an abscess complicating earlier multiple rib fractures. Harvey was able to pass three fingers and a thumb through the defect to palpate the heart. He demonstrated this patient to his "serene friend, King Charles" (Charles I) who, for all his notorious shortcomings, was a staunch patron of the sciences. His Majesty acknowledged that "the heart was without sense of touch, for the youth never knew when we touched his heart except by sight, or by sensation he had through the integument" (Figure 12).

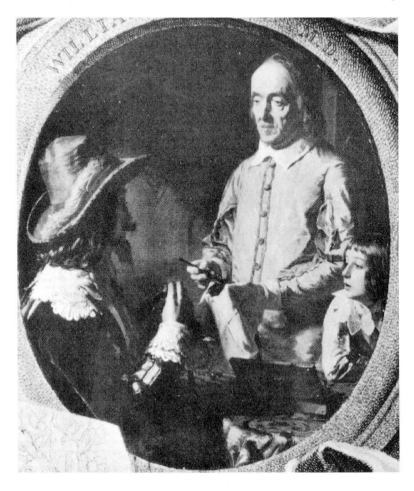

Figure 12. *A painting by Robert Hannah depicting William Harvey explaining his theory of circulation of the blood to his patron King Charles I. Harvey was physician to the royal household and held the same position in the court of Charles' father, James I. Both monarchs were patrons of the sciences, and it was customary for eminent men of science to demonstrate their experiments in front of the King at Court. One can imagine that on the occasion when William Harvey demonstrated that heart and pericardium do not perceive painful stimuli and touch, his distinguished patron watched with interest.* (From Bettmann: A Pictorial History of Medicine. Charles Thomas, 1956, Springfield, IL).

Spodick *(1959)* summarized the available data in his monograph on acute pericarditis, concluding that only one sixth of the pericardial surface is directly responsive to painful stimuli and that pain is transmitted via the phrenic nerve, which enters the spinal cord at segment C4-C6. The importance of the stellate ganglion in pericardial innervation is highlighted by the observation that stellate ganglion block can relieve pericardial pain (*Weissbein and Heller, 1961*).

2.2.3   Possible relation to the pain of myocardial ischemia

It has been suggested (*Fisch, 1980*) that myocardial ischemic pain is caused by abnormalities in regional left ventricular wall motion that cause the ventricle to push against the pericardium, producing angina or the pain of acute myocardial infarction. The currently prevailing theory that pain arises when abnormal metabolites stimulate cardiac nerve endings has never been proven, and fails to account for painless ischemia or relief of angina by sham operations or in spite of graft closure. Nevertheless, I do not think this challenge to the prevailing theory will prevail, but it offers an interesting alternative and has the virtue of being iconoclastic and thus a stimulus for research.

2.2.4   Reflexes

Numerous reflexes elicited by stimulation of the pericardium have been described (*Holt, 1970; Sleight, 1964*). Nicotine applied to the pericardium slows the heart rate and lowers blood pressure. Stimulation of the pericardium of the anaesthetized dog lowers arterial pressure and causes the spleen to contract (*Krichevskaya, 1962*). Action potentials have been recorded from the afferent fibers of pericardial mechanoreceptors in the dog (*Sleight and Widdicombe, 1965*).

2.3   Blood supply

The human pericardium is supplied by small branches of several vessels: the internal mammary arteries, the musculo-phrenic arteries, and the aorta. For a short period, these branches of the internal mammary artery were utilized as a source for myocardial revascularization as treatment of angina pectoris (*Bettezzati, Tagliaferro, De Marchi 1955*). It was believed that ligation of the internal mammary arteries would dilate its pericardial branches and thus increase blood supply to the epicardium, and eventually the deeper layers of myocardium. This rationale was fatally undermined by sham operations in which only half the patients underwent the ligation and the other half received the same local anaesthesia and the same incision but no ligature on the internal mammary artery (*Dimond, Kittle, Crockett 1960*). At the present time, a clinical study of this design would be considered scientifically correct, but ethically unacceptable.

References

Alexander J, Macleod AG, Barker PS. Sensibility of the exposed human heart and pericardium. Arch Surg 1929; 19:1470-1480.

Ando M, Imai Y, Takanashi Y, Hoshino S, Seo K, et al. Fate of trileaflet equine pericardial extracardiac conduit used for the correction of anomalies having pulmonic ventricle-pulmonary arterial discontinuity. Ann Thorac Surg 1997; 64:154-158.

Battezzati M, Tagliaferro A, De Marchi G. The ligature of the internal mammary arteries in disorders of vascularization of the myocardium. Minerva Med 1955; 46 (part 2):1178-1188.

Boulanger B, Yuan Z, Flessner M, Hay J, Johnston M. Pericardial fluid absorption into lymphatic vessels in sheep. Microvasc Res. 1999; 57:174-186.

Braile DM, Soares MJF, Souza DRS, Ramirez VDA, Suzigan S, et al. Mapping of bovine pericardium: Physical and histopathologic tests. J Heart Valve Dis 1988; 7:202-206.

Bull RK, Edwards PD, Dixon AK. CT dimensions of the normal pericardium. Brit J Radiol 1998; 71:923-925.

Choe YH, Im JG, Park JH, Han MC, Kim CW. The anatomy of the pericardial space: a study in cadavers and patients. AJR Am J Roentgenol 1987; 149:693-697.

Columbus, Realdus (1599). De Re Anatomica

Courtice FC, Simmonds WJ. Physiological significance of lymph drainage of the serous cavities and lungs. Physiol Rev 1954; 34:419-448.

Dimond EG, Kittle CF, Crockett JE. Comparison of internal mammary artery ligation and sham operation for angina pectoris. Am J Cardiol 1960; 5:483-486.

Drinker CK, Warren MF, Maurer FW, McCarrell JD. The flow, pressure and composition of cardiac lymph. Am J Physiol 1940; 130:43-55.

Duran C. The pericardial heart valve: An open question. Replacement Cardiac_Valves. Bodnar E and Frater RWM, eds. Pergamon Press Inc., New York, 1991. pp 277-285.

Elias H, Boyd LJ. Notes on the anatomy, embryology and histology of the pericardium. J New York Med Coll 1960; 2:50-75.

Eliskova M, Eliska O, Miller AJ. The lymphatic drainage of the parietal pericardium in man. Lymphology 1995; 28:208-217.

Ferrans VJ, Hilbert SL, Jones M. Biomaterials. Replacement Cardiac_Valves. Bodnar E and Frater RWM, eds. Pergamon Press Inc., New York, 1991. pp 49-76.

Fineberg MH. Functional capacity of the normal pericardium. An experimental study. Am Heart J 1936; 11:748-751.

Fisch S. On the origin of cardiac pain: A new hypothesis. Arch Intern Med 1980; 140:754-755.

Gibson AT, Segal MB. A study of the composition of pericardial fluid with special reference to the probable mechanism of fluid formation. J Physiol (London) 1978; 277:367-377.

Groell R, Schaffler GJ, Rienmueller R. Pericardial sinuses and recesses: findings at electrocardiographically triggered electron-beam CT. Radiology 1999; 212:69-73.

Herman AG, Claeys M, Moncada S, Vane JR. Prostacyclin production by rabbit aorta, pericardium, pleura, peritoneum and dura mater. Arch Int Pharmacodyn Ther 1978; 236:303-304.

Hollenberg M, Dougherty J. Lymph flow and ^{131}I-albumin resorption from pericardial effusions in man. Am J Cardiol 1969; 24:514-522.

Holt JP. The normal pericardium. Am J Cardiol 1970; 26:455-465.

Holt JP, Rhode EA, Kines H. Pericardial and ventricular pressure. Circ Res 1960; 8:1171-1181.

Hort Von W, Braun H. Untersuchungen uber Groesse, Wandstarke und mikroskopischen Aufbau des Herzbeutels unter normalen und pathologischen Bedingungen. Arch Kreislaufforsch 1962; 38:1-22.

Ishihara T, Ferrans VJ, Jones M, Boyce SW, Kawanamni O, Roberts WC. Histologic and ultrastructural features of normal human parietal pericardium. Am J Cardiol 1980; 46:744-753.

Johansen K, Lenfant C, Hanson D. Cardiovascular dynamics in the lungfishes. Vergleichende Physiol 1968; 59:157-186.

Kagramanov II, Kokshenev IV, Dobrova NB, Kastava VT, Serov RA, et al. Comparative assessment of hepatic Glisson's capsule and bovine pericardium in heart valve bioprostheses. J Heart Valve Dis 1998; 7:273-277.

Kampmeier OF. On the lymph flow of the human heart, with reference to the development of the channels and the first appearance, distribution, and physiology of their valves. Am Heart J 1928-1929; 4:210-222.

Kinney E, Wynn J, Hinton DM, Demers L, O'Neill M, et al. Pericardial-fluid complement: normal values. Am J Clin Pathol 1979; 72:972-974.

Krichevskaya IP. The effect of reflexes from receptors in the pericardium on blood filling in the spleen. Bull Exp Biol Med 1962; 52:1119-1121.

Kubota H, Sato C, Ohgushi M, Haku T, Sasaki K, et al. Fluid collection in the pericardial sinuses and recesses. Thin-section helical computed tomography observations and hypothesis. Investigative Radiology 1996; 31:603-610.`

Kuwahara M, Kuwahara M. Pericardial mesothelial cells produce endothelin-1 and possess functional endothelin ET_B receptors. Euro J Pharmacol 1998; 347:329-335.

Leeds SE, Uhley HN, Meister RB, McCormack KR. Lymphatic pathways and rate of absorption of ^{131}I-albumin from pericardium of dogs. Lymphology 1977; 10:166-172.

Maurer FW, Warren MF, Drinker CK. The composition of mammalian pericardial and peritoneal fluids. Am J Physiol 1940; 129:635-644.

Miller, AJ. Lymphatics of the Heart. Raven Press, New York, 1982.

Miller AJ, Ellis A, Katz LN: Cardiac lymph. Flow rates and composition in dogs. Am J Physiol 1964; 206:63-66.

Miller AJ, Pick R, Johnson PJ. The production of acute pericardial effusion. The effects of varying degrees of interference with venous blood and lymph drainage from the heart muscle in the dog. Am J Cardiol 1971; 28:463-466.

Miller AJ, Pick R, Katz LN. Lymphatics of the mitral valve of the dog. Demonstration and discussion of the possible significance. Circ Res 1961; 9:1005-1009.

Mills SA. Complications associated with the use of heterologous bovine pericardium for pericardial closure. J Thorac Cardiovasc Surg 1986; 92:446-454.

Patek PR. The morphology of the lymphatics of the mammalian heart. Am J Anat 1939; 64:203-249.

Pegram BL, Bishop VS. An evaluation of the pericardial sac as a safety factor during tamponade. Cardiovasc Res 1975; 9:715-721.

Quintero LJ, Lohre JM, Hernandez N, Meyer SC, McCarthy TJ, et al. Evaluation of in vivo models for studying calcification behavior of commercially available bovine pericardium. J Heart Valve Dis 1998; 7:262-267.

Rabkin SW, Ping HH. Mathematical and mechanical modeling of stress strain relationship of pericardium. Am J Physiol 1975; 229:896-900.

Rubanyi GM, Polokoff MA. Endothelins: molecular biology, bio-chemistry, pharmacology, physiology, and pathophysiology. Pharmacol Rev 1994; 46;325-415.

Sacks MS, Chuong CJC, More R. Collagen fiber architecture of bovine pericardium. ASAIO Journal 1994; 40:M632-M637.

Sacks MS, Chuong CJ. Orthotropic mechanical properties of chemically treated bovine pericardium. Ann Biomed Engineering 1998; 26:892-902.

Santamore WP, Constantinescu MS, Bogen D, Johnston WE. Nonuniform distribution of normal pericardial fluid. Basic Res Cardiol 1990; 85:541-549.

Shabetai R, Abel DC, Graham JB, Bhargava V, Keyes RS, et al. Function of the pericardium and pericardioperitoneal canal in elasmobranch fishes. Am J Physiol 1985; 248:H198-H207.

Shimada K, Fujii M, Sato H, Tanaka T, Murakami G, et al. Lymphatics of the thoracic surface of the diaphragm especially located around the inferior surface of the pericardial sac. J Anatomy 1995; 70:11-19.

Sleight P. A cardiovascular depressor reflex from the epicardium of the left ventricle in the dog. J Physiol 1964; 173:321-343.

Sleight P, Widdicombe JG. Action potentials in afferent fibers from pericardial mechanoreceptors in the dog. J Physiol 1965; 181:259-269.

Soliman MK, El Amrousi S, Youssef LB. Physico-chemical properties of pericardial fluid of healthy camels. Indian J Exp Biol 1966; 4:175-176.

Spodick DH. Acute Pericarditis. New York, Grune & Stratton, 1959.

Symbas PN, Schlant RC, Gravanis MB, Shepherd RL. Pathologic and functional effects on the heart following interruption of the cardiac lymph drainage. J Thorac and Cardiovasc Surg 1969; 57:577-584.

Szokodi I, Horkay F, Kiss P, Selmeci L, Merkely B, et al. Characterization and stimuli for production of pericardial fluid atrial natriuretic peptide in dogs. Life Sci 1997; 61:1349-1359.

Tanaka T, Hasegawa K, Fujita M, Tamaki S-I, Yamazato A, et al. Marked elevation of brain natriuretic peptide levels in pericardial fluid is closely associated with left ventricular dysfunction. J Am Coll Cardiol 1998; 31:399-403.

Thanikachalam S, Rajaram PC, Namachivayam A, Elangovan D, Viswanathan TR, et al. Lymphatic drainage of the heart muscle and pericardial sac in the dog. Indian Heart J 1978; 30:287-292.

Tysall GJ, Segal MB. The formation of a pericardial-like fluid from the epicardial surface of the isolated, perfused rat heart. J Physiol (Lond) 1979; 293:17P-18P.

Uhley HN, Leeds SE, Sampson JJ, Friedman M. The cardiac lymphatics in experimental chronic congestive heart failure. Proc Soc Exp Biol Med 1969; 131:379-381.

Weissbein AS, Heller FN. A method of treatment for pericardial pain. Circulation 1961; 24:607-612.

White CS. MR evaluation of the pericardium. Topics in Magnetic Resonance Imaging 1995; 7:258-266.

Chapter 2

PHYSIOLOGY
Pathophysiology

How can evolution have preserved the Starling mechanism if it is not used by the natural heart? Adding a few years of life to people with heart disease, most of whom have passed the reproductive age, would seem irrelevant to the evolutionary process. W.F. Hamilton 1955

1.   HISTORICAL BACKGROUND

The function of the pericardium has interested physiologists and clinicians alike from antiquity to the present. Hippocrates rightly described the pericardium as a "smooth mantle surrounding the heart and containing a small amount of fluid resembling urine" (*Boyd and Elias 1955; Spodick 1970*). Galen considered the pericardium to be a protective structure for the heart.

1.1   Prevention of distension of the heart

Barnard *(1898)* presented to the Physiological Society and published in their journal a series of experiments designed to answer the question whether the pericardium limits the volume of the heart. He subjected pericardial strips to traction and found them "practically inextensible." He also raised the pressure in an excised heart with the pericardium intact with a bicycle pump until the heart and pericardium ruptured. The pericardium gave way from its attachments to the great vessels at a pressure of 1.25 atmospheres. The "fundus" of the pericardium did not rupture at a pressure of two atmospheres, a pressure sufficient to rupture the thick rubber tubes in the preparation. A heart unsupported by a pericardium ruptured at a pressure between 0.75 and 1.0 atmosphere. The left "auricular" (atrial) appendage was the weak spot, a finding that will not surprise cardiologists trained in transseptal catheterization of the left atrium. In another experiment, Barnard showed that distension of a postmortem canine heart with a pressure of 20 cm H_2O required 12 ml of saline; upon removal of the pericardium, 11 more ml were required to fill the heart to the same pressure. From these results, Barnard concluded that the pericardium exerts a significant restraining influence on the heart. This conclusion subsequently found widespread support *(Kuno 1916; Carleton 1929; Holt, Rhode, Kines 1960)*. Quantification of pericardial restraint when the heart is normal and when it is acutely or chronically dilated remains a subject of research and is discussed in subsequent sections of this chapter. The extent of pericardial restraint and how it is best measured remains controversial to this day.

2.   THE PERICARDIUM AND CARDIAC CHAMBER INTERACTION (INTERDEPENDENCE)

The volume and pressure of a cardiac chamber influences the volume and pressure of other cardiac chambers. Interaction between the two ventricles, especially in diastole, has been the most thoroughly investigated of these interactions, although atrial and atrio-ventricular interaction also occur. These interactions, which are weak in the absence of the pericardium, as the studies of Barnard would suggest, become stronger when the pericardium is intact, and very marked in cardiac tamponade and constrictive pericarditis (see Chapters 4, 6 and 7). Pericardial enhancement of interventricular action helps provide the means whereby the stroke volume of the two ventricles is continuously adjusted by operation of the Frank-Starling mechanism to provide equal left and right heart output *(Wiggers 1962)*. W.F. Hamilton *(1955)*, working at the Medical College of Georgia, and better known for the Stewart-Hamilton equation for calculating cardiac output from indicator dilution curves, strongly supported this concept. Henderson and Prince (1914), four years before Starling *(1918)* published his brilliant Linacre lecture on the law of the heart, showed that the output from the two sides of the heart was integrated by the response of left ventricular output to its distending pressure (Figure 1). They predicted that when venous return to the right ventricle increases, the interventricular septum must bulge from right to left. Their observations have been largely forgotten in the spate of more recent literature on ventricular interaction, so, in view of its current relevance to the present era, are quoted here.

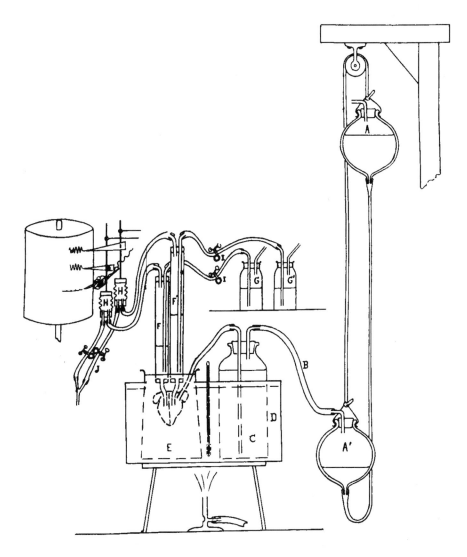

*Figure 1.*Apparatus used by Henderson & Prince to record the influence of various diastolic distending pressures in the right and left ventricles upon their respective stroke volumes. (*From Henderson and Prince, in Heart 1914, with permission*)

"*If, for even a few moments at a time, the right heart pumps more blood into the pulmonary vessels than the left heart pumps out of them, congestion of the lungs must result. If, on the other hand, the left heart pumps out more than the right pumps in, an acute depletion of the lungs would be produced. It is wonderful, not that pulmonary congestion sometimes occurs, but rather that it is not a common occurrence. It is still more remarkable that a condition of pulmonary depletion, except as a result of exsanguination is unknown either to physiology or clinical medicine."* (The last sentence, however, is incorrect, as depletion occurs in congenital heart disease and with pulmonary embolism.) *"During health the two sides of the heart must propel exactly the same volume of blood per minute. As they execute the same number of beats their systolic discharges must therefore **on average*** (author's emphasis) *be absolutely equal. And as the heart (that is the ventricle) is a somewhat shapeless muscular bag divided into two compartments, which appear rather unequal in size, it is a problem to determine the nature of the adjustment by which the exact equivalence of their systolic discharges is effected."*

To demonstrate ventricular interaction *in vitro,* Henderson and Prince used an ingenious device to maintain one ventricular distending pressure constant while the opposite ventricular distending pressure was progressively increased (Figure 1). While conceding that pulmonary hypertension is the usual reason for right heart failure complicating left heart failure, with remarkable prescience they went on to state that *"The behaviour of the heart here noted suggests that the congestion may sometimes be, so to speak, short circuited through the heart itself by displacement of the ventricular septum during diastole. This interdependence between the two ventricles would be considerably weaker, were not the whole heart enclosed within the pericardial sac."*

2.1   Classic studies: mid 20th Century

The middle years of the 20th Century witnessed intense research on cardiac chamber interaction and interdependence. It was during this epoch that direct or parallel interaction, due to the influence of right heart pressure and volume on those of the left heart, was defined and distinguished from series interaction, that is, the interaction attributed to the series arrangement of the circulation.

The right and left ventricles of the heart are related by the common interventricular septum, circumferential and spiral muscular bundles that encircle both of them and the pericardium. From this anatomical arrangement, it is predictable that the extent of filling of one ventricle should alter the distensibility of the other (Figure 2). The ventricles of the canine heart are more distensible when filled individually than when both chambers are filled simultaneously with equal volumes. Taylor, Covell, Sonnenblick *(1967)* studied ventricular interaction in a canine model. Starting with *in vivo* experiments, they measured right ventricular diastolic pressure while altering that of the left ventricle. They then arrested the heart *in situ* in diastole and determined the diastolic pressure-volume curve of the left ventricle with the right ventricle filled to various volumes determined by the *in vivo* experiments in which the pericardium had been removed. The volume of the right ventricle had little effect on the distensibility of the left ventricle at physiological levels of left ventricular diastolic pressure, but became significant as left ventricular diastolic volume and pressure were progressively elevated.

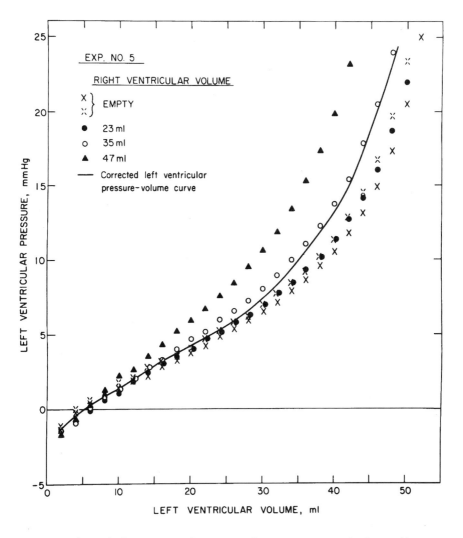

Figure 2 Left ventricular pressure-volume curves from postmortem canine heart with open pericardium to demonstrate ventricular interdependence. *(From Taylor, Covell, Sonnenblick 1967, with permission.)*

Simultaneous infusion into both ventricles of the fresh postmortem canine heart, compared with infusion into one ventricle at a time results in a considerably larger left ventricle when its diastolic pressure is 10 mm Hg *(Laks, Garner, Swan 1967)*. Ventricular interaction was also studied using an elaborate system of pumps and reservoirs to permit independent control of both filling and emptying of the left and right sides of five isolated feline hearts, thereby breaking the normal series arrangement of the two pumps *(Elzinga, Van Grondelle, Westerhof 1974)*. When the filling of one atrium was increased, output of the opposite side decreased. This effect, although demonstrable when the pericardium was widely open, was more pronounced after the pericardium had been reapposed, and was ascribed to reduced compliance of the opposite ventricle. Subsequent investigators have pointed out that when the pericardium is resutured, its hemodynamic influence is exaggerated and therefore the hemodynamic effects of the pericardium are more appropriately evaluated using experimental models in which pericardial integrity is maintained. Nevertheless, the design of this study enabled the authors to separate the *direct* relationship between the two ventricles, which is a consequence of the fact that the two pumps comprise a single organ with a common septum and muscle bundles, from the *indirect* relationship that results from the series arrangement of the two pumps, whereby decreased output from one pump decreases input to the other.

Santamore, Lynch, Meier *(1976)* also studied the alterations in ventricular pressure-volume relationships and ventricular geometry caused by varying the volume of the opposite ventricle. They used an isolated heart preparation to remove all neural, hormonal, and pulmonary circulatory influences from the heart. When the investigators varied left ventricular volume in the beating heart, they caused an acute change in the right ventricular diastolic pressure-volume relationship. Increasing left ventricular volume caused an increase in right ventricular diastolic pressure, whereas decreasing left ventricular volume caused a decrease in right ventricular diastolic pressure. They demonstrated that left ventricular diastolic pressure can be elevated not only by directly increasing right ventricular volume, but also by constriction of the pulmonary artery, which distends the right ventricle causing the interventricular septum to bulge from right to left.

Experiments in which the right heart was either bypassed or distended were carried out by Moulopoulos, Sarcas, Stamatelopoulos *(1965)*, to examine the question of whether the degree of filling of the right ventricle changes left ventricular performance by a direct mechanical contiguous effect, or, indirectly, by altering flow into the left ventricle. These studies were performed at constant heart rate and after sympathectomy, and showed that when left ventricular filling and resistance to emptying were held constant, and the right ventricle was filled until diastolic pressure rose to 10 mm Hg, left ventricular diastolic pressure began to rise and increased even more when right ventricular pressure exceeded 10 mm Hg. These authors also showed that left ventricular function curves deteriorated. Developed left ventricular isovolumic pressure declined when the right ventricle was overdistended. These studies were performed with the pericardium wide open.

Bemis, Serur, Borkenhagen *(1974)* sutured the pericardium loosely around isolated dog hearts and evaluated the influence of right ventricular filling pressure on left ventricular pressure and dimensions. The experimental model was such that right ventricular pressure and volume could be varied while inflow to the left ventricle, peak left ventricular pressure, arterial blood pressure, and heart rate were held constant. In addition to measuring pressure, the authors measured left ventricular dimensions by means of two pairs of radio-opaque markers, one on the septum and free wall of the left ventricle, and the other on the anterior and posterior walls. Increased right ventricular filling pressure was associated with a reduction in the septum-to-free-wall hemi-axis of the left ventricle and corresponding increase in the anterior-posterior axis. Thus, right ventricular filling was associated with elongation and narrowing of the left ventricular cavity. The magnitude of this shape change was small, but it was nevertheless accompanied by a substantial increase in left ventricular filling pressure and decreased compliance.

The experimental studies cited suggest that when the pericardium is absent, right ventricular filling exerts a major effect on left ventricular diastolic pressure and compliance only at elevated levels of left ventricular diastolic pressure. On the other hand, the data of Bemis et al. demonstrated alterations in left ventricular geometry and pressure over the entire range of right and left diastolic pressures they studied. We ascribe this difference to the pericardium that was sutured closed after instrumentation was completed. The authors emphasized that the pericardial closure was accomplished without overlap using loose sutures. Nevertheless, one cannot regard a pericardium sutured together, however carefully, as normal. Indeed, when considering the literature on ventricular interaction, it is important to separate studies in which the pericardium had been widely excised (and therefore could not exert any influence) from studies performed with the pericardium intact, in which the normal function of the pericardium can become evident, but also from studies in which the pericardium was incised and resutured, in which pericardial effects are doubtlessly considerably exaggerated. The differences in experimental results with the pericardium truly intact compared with after resuture were pointed out by Gibbon and Churchill (1931) and have since been documented by Stokland, Miller and Lekven, *(1980)*.

Leftward bulging of the interventricular septum in humans has been recognized as a useful echocardiographic finding in right ventricular

overload since the studies of Brinker, Weiss, Lappe (1980) (Figure 3).
Using two-dimensional echocardiography during the Müller manoeuvre to
study the effects of acute right ventricular loading on the left ventricle in
nine normal human subjects, they noted a substantial increase in the radius
of curvature of the interventricular septum indicating flattening. This change
resulted in displacement of the septum from the right to the left ventricle
(Figure 3) and a corresponding decrease in left ventricular volume.

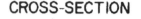

CROSS-SECTION

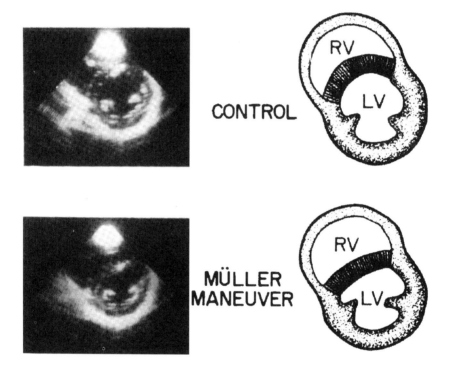

Figure 3 An early echocardiographic study of ventricular interaction. Diastole at top, systole
at bottom. The changed angle of curvature of the ventricular septum (shaded) with right heart
volume loading, illustrated ventricular interaction mediated by the septum. (*From* Brinker,
Weiss, Lappe 1980, with permission)

    The literature does not reflect unanimity of opinion regarding ventricular
interaction or the extrapolations therefrom that, in health, reciprocal changes
occur in the dimensions of the two ventricles, and that changes in the
hemodynamic events in the pulmonary and systemic circulation should be

180 degrees out of phase. In one study (*Franklin, Van Citters, Rushmer, 1962*), phasic aortic and pulmonary arterial blood pressure and flow were measured in instrumented conscious dogs, breathing quietly and spontaneously. Observations were made following changes of posture and while the dogs ran on a treadmill. In these experiments, respiratory variations in the systemic and pulmonary circulation were almost *in phase.* The authors attributed this difference in their results compared with those that demonstrate ventricular interaction to studying intact fully conscious animals with unimpaired reflex responses and physiological heart rates.

Systolic ventricular interaction was studied less than diastolic during this time, although it was noted that shape and compliance changes of the left ventricle caused by right ventricular distension may affect left ventricular systolic performance *(Bemis, Serur, Borkenhagen 1974; Elzinga, Piene, DeJong 1980).* These investigators obtained right and left ventricular function curves in isolated ejecting feline hearts in which the natural series arrangement of the two sides of the heart was broken. Isovolumic beats on the left side of the heart enhanced right ventricular pump function, but right ventricular isovolumic systoles had practically no effect on left ventricular systolic function. Thus it appeared that the major effect of systolic interaction is that left ventricular contraction augments right ventricular function.

Janicki and Weber *(1980)* studied the influence of the pericardium on systolic and diastolic ventricular interaction and on ventricular dimensions. They employed an areflexic isolated paced canine heart preparation in which they could measure and control the pressure and volume of each ventricle. The ventricles were uncoupled by this type of preparation, and isovolumic beats were used to study ventricular interaction throughout the cardiac cycle before and after removal of the pericardium. In all experiments both the right and left ventricular pressure volume relationships were shifted downward or to the right after removal of the pericardium, and this effect was most pronounced at high ventricular volumes.

Diastolic interaction, consisting of an elevation in the filling pressure of one ventricle as the filling pressure of the other ventricle was increased, was found in all experiments, and the magnitude of this interaction was always greater with the pericardium intact than after its removal. The data concerning systolic interaction, that is, alteration in the developed isovolumic pressure of one ventricle as the filling pressure of the opposite ventricle was varied, were inconstant but, in general, systolic interaction was more pronounced when the pericardium was preserved. Indeed, it has long been appreciated that the pulmonary circulation is highly dependent on the left ventricle. Major damage to the left ventricle impairs right ventricular performance, and ever since the dramatic experiments of Starr, Jeffers, Meade *(1943)*, we have known that cardiac output can be maintained without elevation of the venous pressure after extensive cauterization of the free wall of the right ventricle.

Open heart surgery provides an opportunity for studying the function of the human pericardium, although there are obvious limitations to the experimental models that can be applied. Mangano *(1980)* constructed ventricular function curves in 20 patients who underwent pericardiectomy as a preliminary to coronary artery bypass surgery. The function curves were generated before and after opening the pericardium by changing body position to create large alterations of systemic and pulmonary venous pressures. In this study, pericardiectomy altered neither the relationship between left ventricular stroke work and pulmonary wedge pressure nor the relationship between right ventricular stroke work and the central venous pressure. Furthermore, pericardiectomy did not change the ratio of central venous pressure to pulmonary venous pressure. Thus, in this investigation, no effect of the pericardium either on systolic function of the ventricles or on ventricular interaction was demonstrated. A major limitation of this study is that it was not possible to measure cardiac dimensions.

Spotnitz and Kaiser *(1971)* used a canine model to quantify the pericardial influence on the left ventricle. They calculated that 46 percent of ventricular pressure at 10 cm H_2O and 34 percent at 20 cm H_2O were contributed by the pericardium, and that absolute increases in pressure caused by the pericardium were 4.6 cm H_2O and 6.8 cm H_2O respectively. Volume increases associated with removal of the pericardium were 6.2 ml/100 g left ventricular weight at 10 cm H_2O, and 7.2 ml/100 g at 13.6 cm H_2O. To obviate the possibility of artifact owing to the use of intraventricular balloons, these investigators confirmed their results using left ventricular pressure-volume curves. Their results support the view that in normal diastole the heart is gently compressed by the pericardium, and suggest that the elastic limits of the pericardium are not reached with left ventricular diastolic pressures up to 20 cm H_2O. More recent studies place this threshold nearer to 10 mm Hg.

I have not attempted a comprehensive review of the complex subject of ventricular interaction. Rather, I have selected contributions to show that, under appropriate circumstances, ventricular interaction can be consistently demonstrated and that this interaction is significantly stronger in the presence of an intact pericardium. The importance of ventricular interaction in the normal healthy subject has not yet been finally established, but in the experimental situation and in disease of the pericardium ventricular interaction is important. It is also important in several cardiac disorders, leading us to a broader question, How and to what extent does the pericardium restrain the size of the normal heart?

2.2 Recent studies

The pace of research on the physiology of ventricular interaction has slowed since publication of the examples cited. A number of more recent studies have been published, and the proportion addressing systolic interaction has increased. Beloucif, Takata, Shimada *(1992)* studied "vertical chamber interdependence" (atrioventricular) in open chest dogs with special reference to the influence of cardiac tamponade or pericardiectomy. When the pericardium was intact, pericardial fluid volume was assumed to be low, such that over some regions of the heart the pericardium would directly contact the myocardium and therefore regional variations in the pericardial contact force could exist (see discussion of contact force, below). Systemic and pulmonary venous return occurred in both systole and diastole; therefore, during systole, the volume of ventricular filling contributed by the atrium was less than the volume ejected by the ventricle, in other words, atrioventricular coupling (interdependence) was weak. Pericardiectomy increased the diastolic component of venous return to a small extent, indicating a slight decrease in the existing mild interdependence. Descent of the closed atrioventricular valves during the ejection period was considered the main driving force for venous return on both sides of the heart. The other effect of pericardiectomy was to lower atrial pressure a little, but not diastolic pressure, in the ventricles. This difference would mean that, under normal conditions, pericardial restraint is weak and exerted on the atria, but not the ventricles.

Increasingly severe cardiac tamponade elevated and equalized pericardial and atrial pressures, eventually reducing transmural cardiac pressures to zero, ensuring equal pericardial diastolic pressure over the entire heart. Under these conditions, systemic venous return was confined to systole and the diastolic component of pulmonary venous return was greatly diminished, though not entirely absent. Thus atrial filling and ventricular ejection volumes were equal and simultaneous. Total cardiac volume remained invariant throughout the cardiac cycle. The heart was behaving as two reciprocating pumps and vertical interaction was 100 percent.

In the dogs with cardiac tamponade, the *y* descent of right atrial pressure, as would be expected, was abolished, but the *y* descent in the pulmonary venous pressure curve persisted, because the left heart is less compliant than the right. The steeper left heart diastolic pressure-volume relation would lower left atrial luminal pressure, thereby providing a driving pressure for pulmonary venous, but not systemic venous diastolic flow.

Several publications by Farrar and Chow have reported on the effect of the pericardium on both systolic and diastolic ventricular interactions. In the paced canine model of dilated cardiomyopathy, Farrar, Chow and Brown

(1995) demonstrated that the pericardium increased diastolic, but not systolic interaction. To procure isolated systolic and diastolic interaction, they used a ventricular assist device in which the inflow and outflow valves had been removed and the outflow port blocked off. A cannula connected the cardiac apex to the inflow port. The setup enabled rapid filling of the assist device during a single systolic or late diastolic interval. Mean ventricular systolic interaction gain was calculated as the interventionally induced change in mean right ventricular systolic pressure divided by that in mean systolic left ventricular pressure. Gain in diastolic interaction was calculated in a comparable manner. Systolic interaction significantly contributes to right ventricular performance except in the instance of right or left ventricular hypertrophy in which septal elastance is increased. Pericardiectomy slightly decreased systolic interaction but, as would be anticipated, the increase in diastolic interaction was considerably greater. Volume loading increased interaction in both systole and diastole.

Cardiac output can be maintained with low systemic venous pressure when the right ventricular free wall of a dog has been destroyed by cauterisation *(Starr, Jeffers and Mead, 1943)*. Likewise, circulation can be maintained when the right heart is bypassed, as in the Glenn and Fontan procedures. The clinical implications of these findings and subsequent studies confirming the ability of the heart to maintain the circulation when the right ventricle is akinetic or severely hypokinetic stimulated Hoffman, Sisto, Frater *(1994)* to study systolic interaction in a canine preparation in which the right ventricular free wall had been replaced by a pericardial xenograft patch. The preparation allowed data acquisition with the non-contractile right ventricle empty or filled with increasing volumes. The left ventricle generated satisfactory cardiac output via ventricular systolic interaction, augmenting right ventricular systolic function as long as right ventricular volumes were kept low, and the output rose in proportion to the left ventricular diastolic pressure (Starling effect on the left ventricle). The deleterious effects of right ventricular volume overload or raised pulmonary vascular resistance on cardiac output, however, could not be overcome by ventricular interaction.

When the pericardium was resutured, the heart, in order to perform a given amount of work, required a higher venous pressure than after the pericardium had been opened. When the venous pressure was normal, however, the heart could perform as much work as the heart without a pericardium and it did so without causing myocardial hemorrhage or tricuspid incompetence.

When the pericardium was open, however, it was difficult to increase the work of the heart above its normal level without producing myocardial hemorrhage and tricuspid incompetence. In two of the dogs, left ventricular pressure circumference curves were constructed during stepwise hemorrhage and transfusion with the pericardium open, and were repeated after the pericardium had been repaired. After the repair, the slope of the pressure-volume relationship increased. This exaggerated response again illustrates the different pressure-dimension changes of the left ventricle obtained when results with open pericardium are compared with a resutured rather than a genuinely intact pericardium.

Right ventricular volume was acutely and substantially increased by inducing right ventricular infarction, and then reduced by opening a modified Glenn shunt in eight pigs *(Danton, Byrne, Flores, 2001)*. Right ventricular dilation reduced left ventricular elastance and lengthened *tau*. These adverse changes were ameliorated when the Glenn shunt was opened. Similarly, when biventricular pressure-volume loops were obtained in conscious dogs in which reflex activity was blocked pharmacologically *(Karunanithi, Michniewicz, Young, 2001)*, left ventricular afterload was increased by aortic constriction. The relation of right ventricular stroke work and end-diastolic volume, although remaining linear, was thereby decreased without change in the length-axis intercept. The same effect was observed in right ventricular regional systolic function. Right ventricular mean ejection pressure was not changed; thus, the authors attributed impaired right ventricular performance to ventricular interaction.

A case of severe pulmonary valvular stenosis with biventricular dysfunction responded to valvuloplasty with a prompt improvement in right ventricular function, but the recovery of left ventricular function was delayed *(Patel, Hatle, Mimish 1999)*. Although left ventricular dysfunction was likely due in part to ventricular interaction, an intrinsic left ventricular myopathy would best explain the prolonged course of left ventricular recovery. Left ventricular dysfunction is therefore not a contraindication to pulmonary balloon valvuloplasty.

Several studies had implicated the pericardium as playing a role in left ventricular dysfunction following right ventricular infarction (*Goldstein, Vlahakes, Verrier* 1982; *Burger, Straube, Behne 1995*). Simulation of the pattern of constrictive pericarditis by right ventricular infarction is a well recognized clinical phenomenon, explained by ventricular interaction due to acute ventricular dilation, sufficient both to compress the left ventricle and cause the heart to engage the pericardium (*Cohn, Guiha, Broder 1974*). The contribution of the pericardium to ventricular interaction after right ventricular infarction and the intricacies of volume expansion as treatment were re-investigated long after its empirical use was established *(Calvin, 1991)*. Calvin postulated a delicate balance between a therapeutic and deleterious result. In a canine right ventricular infarct model studied with the pericardium either intact, partially opened in order to free the right atrium, or widely open, he found that volume loading increased the pressure referred to atmospheric, but not the transmural diastolic pressure of both ventricles. He concluded that the pericardium augments a weak atrio-ventricular interaction and a much stronger interaction between the two ventricles.

2.3   Clinical importance of ventricular interaction

We have seen that ventricular interaction can be easily demonstrated in fresh postmortem hearts and *in vivo* experiments in which the input to and the output from the two sides of the heart can be regulated. Ventricular interaction is readily apparent in studies using volume loading of the heart, in cardiac tamponade and constrictive pericarditis, right ventricular infarction, acute tricuspid regurgitation and, in some cases, of cor pulmonale and acute massive pulmonary embolism. Raised central venous pressure in patients with left ventricular disease is usually and correctly attributed to a combination of water and salt retention and right heart failure consequent upon pulmonary hypertension. The experimental studies cited on ventricular interaction and its enhancement by the pericardium show that right ventricular failure complicating left ventricular failure may also in part be a direct mechanical effect.

Manifest ventricular interaction, as documented by exaggerated respiratory variation of transatrio-ventricular inflow velocity, is a highly sensitive sign of raised pericardial pressure, but does not indicate the degree of elevation *(Shaver, Reddy, Curtiss, 2001)*. Thirty-three (33) patients, in 13 of whom pericardial pressure was elevated, underwent invasive study. EchoDoppler evidence of ventricular interdependence was observed when the elevated pericardial pressure remained lower than pressure in both atria, was the same as right atrial, but less than left atrial pressure, and when all three pressures were equal (overt tamponade).

The clinical syndrome of right heart failure, "out of proportion to the severity of left heart failure," has been recognized for many years (the Bernheim syndrome) *(East and Bain 1949)*. The early speculation that bulging of the septum may be the underlying mechanism is supported by the experimental results obtained from animal studies of ventricular interaction.

The question of how cor pulmonale may induce left ventricular failure remains unsettled. The mechanisms that have been proposed include increased left ventricular work secondary to intrapulmonary arteriovenous shunting, hypoxia and acidosis, and bulging of the interventricular septum into the left ventricle (reversed Bernheim syndrome), which has been shown to decrease the apparent compliance of the left ventricle and to impair its contractile performance *(Scott and Garvin 1941)*. Inasmuch as the pericardium reinforces ventricular interaction, it plays a part in modifying left ventricular function in cor pulmonale. Increased negative pressure in the thorax contributes by significantly increasing left ventricular afterload. In these patients, left ventricular volumes may not decrease during inspiration, but instead actually become larger.

Left ventricular pacing, like biventricular pacing, is an adjunctive therapy for heart failure in patients with increased QRS duration (see a subsequent section in this chapter). The rationale is that decreased duration of electrical activation improves the synchrony of ventricular contraction and relaxation. An alternative explanation for the benefit of left ventricular pacing is that, by delaying right ventricular filling, it decreases ventricular interaction, thereby improving left ventricular function *(Morris-Thurgood, Turner, Nightingale, 2000)*. Whether this explanation will stand further scrutiny remains to be seen, but it merits attention from students of ventricular interdependence.

Investigations using the canine heart in which the right ventricle was isolated by an electrical technique *(Goldstein, Harada, Yagi, 1990)* confirmed the importance of left ventricular contraction in maintaining right ventricular function when the right ventricular free wall was acutely akinetic. After the right ventricle was isolated, pacing electrodes were affixed to both atria and the left ventricle, and the sinus node was crushed. Short axis and apical four chamber echocardiograms were obtained along with high fidelity ventricular pressures. The dogs were studied during atrio-biventricular pacing, then during right hypokinesis of the free wall of the right ventricle obtained by discontinuing right ventricular pacing. The atria were paced at the same rate and AV interval as previously. Finally, the dogs were studied during isolated left ventricular pacing, also at the same rate as before. The results showed that dysfunction of the free right ventricular wall caused systolic and diastolic right ventricular dysfunction, the latter partly compensated for by enhanced right atrial contraction and maintaining constant atrio-ventricular conduction time. Septal rightward motion significantly augmented right ventricular systolic function (Figure 4).

3.   PERICARDIAL RESTRAINT

Interaction and restraint are closely related phenomena and we have seen that most experiments designed to evaluate ventricular interaction also demonstrate that the pericardium restrains the volume of the heart. Kuno *(1916)* published the results of a long series of experiments designed to elucidate the function of the pericardium and, in particular, to test the hypothesis that the pericardium prevents overdistension of the heart.

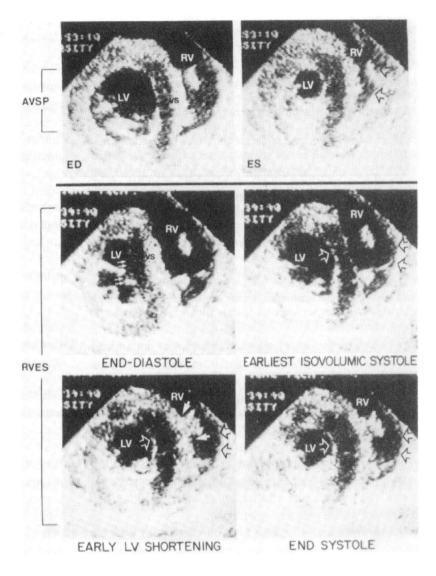

Figure 4 Short axis images during atrio-ventricular sequential pacing (AVSP) demonstrate
normal end-diastolic (ED) orientation of the ventricular septum (VS) and normal right
ventricular wall motion (open arrows) at end systole (ES). During right ventricular electrical
silence (RVES) (lower four panels) the frame-by-frame sequence demonstrates reversed
septal curvature (small arrows) from the dilated right ventricle to the volume-deprived left
ventricle. During earliest isovolumic systole, with minimal left ventricular-septal thickening,
the septum (open white arrows) moves paradoxically into the right ventricle, the free wall of
which is non-contractile (solid white arrows), reducing right ventricular volume despite right
ventricular free wall non-contractility (open black arrows). With peak end-systolic left
ventricular septal shortening, the septum has moved posteriorly toward the left ventricle (open
white arrow). *(From Goldstein, Harada, Yagi 1990, with permission)*

Some of the experiments were performed using the Starling heart-lung preparation, and others were conducted in open-chest dogs. The basic design of all the studies was that observations were made both with the pericardium widely open and after it had been resutured. Kuno found that when the pericardium was intact, the heart, in order to perform a certain amount of work, required a higher venous pressure than when the pericardium was open. When the venous pressure was normal, however, the heart could perform as much work as the heart without a pericardium, and did so without causing myocardial hemorrhage or tricuspid regurgitation. In the absence of the pericardium, it was difficult to increase the work of the heart above the normal level without causing both these lesions.

Dauterman, Pak, Maughan *(1995)* avoided the use of pharmacological agents to assess external restraint, because they exert multiple cardiovascular effects. Also, being a clinical study, pericardial pressure was not measured, which was fortunate in view of the problems surrounding measurement of pericardial pressure or contact force *(vide infra)*. To assess the external constraining forces on the pericardium, they instead employed balloon occlusion of the inferior vena cava that abruptly dropped the right ventricular diastolic pressure to near zero. Using a conductance catheter and high fidelity pressure measurements, they obtained left ventricular pressure-volume curves. A critically important advantage of their study design is that immediately after right ventricular diastolic pressure dropped to almost zero, the left ventricle continued to fill for several more cardiac cycles. Obtaining sequential left ventricular pressure-volume loops before and during occlusion of the inferior vena cava permitted the investigators to measure changes in left ventricular diastolic pressure and volume, both early, when only right ventricular pressure and volume were reduced and left ventricular volume was little changed, and subsequently, when left ventricular filling was also reduced. The early changes were attributed to lessening constraint on the left ventricle by the right ventricle and pericardium (Figure 5).

The study population comprised patients with documented normal left ventricular systolic function and diastolic pressure under 20 mm Hg, patients with idiopathic dilated cardiomyopathy, hypertension with left ventricular hypertrophy, and patients with left ventricular dysfunction secondary to coronary artery disease. In the latter group, the pericardium likely had stretched, reducing its contribution to external restraint. The study showed that 30 to 40 percent of measured left ventricular diastolic pressure is generated by external forces and this percentage was similar in all the patient groups. Below a left ventricular diastolic pressure of 6 mm Hg, external constraint on the left ventricle was negligible, but at higher pressures, only one third of measured left ventricular diastolic pressure reflects the intrinsic mechanical properties of the left ventricle (Figure 5). With characteristic prescience, Braunwald and Ross *(1963)* editorialised that elevated left ventricular diastolic pressure does not necessarily imply classic heart failure, but can be due to diastolic dysfunction, volume overload or pericardial restraint.

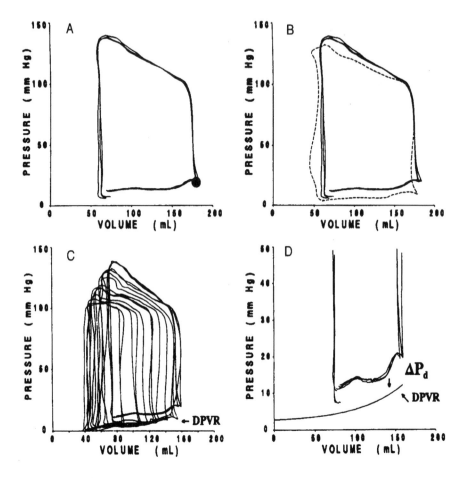

Figure 5. Left ventricular pressure-volume relation **(A)** before and **(B)** immediately after initiating occlusion of the inferior vena cava, and **(C)** during sustained occlusion. **A:** control, the loop is stable. **B:** Systemic venous return is severely reduced; therefore, right heart volume shrinks. Pulmonary venous return is not yet affected; therefore, the left heart continues to fill. The dashed loops show a downward shift of diastolic pressure caused by withdrawal of normal external restraint, but no decline in left ventricular pressure. **C:** With more prolonged caval occlusion, pulmonary venous return falls, causing left ventricular pressure to decrease. The loop is shifted progressively leftward. The diminishing height and width of successive loops indicates falling systolic pressure and stroke volume. **D:** the contribution of external restraint to the left ventricular diastolic pressure-relation. **DPVR:** diastolic pressure volume relation of the left ventricle. ΔP_d: difference in diastolic pressure. *(Modified from Dauterman, Pak, Maugham 1995, with permission).*

4. ROLE OF THE PERICARDIUM IN HEART FAILURE

Acute heart failure and volume overload increase pericardial constraint with the result that much of the increase in ventricular diastolic pressures is borne by the pericardium, such that the increase in ventricular transmural pressure is considerably less than that of pressure referred to atmospheric.

The pericardium also plays a role in the pathophysiology of chronic heart failure. In the past, pericardiectomy was considered a possible treatment for heart failure unresponsive to other treatment. The underlying idea was that the procedure would lower ventricular diastolic pressure by removing pericardial constraint, and that further pressure increase, were the heart to continue to dilate, would be limited. Although some pericardiectomies were performed with this rationale in mind, they no longer are. The opposite approach is now under investigation, namely to place a cardiac restraining device over the left ventricle in order to prevent continued dilation. Myocardial stretch is a potent source of signalling that leads to cardiac remodelling with subsequent heart failure. By inhibiting this process, cardiac restraining devices hold promise to become an effective therapeutic adjunctive therapy for chronic dilated heart failure (*vide infra*).

The background necessary to appreciate the role of the pericardium in heart failure includes ventricular interaction, forces responsible for pericardial restraint on the heart, assessment of diastolic function, the biomechanics of the pericardium, and the nature and measurement of pericardial pressure.

4.1 Ventricular diastolic function

Before describing experimental methods that have been used to evaluate how the pericardium influences the hemodynamics of heart failure, it will be helpful to review, very briefly, ventricular diastolic function in normal hearts, in heart failure and in the presence of pericardial diseases that compress the heart. Most of the available data pertain to the left ventricle, but most likely apply in large measure to the right ventricle as well.

Although the word diastole implies a passive or inactive state, in reality the only passive portion of the cardiac cycle is the diastasis that occurs between the early rapid filling period and the onset of atrial contraction. When the heart rate increases, it does so at the expense of diastasis, which is eliminated when tachycardia is sufficiently severe. Early rapid filling is an energy and calcium dependent process that causes the ventricle to relax and thereby increase in volume. During this time, ventricular diastolic pressure drops below atrial pressure and the ventricle therefore sucks blood from the atrium and pulmonary veins. The basic underlying mechanism is removal of calcium from the active contraction site of the myocyte back to the sarcoplasmic reticulum where it is stored. The complex details of the responsible calcium cycling will not be discussed here, but are readily available elsewhere *(Gillebert and Sys 1994)*. Pericardial disease can adversely affect relaxation and compliance.

4.1.1   Recognition of the phases of diastole

EchoDoppler cardiography is the most available and commonly used means to identify the different phases of diastole. Doppler measurement of transmitral and trans-tricuspid blood flow velocity registers the E wave that identifies early rapid filling. This E wave is taller than the A wave depicting blood flow velocity consequent on atrial contraction. Impaired early diastolic relaxation reverses the ratio of the E and A velocities and increases the deceleration time of early rapid filling that marks equilibration of the atrial and ventricular diastolic pressures (Figure 6). This abnormality is caused by myocardial disease and may be seen in cardiac tamponade.

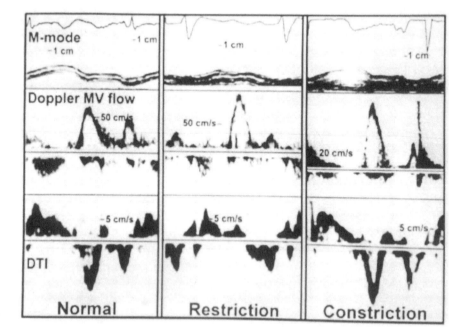

Figure 6. Echo Doppler parameters of diastolic function. For description, see the text. *(Oh, Hatle, Mulvagh, 1993. Reprinted with permission.)*

Reduced left ventricular compliance, on the other hand, has the opposite effect; here, the normal ratio of E to A peak velocities is exaggerated. The E wave is very tall and its deceleration is very short; the A wave is diminutive. Less commonly, apparent diminution of ventricular compliance may be caused by constrictive pericarditis. Tissue Doppler, which measures the velocity of motion of the mitral annulus, serves to distinguish between these two causes of what is sometimes referred to as a "restrictive filling pattern." When the pathology resides in the myocardium, annular motion is slow, whereas when it resides in the pericardium, myocardial velocity, like transmitral velocity, is very rapid (see Chapter 4).

4.2   Pericardial restraining forces in heart failure

Barnard (1898), whose work was discussed at the beginning of this chapter, concluded from his experiments:

"When a relaxed heart is subject to a venous pressure of from 10 to 20 mm Hg, the pericardium takes the strain and prevents dilatation of the heart beyond a certain point."

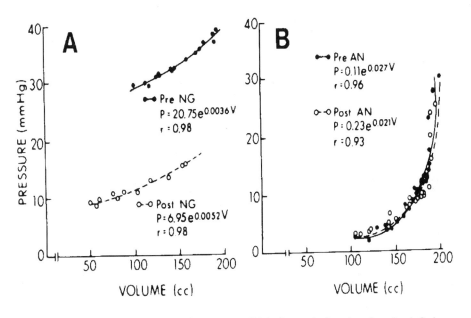

Figure 7 Left ventricular pressure-volume curves (**A**) before and after nitroglycerine infusion and (**B**) before and after amyl nitrite inhalation. Significant downward and leftward displacement of the pressure-volume curve occurs after nitroglycerine. In contrast, the data points of the diastolic pressure-volume curves before and after amyl nitrite fall on the same curve. (*From Ludbrook, Byrne, McKnight 1979, with permission*)

The effect of vasodilator administration to patients with acutely decompensated heart failure shed unanticipated light on the contribution made by the pericardium to elevated left ventricular diastolic pressure (*Ludbrook, Byrne, McKnight 1979*). High fidelity pressure measurements and left ventricular volumes determined by ventriculography were used to construct the diastolic pressure-volume relation before and after the sequential administration of nitroglycerine and amyl nitrite. The effects of the two drugs were in striking contrast. The venodilator nitroglycerine displaced the entire curve down on the pressure ordinate, whereas, the arteriolar dilator, amyl nitrite, lowered ventricular diastolic pressure along the control curve. We postulated that nitroglycerine shrank cardiac volume such that the heart disengaged from the pericardium, thereby removing the contribution the pericardium made to elevated ventricular diastolic volume. The arteriolar dilator did not shrink cardiac volume significantly, but allowed pressure to drop following coordinates on the control curve (Figure 7).

Our hypothesis was that in those patients with severe heart failure, much of the ventricular diastolic pressure was borne by the pericardium, and had it been possible to measure pericardial pressure, it would have been high, such that transmural ventricular pressure would have been substantially lower than pressure recorded in the standard manner. A precedent for this idea is found in the work of Holt, Rhode, and Kines *(1960)* who, in a seminal work, had shown that the increase in right atrial and biventricular diastolic pressures after a large and rapid infusion of dextran also increased pericardial pressure and therefore the increase in transmural cardiac pressures was quite small. A reasonable extrapolation is that in acute heart failure the same relationship between ventricular diastolic pressures referred to atmospheric pressure, pericardial pressure, and transmural ventricular diastolic pressure would be found (Figure 8).

Acute heart failure due to spontaneous rupture of chordae tendiniae furnishes a clinical example (*Bartle and Hermann 1967*). Hemodynamic studies demonstrated the anticipated tall narrow peak of left ventricular pressure during ventricular systole. Germane to the present context, the authors observed equilibrium between the elevated left and right ventricular pressures with each other and with right atrial pressure (Figure 9). The waveform of right and left atrial pressure was characteristic of pericardial constriction. In these cases, acute volume overload produced a strong distending force that was resisted by the tightly stretched, and therefore non-compliant pericardium. It is tempting to speculate that incision of the pericardium would have caused a prompt and substantial fall in ventricular diastolic pressure and relief of pulmonary congestion.

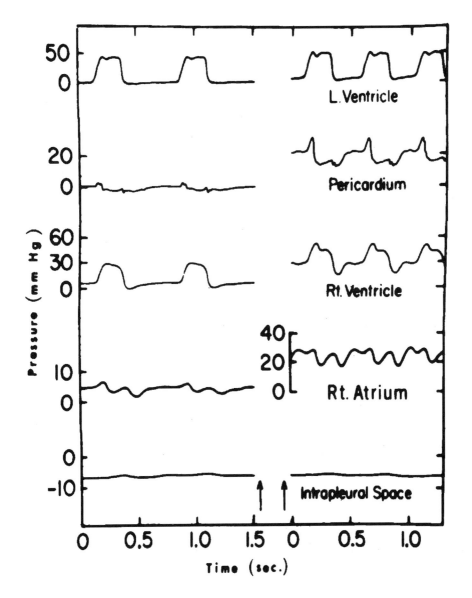

Figure 8 Pressure responses to rapid large volume infusion to the normal dog. Pericardial pressure was measured with a flat balloon three fourths of which lay on the surface of the right ventricle and one fourth on the right atrium. Between the arrows, 1000 ml. of Dextran was infused over a period of a few minutes. All pressures except pleural rose. The increased pericardial pressure lessens the effect of acute hypervolemia on transmural ventricular diastolic pressures. Note the accentuated decline of pericardial pressure accompanying ejection in the acute hypervolemic state.

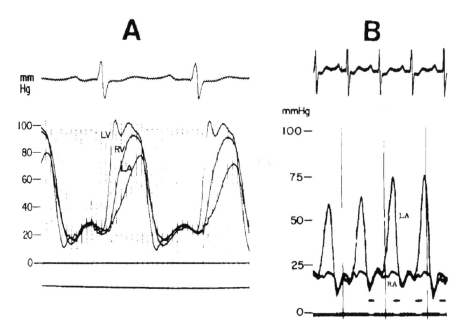

Figure 9 (A): Left ventricular, right ventricular and left atrial pressures recorded in a case of acute mitral regurgitation. Diastolic pressures from these sites are elevated and equal. **(B):** Simultaneous left and right atrial pressures from the same patient. Note equalization and prominent *y* descent of atrial diastolic pressures. The left atrial pressure pulse is characterized by tall, narrow systolic waves, characteristic of acute mitral regurgitation. (*From Bartle and Hermann, 1967, with permission*)

To test our speculation that the differing results of venous versus arteriolar dilation on severely exacerbated heart failure obtained by Ludbrook, Byrne, McKnight *(1979)* could best be explained in terms of pericardial restraint, we performed the following animal experiments. In chronically instrumented dogs we measured ventricular segment length with ultrasonic crystals as a surrogate for volume together with high fidelity pressure measurements starting at the end of the early rapid filling period and ending at the onset of atrial systole, that is, throughout diastasis. We then rapidly infused a liter of dextran. This intervention caused a dramatic upward shift along the pressure axis of the *entire* pressure-volume relation. We then infused nitroprusside, which caused a dramatic fall of the entire curve back down the pressure axis (Figure 10). We also measured pericardial pressure to confirm the observations of Holt, Rhode, and Kines *(1960)* that pericardial pressure rises during acute massive volume overload. Pericardial pressure fell in parallel with ventricular diastolic pressure during nitroprusside administration. Pericardiectomy was performed and the animals were restudied several days later, after full recovery from surgery.

Dextran infusion produced a large increase in ventricular diastolic pressure, but this time not by shifting the whole curve upwards, but by adding higher pressure points to the control curve. Likewise, nitroprusside infusion subsequently restored lower diastolic pressure by adding lower points to the control curve, not by shifting the entire curve down on its pressure axis.

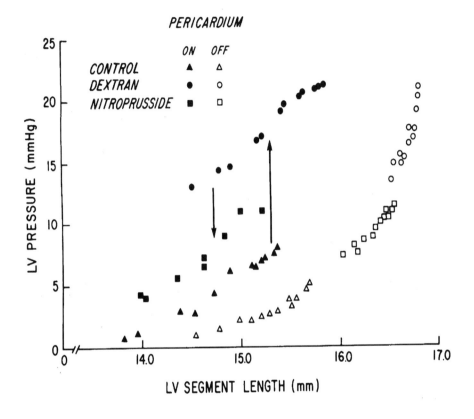

Figure 10 Left ventricular diastolic pressure-segment length relation before and after pericardiectomy. Dextran infusion shifted the entire curve upwards, nitroprusside lowered the curve toward control. The same interventions after pericardiectomy did not shift the curve, but the new data points fell along the original curve. *(From Shirato, Shabetai, Bhargava 1978, by permission of the American Heart Association, Inc.)*

When, in animals studied before pericardiectomy, we subtracted pericardial from ventricular diastolic pressure to obtain ventricular transmural pressure, and plotted that against volume, the curves appeared similar to those after surgical pericardiectomy (mathematical or virtual pericardiectomy) (Figure 11). In summary, the studies confirmed the important hemodynamic role of the pericardium in acute volume overload states relevant to acute heart failure.

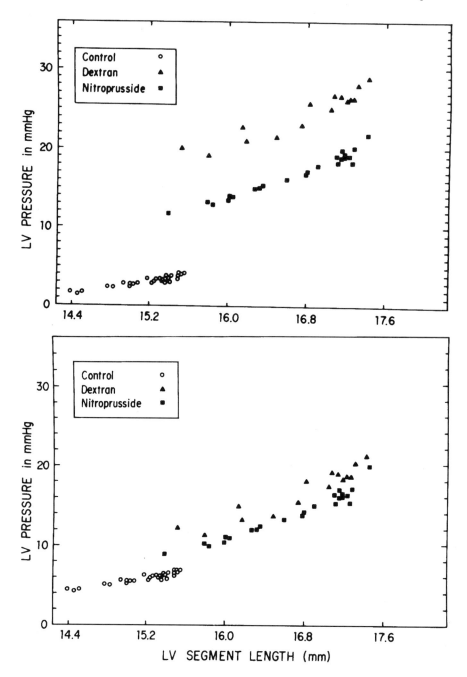

Figure 11 Pressure-segment length data response to dextran infusion followed by nitroprusside infusion. In the bottom panel, transmural ventricular diastolic pressure replaces cavity pressure. This manipulation has the same effect as pericardiectomy. *(From Shirato, Shabetai, Bhargava 1978, by permission of the American Heart Association, Inc.)*

The diagram in Figure 12 represents the two sides of the heart as water-filled balloons in a rigid, fluid-filled box (the pericardial cavity). (Modified from *Tyberg, Misbach, Glantz, 1978*)

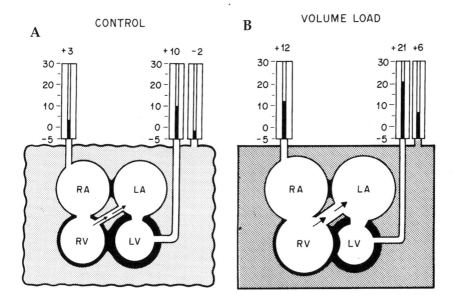

Figure 12 Ventricular interaction, acute volume overload and pericardial pressure. Schematic hydraulic model of the series arrangement but parallel juxtaposition of the left and right series of the heart surrounded by the fluid-filled, less compliant pericardium. **(Left) Control**: The diastolic pressures are higher on the left than on the right and exceed pericardial pressure. The ventricles and atria are separated by common septa, and right ventricular output is fed to the left atrium. The pericardium is lax and its pressure slightly negative, right atrial pressure 3, left 10. **(Right) Volume overload.** The heart, especially the more distensible atria and right ventricle is dilated. This expanded cardiac volume is not met by commensurate stretching of the pericardium; pericardial pressure is therefore increased from –2 to +6. The ventricular septum now bulges from right to left. Increased cardiac output is indicated by the wider channel connecting right ventricular output to the left heart. Right atrial pressure has risen to 12, left to 21.Transmural right and left cardiac pressures increased respectively, from 5 to 6 and 12 to 15. A portion of the increased cardiac pressures is thus borne by the pericardium. Septal bulging and increased cardiac output contribute the rest. *(Modified from Tyberg, Misbach, Glantz 1978).*

To address the question of more chronic volume overload that would be applicable to most instances of heart failure, investigators in our laboratory employed a surgical infrarenal aorto-caval anastomosis. They compared the effect of immediate pericardiectomy on the left ventricular end-diastolic pressure-segment length relation over a large range of ventricular diastolic volumes obtained by balloon occlusion of the inferior vena cava, followed by gradual release and subsequent dextran infusion *(LeWinter and Pavelec 1982).*

Dogs in which the shunt had functioned for only a matter of days showed a rightward shift along the volume axis after pericardiectomy, whereas in those studied after several weeks, this effect was greatly attenuated or absent, indicating that abnormal pericardial restraint was no longer present (Figure 13). This result demonstrated that, given time, in response to chronic volume overload, the pericardium creeps, thereby becoming more compliant. This result is relevant to chronic heart failure without a recent acute exacerbation. As is the case with myocardium, it was found that, by weighing the pericardium and measuring its thickness with a micrometer postmortem, the chronic stretch initiated hypertrophy. To elucidate the consequences of pericardial adaptation to stretch *in vivo*, pericardial pressure volume curves obtained in dogs with a chronic aorto-caval shunt were compared with those of control dogs. The curve was shifted far to the right as a consequence of chronic cardiac enlargement *(Freeman and Lewinter 1984)* (Figure 14).

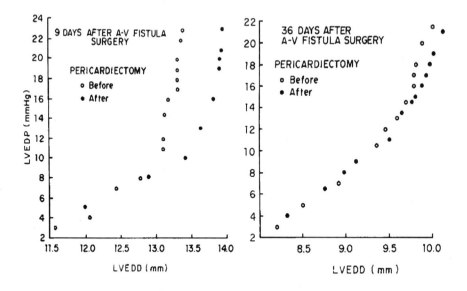

Figure 13. Left ventricular end-diastolic pressure-segment-length relation before and after pericardiectomy. The animals were studied either several days **(left)** or several weeks **(right)** postoperatively. In the dogs studied early, pericardiectomy demonstrated pericardial restraint by a rightward shift of the curve after pericardiectomy. This effect was lost in dogs studied later. *(From LeWinter and Pavelec 1982, with permission)*

To address whether increased pericardial compliance resulted from a change in intrinsic tissue compliance or was merely due to altered geometry of the pericardial sac, stress-strain curves were also generated, but they were not changed by pericardiectomy (Figure 14). The problem with this method, often satisfactorily used to calculate myocardial stress-strain relations, is that it is difficult to apply to the pericardium, because pericardial thickness is so much less than myocardial. This component of the stress equation is therefore not measured accurately in the case of the pericardium. We were unwilling to conclude that we had the evidence to state that the intrinsic mechanical properties of pericardium are not changed by chronic cardiac dilation. These were *in vivo* experiments, therefore the strong pericardial ligaments that attach the pericardium to the sternum, diaphragm and vertebrae remained intact, contributing to pericardial compliance; thus, even a stress-strain curve would not reflect the compliance of pericardial tissue; that would require an *in vivo* measuring technique *(Freeman and Little 1986)*.

To compare the compliance of the pericardium before and after chronic volume loading in intact dogs, we therefore studied the biomechanical properties of pericardium by biaxial stretching pieces of pericardium obtained from dogs with and without a chronic aorto-caval fistula *(Lee, LeWinter, Freeman, 1985)*. The curves from shunted dogs were shifted to the right (Figure 15).

4.2.1   Pericardial biomechanics

We acquired pericardial tissue compliance by excising a piece of pericardium about one centimetre square and performing biaxial stretching with the tissue oriented as it had been *in vivo*. The specimens needed for this purpose were obtained from dogs *(Lee, Lewinter, Freeman, 1985)*, but for comparative studies, we also obtained specimens from patients without cardiac enlargement during coronary arterial surgery *(Lee, Fung, Shabetai, 1987)*. Cyclical strain was applied to one axis while the tension of the orthogonal axis was held constant. Stress-strain curves of specimens from dogs with chronic volume overload were shifted to the right compared with those from control dogs, indicating pericardial creep (Figure 15). This change in *tissue* compliance underlies the parallel shift in pericardial *chamber* compliance we observed in dogs with sustained volume overload and confirmed that we had been unable to obtain pericardial stress-strain curves *in vivo*.

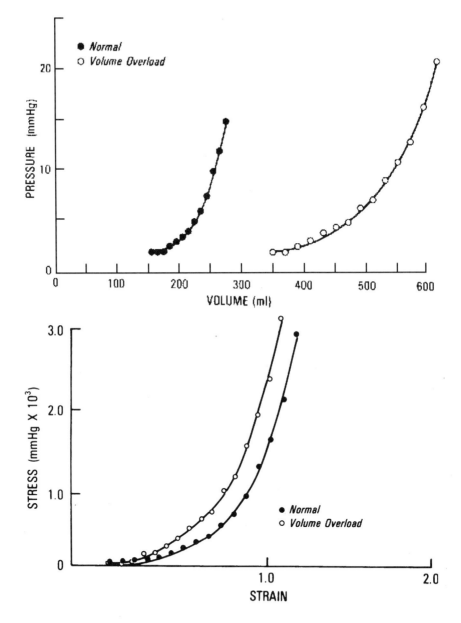

Figure 14 **Top:** Pericardial end-diastolic pressure-segment-length relation of a dog with a chronic aorto-caval shunt and cardiomegaly compared with a normal dog, showing marked right shift in the volume loaded animal. **Bottom:** Stress-strain curves done to determine whether the increased compliance observed in the left panel was due to altered geometry or a true increase in tissue compliance. The pericardium was too thin to allow measurement of changed stress. (*Reproduced from Freeman and LeWinter 1984, with permission*)

Canine pericardium proved highly anisotropic. It stretches easily along the horizontal axis, but is very noncompliant along the base-to-apex axis as had been shown *in vivo* earlier *(Mann, Lew, Ban-Hayashi, 1986)*. Both canine and human pericardium develop large deformations near the beginning of loading; then, as load is increased, become increasingly stiff and, finally, almost inextensible. Common to both species is hysteresis and that the tension stretch-relationship is insensitive to loading frequency, and stress relaxation is substantial, but creep is insignificant. Unlike canine pericardium, human pericardium is nearly isotropic and almost three times thicker. The human curve is left shifted compared with the canine, indicating that it is less extensible.

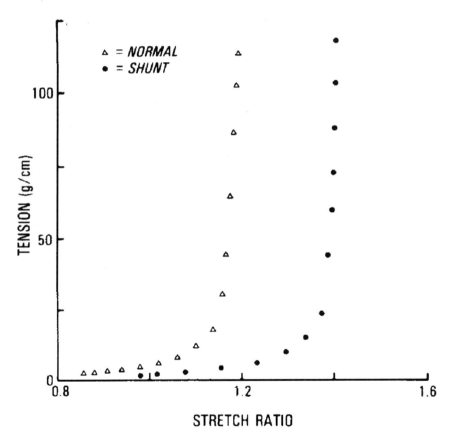

Figure 15 Stress-strain relation of pericardium, obtained by biaxial tissue stretching, from a normal dog and from a dog with chronic volume overload. The sample from the chronically volume overloaded dog is shifted to the right, indicating the tissue compliance has increased. *(From Lee, LeWinter, Freeman, 1985, with permission)*

4.2.2   Other components of cardiac restraint

Up to this point, we have considered cardiac restraint in terms of the compliance of the pericardial sac and that of pericardial tissue, but there are other components that will be discussed in the following section. Furthermore the constraints placed solely on the left ventricle rather than those affecting the whole heart are of physiological importance.

4.2.2.1   Pericardial attachments

The attachments of the pericardium to the diaphragm, sternum and great vessels were described in Chapter 1. The influence of pericardial attachments on the *in vivo* pericardial compliance was identified by comparing the *in situ* and *in vitro* pericardial pressure-volume relation in dogs (*Freeman and Little 1986) (Figure 16)*. Pericardial pressure-volume curves with the heart completely evacuated of air or fluid were generated using a Harvard pump for filling and emptying the sac *(in situ)*. The intact pericardium was then removed and mounted as shown in Figure 16. *In vitro* curves were then obtained and compared with the *in vivo* curves. The *in vitro* curves showed a more abrupt transition from the shallow to the steep portion of the curve, and the slope of the steep portion was increased. This result shows that tissue compliance determines pericardial compliance and the resulting cardiac restraint. The principal reason for the difference in *in vivo* and *in situ* pericardial pressure-volume is that when pericardial pressure-volume relations are studied *in vivo*, the attachments (the compliance of which is unknown) decrease its apparent compliance.

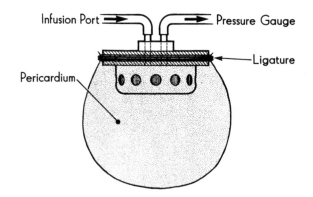

Figure 16 Diagram of the apparatus for *in vitro* tests of pericardium *(From Freeman and Little, 1986, with permission)*

The pericardium is not the sole external restraint on the heart which is a mediastinal structure encased (in good hands) by the lungs in what has been termed the cardiac fossa *(Butler 1983; Grant, Kondo, Maloney 1994)*. The effective surface pressure acting on the left ventricle is a function of both pericardial pressure and right ventricular pressure weighted to the respective surface areas over which they apply. The interventricular septum constitutes approximately one third of the left ventricular surface; therefore, the effective external pressure equals approximately two thirds the pericardial pressure plus one third right ventricular diastolic pressure (M*irsky and Rankin 1979)*.

In a canine model of acute ischemic left ventricular failure, changes in preload, afterload and circulating blood volume shifted diastolic pressure-volume relations by stretching or relaxing the pericardium, which in turn reduced ventricular pressure. Changes in transmural ventricular diastolic pressure were absent or minimal. *(Smiseth, Refsum, Junemann, 1984)*.

Less research has been done on constraint of the right ventricle, but downward and rightward shifts of the right ventricular pressure-volume relation are known to follow pericardiectomy *(Assanelli, Lew, Shabetai, 1987; Traboulsi, Scott-Douglas, Smith, 1992; Janicki and Weber, 1980)*.

Twenty patients were studied during operation for coronary arterial disease. Right ventricular volumes and ejection fraction were assessed by thermodilution. *(Burger, Straube, Behne 1995)*. After determining control values, the pulmonary artery was compressed digitally through a small pericardial incision, increasing the pulmonary arterial pressure to approximately 40 mm Hg. The pericardium was then widely opened and the measurements were repeated.

Compression with the pericardium intact (except for the small incision) over the pulmonary artery reduced systemic arterial pressure and the ejection fraction of the right ventricle. Right atrial, right ventricular pressures and end-systolic volume increased. After pericardiotomy, pulmonary arterial compression caused right ventricular end-diastolic and end-systolic pressures to increase and a fall in its ejection fraction. The decline in left heart hemodynamics observed with the intact pericardium was no longer seen. The right ventricular pressure-volume curve was shifted to the right. Pericardiotomy did not change right ventricular diastolic volume in the control setting. During acutely elevated right ventricular afterload, pericardial restraint of the right ventricle became manifest.

Acute pulmonary embolism furnishes a dramatic example of the deleterious effects of severe acute increase in right ventricular afterload that ensues. The left ventricle is underfilled by the intense series and parallel ventricular interaction, and pericardial restraint also becomes intense because of the massive dilation of the right heart and intrapericardial pulmonary artery. The initial life saving manoeuvre in this critical situation may be extensive pericardiotomy (*Belenkie, Dani, Smith, 1992*).

4.2.2.2   Pericardial restraint during exercise in heart failure

During exercise, the ventricles of the failing heart dilate sooner and to a greater extent than the ventricles of a normal heart. Janicki *(1990)* posited that in patients with heart failure, cardiac dilation may cause the heart to engage the pericardium with the result that ventricular interaction would be enhanced, much as it is in acute volume overload or constrictive pericarditis. To test this hypothesis, he performed upright exercise studies in patients with heart failure. With heart failure in the absence of significant pericardial restraint, pulmonary wedge pressure rose more steeply than right atrial pressure and cardiac output increased until maximal effort had been achieved.

Three different responses were found in heart failure (Figure 17). The first response was that, in the early stage of exercise, pulmonary wedge pressure rose steeply, but right atrial pressure rose only slightly and stroke volume increased for the duration of exercise (C1). The second response was that, in the early stage of exercise, left atrial pressure rose faster than right and stroke volume increased, but in the later stage of exercise, the two slopes were parallel and stroke volume was invariant (C2). The third response was an equal slope of pressure increase in wedge (PCW) and right atrial pressures (RAP) and a fixed stroke volume throughout exercise (C3). In our laboratory, we perform cycle exercise with measurements of cardiac output and right heart pressures in candidates for cardiac transplantation, but have not observed an equal slope of increase in pulmonary wedge and right atrial pressure in any patient.

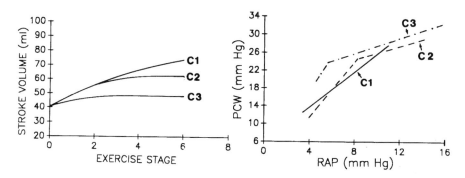

Figure 17. Pericardial restraint becomes evident during upright exercise in patients with heart failure. Explanation in text. (From *Janicki (1990), with permission*)

4.2.2.3   Pericardium and exercise without heart failure

Evidence has been published favouring the development of cardiac restraint during treadmill exercise in normal animals. One of the most interesting was that of Stray-Gundersen, Musch, Haidet (1986) in which they reported that removing the pericardium of the greyhound allowed a 25 percent increase in maximal oxygen uptake and cardiac output. We have confirmed this observation for the pig (*Hammond, White, Bhargava, 1992*), observing a similar increase in both parameters. Our studies also showed that in the weeks following pericardiectomy, a progressive increase in ventricular volume takes place, and furthermore, its pressure-volume relation is shifted rightwards along the volume axis. End-systolic volume did not decrease, indicating that in normal animals the increased cardiac performance results, not from increased contractility as would be expected, but via the Frank-Starling mechanism. Confirming this interpretation for any given workload, the heart rate after pericardiectomy was lower than with the pericardium intact.

4.2.3   Summary

Pericardial restraint is apt to become manifest in heart failure. This constraint may be evident at rest, particularly in acute or recently decompensated heart failure. An important manifestation is downward displacement of the left ventricular diastolic pressure-volume curve in response to reducing cardiac volume with a venodilator. In some patients, pericardial restraint is not detected at rest, but develops during exercise and may contribute to limited performance. On the other hand, in acute heart failure the pericardium may play a beneficial role, preventing excessive cardiac dilation. Some decades ago, this concept gave rise to the idea that late stage intractable heart failure could be treated by pericardiectomy, but the idea was quickly abandoned. As often happens in clinical medicine, the exact opposite course, treating heart failure with a cardiac restraining or supporting device, is now in clinical trial.

4.3   Cardiac support devices

4.3.1   Acorn

When the *latissimus dorsi* wrap (cardiomyoplasty) was introduced as adjunctive treatment for dilated heart failure, it was proposed that improved cardiac function would result from regular contractions of the trained, paced muscle wrapped around the heart (*Carpentier and Chachques 1991*). Others, however, questioned this hypothesis, proposing instead that cardiac benefit resulted more from partial reversal of mechanical and electrical remodelling brought about by the added passive constraint. Thus, a study was done in which cardiomyoplasty was performed on 6 of 11 dogs with severe dilated heart failure induced by prior rapid pacing, without ever turning on the stimulator. When the animals with a wrap were compared with controls, less ventricular dilation and a higher ejection fraction were observed in those with the wrap in spite of the absence of electrical stimulation of the muscle wrap (*Capouya, Gerber, Drinkwater 1993*). The authors proposed that increased external restraint contributes to the beneficial effects of cardiomyoplasty traditionally ascribed to augmentation of systolic function by the muscle squeeze provided by the paced muscle wrap. In a clinical study of three patients being treated for heart failure by cardiomyoplasty, left ventricular pressure-volume curves were obtained with the stimulator either turned on or off. Under both conditions, ventricular volume decreased and performance increased, in comparison with control, without evidence for enhanced systolic function (*Kass, Baughman, Pak 1995*). The authors speculated that cardiomyoplasty acting as an elastic girdle around the heart helps to diminish or reverse remodelling. These studies led to the consideration of some kind of cardiac wrap designed to act primarily as a supporting device. The wrap would not be made of muscle, but by an inorganic material. From what has been discussed thus far about pericardial biomechanics, the design of a wrap suitable for this application must have presented formidable engineering and manufacturing problems. Aside from the standard requirements for any bio-prosthesis, the compliance of the device would be critical. If it were too compliant, the device simply would not work; were it not compliant enough, it would induce constrictive physiology.

The Acorn device is presently the most developed of these devices. As its name implies, it fits the heart like an acorn in its cup (Figure 18). It is composed of micro fibers of polyester oriented in multiple directions and its compliance is appropriate for its task. One of the prescribed requirements was that, in addition to containing or reducing cardiac volume, it should decrease the abnormal sphericity characteristic of the dilated ventricle and partly restore the normal ellipsoid configuration. Therefore, the Acorn was designed to be more compliant in its long than its short axis, that is, intentionally the opposite of the anisotropy of the normal canine pericardium. Human pericardium is isotropic. The reactive tissue that forms between the device and the epicardium is soft enough not to impede diastolic function, but sufficient to bond the device to the heart, and does not invade the epicardium.

The device has been successfully applied in many animal models and presently is in several clinical trials. At the present writing, a significant body of evidence supporting its hemodynamic and clinical effects and its mechanism of action is available (*Saavedra, Tunin, Paolocci. 2002*). Constrictive physiology has not been encountered by invasive and non-invasive hemodynamic investigations or clinical outcome after implanting the device.

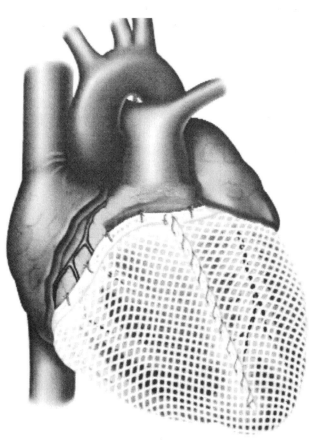

Figure 18. The Acorn cardiac support device

4.4   Mechanisms of action of passive restraint

The hypothesis underlying the development of cardiac support devices was that they would not simply reduce ventricular end-diastolic pressure mechanically, but that, by limiting or preventing progressive dilation, and thus myocardial stretch, they would reduce or turn off signals for ventricular remodelling, the principal reason for the progressive nature of heart failure. It was first established that the devices significantly reduce ventricular diastolic volume and prevent or slow the rate of progressive dilation. Basic studies have established that the remodelling process is indeed checked and cardiac function thereby improved. End systolic ventricular volume, a potent marker of contractility, diminishes. Proteins and their messengers, signalled by stretch, diminish or disappear, myocyte contractility is enhanced, the collagen skeleton of the heart is rearranged to conform to a more normal pattern and the altered ratio of its fiber types are partially restored to normal. The function of the sarcoplasmic reticulum improves and is one of the mechanisms accounting for improved calcium handling. Myocyte hypertrophy and interstitial fibrosis diminish. Physiological studies have shown that diminished preload reserve is partially restored (*Chaudhry, Mishima, Sharov 2000*).

Several mechanisms are responsible for the beneficial effects that ensue after providing passive external support to the failing dilated heart using the Acorn device (*Saavedra, Tunin, Paolocci, 2002*). The investigators recorded left ventricular pressure-volume loops at differing preloads obtained by inflating a balloon in the inferior vena cava, before and three to six months after implanting the device in six dogs. They also evaluated adrenergic and adenylyl cyclase responsiveness to dobutamine infusion. In addition, they measured preload reserve and evaluated the animals for evidence of the development of constrictive physiology after implantation.

End-diastolic volume was reduced by 19 percent and end-systolic dimension by 22 percent. The end-systolic pressure-volume elation was shifted to the left, confirming reverse remodelling, but its slope did not change. Of great importance, the end-diastolic pressure and chamber stiffness were unchanged. With the device in place, dobutamine infusion increased the left ventricular ejection fraction by 55 percent, compared with only 10 percent before implantation. Although the adenylyl cyclase response was heightened after implantation, there was no parallel increase in the density or affinity of the beta-adrenergic receptors. Diastolic compliance was not adversely affected. Dextran infusion almost doubled cardiac output without inducing the square root sign of left ventricular diastolic pressure.

4.5   Required compliance for a cardiac support device

It is apparent that an appropriate value for compliance of these devices is critical, if it is to exert the desired effects on remodelling and yet not cause constrictive physiology. The desired pressure-volume relation of a cardiac restraining device is neither that of the normal pericardium, which is extremely stiff even at small cardiac volumes, or that of the severely dilated heart, in which the diastolic pressure is excessive when cardiac volume is greatly increased (Figure 19). The compliance of the current version of the Acorn device appears to have met these requirements, but the device is still in an early stage of clinical testing and other manufacturers are planning or making comparable devices. The advent of this technology has opened an exciting new chapter in the story of external constraint on the heart. The earlier paragraphs of this chapter have shown that the pericardium is beautifully designed for the normal heart and copes nicely with the early stages of chronic heart failure. In severe or acute heart failure, the pericardium is an obstacle to maintaining a normal or compensated hemodynamic status.

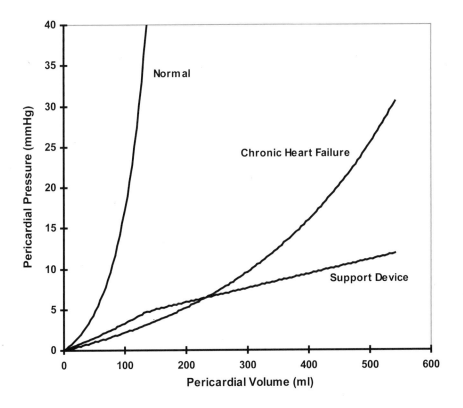

Figure19. Schematic of the desired compliance of a cardiac support device. The device must gently restrain progressive dilation of the heart with an external pressure that does not increase ventricular interaction or ventricular diastolic pressure to a clinically significant degree.

5.   PERICARDIAL PRESSURE AND CONTACT FORCE

We come now to a question to which I have previously alluded; what are cardiac pressure and contact force and how should they be measured?

In the early papers on ventricular interaction reviewed at the beginning of this chapter, pericardial pressure was measured using standard laboratory methods. It has, however, been forcefully and in many ways persuasively argued by many investigators that these methods are not appropriate for the pericardium, because the pericardial space is for the most part potential rather than actual. Thus pericardial fluid is concentrated over the interventricular and interatrial grooves and only a thin fluid film may overlie the flat cardiac surfaces (*Santamore, Constantinescu, Bogen,* 1990). This distribution of pericardial fluid, according to some investigators, vitiates pericardial pressure measurements obtained either using an intrapericardial catheter via its lumen or a transducer at its tip, unless the subject has a pericardial effusion. According to this school of thought, when pericardial fluid is scant or absent, the result of a conventional pressure measurement is an artifact. Instead, contact force should be measured via a flat gas or liquid-filled unstressed balloon introduced between the pericardium and the heart. The difference between pressures measured in these two ways is not trivial. See Table 1.

Table 1. Pericardial pressure versus contact force

Pericardial liquid pressure	Pericardial contact force
Essentially uniform over the heart	Regional variation
Slightly below atmospheric	Equals right atrial pressure
Significant RV diastolic transmural pressure	RV diastolic transmural pressure almost zero
Substantial pressure required to cause significant strain (increase preload)	Very small pressure increments needed to increase preload
Left ventricular (LV) minus pericardial pressure approximates transmural LV pressure	Left ventricular minus right atrial pressure approximates transmural LV pressure

JV Tyberg has pioneered research on measurement of pericardial pressure or, as he prefers to consider it, epicardial radial stress. He proposed that the magnitude of pericardial restraint can be determined by the static equilibrium equation, that is, the drop of left ventricular diastolic pressure upon widely opening the pericardium, measured at the same ventricular volume. He named this value the theoretical pericardial pressure. He and co-workers showed that pericardial pressure measured by balloon was essentially the same as the theoretical pericardial pressure, providing pericardial effusion is absent (*Tyberg, Misbach, Glanz, 1978; Traboulsi, Scott-Douglas, Smith, 1992; Smiseth, Frais, Kingma, 1985*) (Figure 20). When pericardial fluid volume is increased, the difference between balloon and catheter tip measurement progressively diminishes.

The higher pericardial pressure obtained using a balloon has a number of important consequences for cardiac physiology. Before this concept had been advanced, it was assumed that equal external pressure all around the heart prevents regional differences in transmural pressure when the subject is submitted to changing gravitational force (*Banchero, Rutishauser, Tsakiris 1967*).

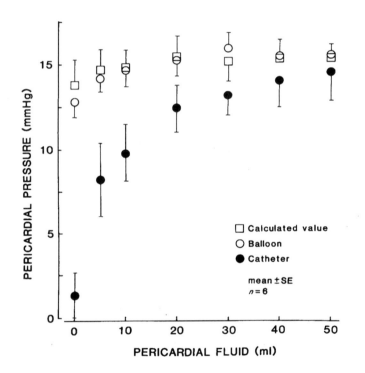

Figure 20. Comparison of theoretical pericardial pressure and pericardial pressure recorded either from a catheter tip or via a flat balloon. *(From Smiseth, Frais, Kingma, 1985, with permission of the American Heart Association, Inc.)*

The authors measured atrial, pericardial, and pleural pressures in dogs subjected to up to 7g by centrifugation in the supine, prone and both decubitus positions. At all levels of g tested, end-expiratory pericardial pressure varied directly with the vertical height of the recording site in the thorax and were unchanged during horizontal acceleration, but were slightly changed by vertical acceleration because of change in the weight of the heart. Simultaneously measured pressures in the pleura and pericardium proved that pericardial transmural pressure was zero at all levels of *g* tested. Transmural right and left atrial pressures were independent of the height of the recording site in the chest and were unchanged by the height of the recording site in the thorax. Balloons were not used for these measurements. These findings, which may at first sight seem rather obscure, are of considerable importance in physiology. They imply that pericardial fluid is present in all regions of the pericardial space, if in places only as a thin film, and hence that pericardial pressure is transmitted equally throughout the space. Thus, even over the flat ventricular surfaces, the function of pericardial fluid is not limited to lubrication, as Santamore stated. In this respect, pericardial liquid pressure is valid.

During day-to-day existence, blood in the cardiac chambers is continuously subject to gravitational hydrostatic forces as well as to inertial forces whenever the body velocity accelerates or changes direction. The function of the heart is aided by virtue of being suspended in a hydrostatic system that automatically applies perfectly compensated pressures to its external surfaces whenever gravitational or inertial forces acting on it change. In another study (*Avasthey and Wood, 1974*), the investigators measured pericardial pressure together with pressure in the venae cavae and right and left heart in dogs during sudden changes from supine to head up or head down body positions. This study also demonstrated that vertical pressure gradients within pericardium, atria and great veins behave as a simple hydrostatic system; therefore, transmural cardiac pressures remained practically constant, independent of body position. Thus, just as cerebrospinal and peritoneal fluid minimise the effects of gravitational and inertial forces on the cerebral and abdominal contents, pericardial liquid pressure plays a comparable role for the heart. Cavity liquid pressure in the pericardium and pleura track faithfully throughout the respiratory cycle, but pericardial pressure varies also with events of the cardiac cycle. The pattern of this variability depends on the location of the intrapericardial catheter, but a sharp decline during ventricular ejection is a constant feature.

Catheter measurement of intraventricular pressure is a function of ventricular volume and distensibility, the hydrostatic level of the catheter tip relative to the zero reference employed, and external constraining forces. On the other hand, pericardial pressure is a function of pleural pressure at the level of the pericardial catheter tip, the distensibility of the parietal pericardium and the hydrostatic level of the catheter tip in the pericardial space (*Holt, 1967*).

Equal transmural pressure at all hydrostatic levels ensures uniform muscle stretch at end diastole and uniform operation of the Frank-Starling law. When the chest is open, however, transmural pressure differs at each hydrostatic level of a particular chamber, and may amount to 9 mm Hg for the dog heart (*Holt, 1967*). Thus, at end diastole, the most dependent fibers may be subject to this increase in transmural pressure which would stretch them and, through the Starling mechanism, increase their force of contraction, while in the basal regions may approach zero with consequent reduction of stretch and contraction.

In summary, conventionally measured cardiac transmural pressure is, strictly speaking, the distending force for filling (*Fowler, Shabetai, Braunstein 1959*), is defined as the difference between cardiac and pericardial pressure, and is independent of gravity. It may be estimated using pleural or oesophageal pressure in place of the less readily available pericardial pressure. When pericardial pressure is measured instead by balloon to assess contact force, none of these considerations apply.

5.1   Non-uniform contact pressure

The prediction that contact pressure would not be uniform around the heart has been proven experimentally (*Smiseth, Scott-Douglas, Thompson 1987*) (Figure 21). When balloons are placed at more than one site in the pericardium, the contact pressures recorded vary somewhat, and this variation is substantially increased by interventions that predominantly affect one side of the heart. Compression of the aorta increases regional contact pressure over the left ventricle, whereas compressing the pulmonary artery increases contact pressure regionally over the right ventricle. Likewise, interventions that decrease the volume of one side of the heart cause regional decrease of contact pressure on that side (*Hoit, Lew, LeWinter 1988; Smiseth, Scott-Douglas, Thompson 1987*). The pericardium restrains the right heart more than the left, and differences are present between the inflow and outflow regions of this geometrically complex chamber (*Assanelli, Lew, Shabetai 1987*).

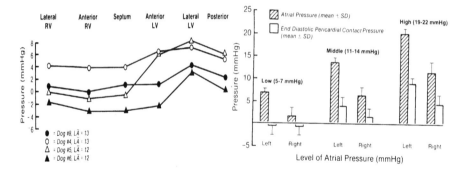

Figure 21. Non-uniform pericardial contact force. **Left:** End-diastolic contact pressures at various sites over the heart for four dogs. The different symbols for each dog are connected. **Right:** Relationship between mean atrial pressure at different levels of filling. As left atrial pressure increases, the proportion of pericardial contact to atrial pressure increases, but it always is more on the left than on the right. (*From Hoit, Lew, LeWinter 1988, with permission*)

5.1.1   Almost zero right ventricular diastolic pressure

In deciding when to use pressure within the pericardial space versus contact pressure to assess restraint by the pericardium on the heart, one of the more difficult issues has been the near zero right ventricular diastolic pressure measured by the latter technique. As we have already noted, the validity of surface pressure measured via an unstressed liquid-filled balloon was established by the static equilibrium equation. This equation states that, at the same chamber volume, the drop in pericardial pressure produced by pericardiectomy is a reliable estimate of pericardial pressure *(Smiseth, Refsum, Junemann, 1984; Smiseth, Kingma, Refsum, 1985)*. The pressures, and still more, the pressure differences between pericardium and ventricle, were low and thus subject to significant error. These errors would be more apt to occur in experiments performed on beating hearts. It therefore appeared to other investigators that errors would be reduced by using an *in situ* post mortem model to evaluate pericardial constraint by static equilibrium *(Slinker, Ditchey, Bell 1987)*. The data show that right ventricular diastolic transmural pressure is not *exactly* zero. Transmural pressure is a term in equations for calculating left ventricular diastolic compliance. It has been suggested that the transmural pressure term be derived from contact pressure *(Smiseth, Refsum, Tyberg 1984)*. This approach would yield a different value for compliance than when the transmural pressure term is based on conventional measurement of pericardial pressure. Thus the appropriate formula for measuring left ventricular diastolic compliance in intact subjects remains controversial.

In spite of the controversy, scrutiny of the data obtained by either method of measuring pericardial pressure lead to the conclusions that right heart transmural pressures are not *exactly* zero. Even at low right atrial pressure the pericardium bears some of that pressure, but this phenomenon becomes physiologically important only at high filling pressure. Experiments in which pericardial pressure is deduced but not directly measured support these conclusions. More recently, a study from Tyberg's laboratory confirmed that the pericardium exerts a strong influence on the right heart chambers, especially the notably compliant right atrium (*Hamilton, Danni, Semlacher, 1994*). Using contact force, not pericardial pressure, does mean that remarkably small changes in pressure are required to change right heart preload.

6. OTHER INFLUENCES OF THE PERICARDIUM ON VENTRICULAR FUNCTION

Pericardiectomy influences the trans-tricuspid and, to a lesser extent, the transmitral blood flow velocity profile. In a combined invasive and echoDoppler study addressing this phenomenon, it was necessary to control or measure confounding variables such as ventricular diastolic volume and pressure, and stroke volume (*Hoit, Dalton, Bhargava, 1991*). Pericardiectomy increased peak transmitral filling velocity and the directly measured pressure gradient at all levels of left ventricular pressure investigated. Both transmitral and tricuspid early velocities were increased by infusion. In the case of the tricuspid orifice, however, pericardiectomy did not increase early filling velocity but, to the contrary, increased atrial velocity, reversing the E/A ratio. This change was exactly mirrored in the directly measured trans-tricuspid pressure gradient, and was therefore attributed to alterations in the determinants of the filling pressure gradient. The different responses on the two sides may be explained by lower left than right atrial compliance. There were significant methodological limitations of this interesting study. These limitations would be insuperable in a clinical echoDoppler investigation.

6.1 Additional sources of external constraint

In addition to the pericardium, other mediastinal structures add to external cardiac constraint. The heart is a mediastinal organ that is situated in the cardiac fossa, formed by the lungs, that also supports and restrains it. The left ventricle is restrained by the right ventricle via the interventricular septum as well as by the pericardium. Based on the relative areas of these two sources of constraint, transmural left ventricular pressure is commonly calculated as left ventricular diastolic pressure minus two thirds of pericardial pressure plus one third of right ventricular diastolic pressure *(Mirsky and Rankin 1979)*. This method would yield a result somewhat different from that obtained by simply subtracting right atrial pressure from left ventricular end-diastolic pressure as has been suggested *(Tyberg and Smith 1990)*, unless pericardial contact stress and right atrial pressures are considered to be nearly equal.

7.   COMPARATIVE PHYSIOLOGY

7.1   Pericardium and the elasmobranch cardiac cycle

The structure and function of the pericardium of fishes are different from those of mammals. We studied the elasmobranch (sharks and rays) after our attention was drawn to the subject by a publication on pericardial structure and function *(Holt, Rhode, Kines 1960)* in which marine biology papers are quoted and an illustration is provided (Figure 22). The classic literature held that elasmobranch filling depends upon a strongly negative pericardial pressure, and that in all fishes atrial systole is the exclusive determinant of ventricular filling. This description of the elasmobranch cardiac cycle went so far as to state that atrial diastolic pressure was lower than ventricular except during atrial systole.

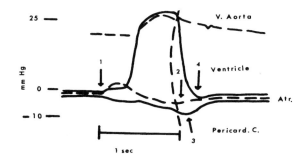

Figure 22. Retouched diagram of the dogfish cardiac cycle. The vertical dashed line indicates the arc of the rectilinear recorder on stationary paper. The numbered arrows refer to points in the cardiac cycle where pressure was measured. Note sub-ambient pericardial pressure throughout the cardiac cycle that decreases further with ventricular systole. Atrial pressure is also sub-ambient except during atrial systole. (From *Sudak, 1965, with permission*)

When we first set out to enquire further into these phenomena, we were surprised to learn that it had long been known that a structure, the pericardio-peritoneal canal, is present in elasmobranchs, but its function had not been described in the literature. On studying this interesting structure, we found that it allows fluid to pass only in the direction of pericardium to peritoneum. Our speculation that it may protect against cardiac tamponade was quickly disproven when we injected fluid into the pericardium until it could be seen exiting the canal. When this expulsion first occurred, adding more fluid to the pericardium failed to increase pericardial pressure further, but severe tamponade ensued that could be relieved only by aspirating pericardial fluid (*Shabetai, Abel, Graham 1985*).

When chronically instrumented submerged elasmobranch are studied, pericardial pressure is ambient, but when the fish is handled or startled, the pressure drops below atmospheric, and returns to ambient, at first rapidly, but requiring several hours to recover fully. The responsible mechanism is expulsion of the pericardial fluid via the canal (*Abel, Graham, Lowell 1986*).

EchoDoppler and direct pressure measurements unequivocally showed bimodal ventricular filling, with E and A waves exactly like those of mammals (Figure 23). Pericardial pressure was ambient, or minimally sub-ambient and atrial pressure exceeded ventricular pressure throughout diastole. As in mammals, early diastolic filling was associated with an increased atrio-ventricular gradient caused by a drop of ventricular pressure during early relaxation. Several other piscine species we subsequently studied also exhibit mammal-like ventricular inflow profiles.

7.2   Structure and function

Unlike the mammalian pericardium which is tightly applied to the surface of the heart, that of the elasmobranch is strongly adherent to the body cartilages, leaving a large fluid-filled cavity between it and the heart. This was the supposed reason for the strongly negative pericardial pressure, the existence of which we have disputed. (*Abel, Graham, Lowell 1986*). The ratio of pericardial to cardiac volume is thus far greater in elasmobranchs than in mammals. Furthermore, pericardial fluid volume can be reduced by expulsion via the pericardioperitoneal canal. The effect of this change is to increase cardiac transmural pressure (preload). This expulsion takes place when the fish is startled or performs burst swimming, and may be a mechanism to increase cardiac output in the absence of a sympathetic innervation of the heart.

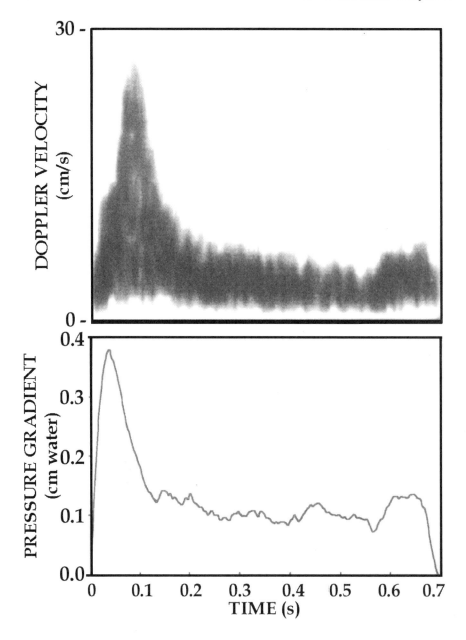

Figure 23. Simultaneously recorded Doppler velocity records of atrio-ventricular inflow with atrio-ventricular pressure gradient obtained by digitised subtraction. *(From Lai, Graham, Bhargava 1996, with permission)*

8. THE EFFECTS OF RESPIRATION ON PRESSURE AND FLOW IN THE CIRCULATION

8.1 Historical background

Ramon Lange attributed the first description of weakening of the pulse in pericardial disease to a paper in the London Journal of Medicine (*Williams 1850*). Boyd and Patras *(1941)* used a cardiometer attached on one side to the heart, and to the pleural space on the other side, to show that during inspiration, the combined left and right ventricular volume increases. This observation was puzzling to Shuler, Ensor, Gunning *(1942),* who wondered, if the heart pumps more blood in inspiration, why should systemic arterial pressure fall? These investigators removed a portion of the ventral chest wall of dogs and affixed paper markers to each ventricle, then resealed the chest with translucent material. When the animal resumed normal respiration, they took motion pictures to record, frame by frame, the areas of the ventricles along with pleural and carotid pressures. They observed increased right ventricular size and stroke volume, but decreased left ventricular size and stroke volume. They concluded that some blood is withheld from the heart until the onset of the next expiration. This is yet another instance of the ingenuity of investigators who lacked the instrumentation available today.

Lauson, Bloomfield, and Cournand (1946) examined the right heart pressure records of 200 patients. At that time, artificial pneumothorax was frequently performed to treat tuberculosis, providing the authors the opportunity to measure pleural pressure and calculate transmural pressure, and to show that transmural right heart pressures increase with inspiration. They noted that the decline of thoracic pressure during inspiration was not of sufficient magnitude to account for the magnitude of the inspiratory drop of systemic arterial pressure, and proposed that pooling in the lung was an additional mechanism. These findings and conclusions confirmed those reported earlier (*Fowler, Shabetai, Braunstein* 1959*). In the chronically instrumented conscious dog with physiological heart rate, transmission of the inspiratory surge of right heart output requires less than two cardiac cycles (*Morgan, Guntheroth, Dillard 1965*). We now know that blood does not pool in the lungs, but there is a finite transit time through the pulmonary circulation.

8.2   Subsequent studies

   The act of respiration induces changes in pulmonary arterial and aortic pressure and flow and on the dimensions of the cardiac chambers. As we have already seen, these changes implicate the pericardium and are exaggerated by respiratory disease or manoeuvres such as the Müller or Valsalva, and by cardiac or pericardial diseases. Inspiration lowers right heart and thoracic and pericardial pressures a few mm Hg, thereby increasing systemic venous return from the extrathoracic great veins. Transmural right heart pressures, however, increase during inspiration. Systemic arterial pressure and flow decrease a few mm Hg with inspiration. The drop in transmural pressure is even less. The several responsible mechanisms include transit time through the lungs, increased afterload; *(Summer, Permutt, Sagawa, 1979; McGregor 1979)* (Figure24), ventricular interaction, and direct transmission of changes in the thoracic pressure to the heart and great vessels. Ventricular interaction is minimal in health, but the increased right heart volume in the presence of the pericardium does slightly reduce left heart volume.

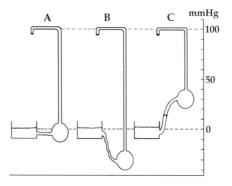

Figure 24. The effects of changing pleural (or pericardial) pressure on right ventricular inflow and left ventricular outflow. **(A):** normal. The heart and lungs are shown as a single pump filled from a venous reservoir at a pressure of 2 mm Hg via *collapsible* tubing. The pump expels blood into the systemic arteries to achieve a pressure-head, equivalent to 100 mm Hg. **(B):** Müller Manoeuvre. Reducing pericardial pressure to minus 30 mm Hg is comparable to lowering the pressures within the heart an equivalent amount with respect to the systemic arterial reservoirs. The left ventricle must develop more force to "raise" the pressure of blood to the previous arterial pressure. Filling of the right ventricle is potentiated by the favourable venous return pressure gradient. **(C):** Valsalva Manoeuvre. Elevation of intrathoracic pressure to 30 mm Hg has the opposite effect. The heart pump is raised relative to the systemic reservoirs. Systemic ejection is facilitated, since less energy is required to raise aortic pressure to the level of the previous arterial pressure. Venous return to the right heart is impeded by the adverse gradient. *(From McGregor, 1979, with permission.)* With normal breathing, these changes are far smaller.

Positive end-expiratory pressure is a commonly employed therapeutic intervention and may induce a drop in cardiac output, unless high cardiac filling pressures are maintained. Causes of the decreased cardiac output include reflexes from pulmonary stretch receptors, impaired systemic venous return, and increased pulmonary vascular resistance. Positive end-expiratory pressure increases the ratio of septal-lateral-to-apical and anterior-posterior axes and raises left atrial transmural pressure (*Scharf, Brown, Saunders, 1979),* shifting the left ventricular pressure-volume curve to the left. The investigators attributed these changes to ventricular interaction enhanced by the pericardium in the face of increased right ventricular afterload.

The pericardium clearly plays a significant role in the way in which respiration affects the circulation in health and disease as will be discussed in Chapters 4, 6, and 7.

References

Abel DC, Graham JB, Lowell WR Shabetai R. Elasmobranch pericardial function. 1. Pericardial pressures are not always negative. Fish Physiol Biochem 1986; 1:75-83

Assanelli D, Lew WYW, Shabetai R, LeWinter MM. Influence of the pericardium on right and left filling in the dog. J Appl Physiol .1987; 63: 1025-1032.

Avasthey P, Wood EH. Intrathoracic and venous pressure relationships during responses to changes in body position. J Appl Physiol 1974; 37: 166-175.

Banchero N, Rutishauser WJ, Tsakiris AG, Wood EH: Pericardial pressure during transverse acceleration in dogs without thoracotomy. Circ Res 1967;20:65-77

Barnard HL. The functions of the pericardium. J Physiol (Lond) (Proc) 1898; 22:xliii-xlviii

Bartle SH, Hermann HJ. Acute mitral regurgitation in man. Hemodynamic evidence and observations indicating an early role for the pericardium. Circulation. 1967; 36:839-851

Belenkie I, Dani R, Smith ER, Tyberg JV. The importance of pericardial constraint in experimental pulmonary embolism. Am Heart J 1992; 733-742.

Belouif S, Takata M, Shimada M, Robotham JL: Influence of pericardial constraint on atrioventricular interactions. *Am J Physiol* 1992; 263 *(Heart Circ Physiol* 32): H125-H134.

Bemis CE, Serur JR, Borkenhagen D, Sonnenblick EH, Urschel CW: Influence of right ventricular filling pressure on left ventricular pressure and dimension. Circ Res 1974; 34:498-504

Boyd JL, Elias H: Contributions to diseases of the heart and pericardium. 1. Historical introduction. Bull NY Med Coll 1955; 18:1-37

Boyd TE, Patras MC. Variations in filling and output of the ventricles with the phases of respiration Am J Physiol 1941; 134:74-82.

Braunwald E, Ross J Jr. The ventricular end diastolic pressure: Am J Med 1963; 34 157 –160

Brinker JA, Weiss JL, Lappe DL, Rabson JL, Summer WR, et al. Leftward septal displacement during right ventricular loading in man. Circulation 1980; 61:626-633

Burger W, Straube M, Behne M, Sarai K, Byersdorf F, et al. Role of pericardial constraint for right ventricular function in humans. Chest 1995; 107: 46-49.

Butler J. The heart is in good hands. Circulation 1983; 67: 1163-1168.

Calvin JE: Optimal right ventricular filling pressures and the role of pericardial constraint in right ventricular infarction in dogs. Circulation 1991, 84: 852-861

Capouya ER, Gerber RS, Drinkwater DC, Pearl JM, Sack JB, et al. Girdling effect of nonstimulated cardiomyoplasty on left ventricular function. Ann Thorac Surg 1993; 56:867-870

Carleton HM: The delayed effects of pericardial removal. Proc Roy Soc London (Series B) 1929; 105:230-247

Carpentier A, Chachques JC. Clinical dynamic cardiomyoplasty: method and outcome. Semin Thorac Cardiovasc Surg 1991; 3:136-139

Chaudhry PA, Mishima T, Sharov VG, Hawkins J, Alferness C, et al. Passive epicardial containment prevents ventricular remodeling in heart failure. Ann Thorac Surg 2000; 70:1275-1280

Cohn JN, Guiha NH, Broder MI, Limas CJ; Right ventricular infarction: Clinical and hemodynamic features. Am J Cardiol 1974; 33: 209-214

Danton MH, Byrne JG, Flores KQ, Hsin M, Martin JS, et al.. Modified Glenn connection for acutely ischemic right ventricular failure reverses secondary left ventricular dysfunction J Thorac Cardiovasc Surg 2001; 122: 80-91

Dauterman K, Pak PH, Maughan WL, Nussbacher A, Arie S, et al. Contribution of external forces to left ventricular diastolic pressure. Implications for the clinical use of the Starling Law. *Ann Intern Med* 1995; 122:737- 742.

East T, Bain C. Right ventricular stenosis (Bernheim's syndrome). Br Heart J 1949; 11:145-154.

Elzinga G, Piene H, DeJong JP. Left and right ventricular pump function and consequences of having two pumps in one heart. Circ Res 1980; 46:564-574

Elzinga G, Van Grondelle R, Westerhof N, van den Bos GC: Ventricular interference. Am J Physiol 1974; 226:941-947

Farrar DJ, Chow E, Brown CD. Isolated systolic and diastolic ventricular interactions in pacing-induced dilated cardiomyopathy and effects of volume loading and pericardium. Circulation 1995; 92:1284-1290.

Fowler NO, Shabetai R, Braunstein JR. Transmural ventricular pressures in experimental cardiac tamponade Circ Res 1959; 7: 733-739.

Franklin DL, Van Citters RL, Rushmer RF. Balance between right and left ventricular output. Circ Res 1962; 10:17-26

Freeman GL, LeWinter MM. Pericardial adaptations during chronic cardiac dilation in dogs. Circ Res 1984; 54: 294 –300

Freeman GL, Little WC. Comparison of *in situ* and *in vitro* studies of pericardial pressure-volume relation in dogs. Am J Physiol 1986; 251 (Heart Circ Physiol 20) H421- H427.

Gibbon JH Jr, Churchill ED: The mechanical influence of the pericardium upon cardiac function. J Clin Invest 1931; 10:405-422

Gillebert TC, Sys SU. Physiologic control of relaxation in isolated cardiac muscle and intact left ventricle. In: Left Ventricular Diastolic Dysfunction and Heart Failure. WH Gaasch and MM LeWinter, eds. Philadelphia, Lea & Febiger, 1994

Goldstein JA, HaradaA, Yagi Y, Barzilai B, Cox JL. Hemodynamic importance of systolic ventricular interaction, augmented right atrial contractility and atrio-ventricular synchrony in acute right ventricular dysfunction. J Am Coll Cardiol 1990; 16:181-189.

Goldstein JA, Vlahakes GJ. Verrier ED, Schiller NB Tyberg JV. The role of right ventricular systolic dysfunction and elevated intrapericardial pressure in the genesis of low output in experimental right ventricular infarction. Circulation 1982; 65: 513-522.

Grant DA, Kondo CS, Maloney JE, Tyberg JV. Pulmonary and pericardial limitations to diastolic filling of the left ventricle of the lamb. Am J Physiol 1994; 266; (Heart Circ Physiol 35): H2327-H2333.

Hamilton DR, Danni RS, Semlacher RA, Smith ER, Kieser TM et al. Right atrial and right ventricular transmural pressures in dogs and humans. Circulation 1994; 90:2492-2500

Hamilton WF: Role of the Starling concept in regulation of the normal circulation. Phys Rev 1955; 35:161-168

Hammond HK, White FC, Bhargava V, Shabetai R. Heart size and maximal cardiac output are limited by the pericardium. Am J Physiol 1992; 263:H1675-1681.

Henderson Y, Prince AL: The relative systolic discharges of the right and left ventricles and their bearing on pulmonary congestion and depletion. Heart 1914; 5:217-226

Hoffman D, Sisto D, Frater RW, Nikolic SD; Left-to-right ventricular interaction with a noncontracting right ventricle. J Thorac Cardiovasc Surg 1994; 107:1496-1502.

Hoit BD, Dalton N, Bhargava B, Shabetai R. Pericardial influences on right and left ventricular filling dynamics. Circ Res 1991; 68: 197-208

Hoit BD, Lew WY, LeWinter M. Regional variation in pericardial contact pressure in the canine ventricle. Am J Physiol 1988; 255 (Heart Circ Physiol 24): H1370-H1377

Holt JP. Ventricular end-diastolic volume and transmural pressure. Cardiologia 1967; 50: 281-290.

Holt JP, Rhode EA, Kines H: Pericardial and ventricular pressure. Circ Res 1960; 8:1171-1181, 1960

Janicki JS. Influence of the pericardium and ventricular interdependence on left ventricular diastolic and systolic function in patients with heart failure. Circulation 1990; 81 (Suppl 111): 111-15 - 111-20.

Janicki JS, Weber KT. The pericardium and ventricular interaction, distensibility and function. *Am J Physiol* 1980; 238:H494-H503.

Karunanithi MK, Michniewicz J, Young JA, Feneley MP. Effect of acutely increased left ventricular afterload on work output from the right ventricle in conscious dogs. J Thorac Cardiovasc Surg 2001; 121: 116-124

Kass DA, Baughman KL, Pak PH, Cho PW, Levin HR, et al. Reverse remodeling from cardiomyoplasty in human heart failure. External constraint versus active assist. Circulation 1995; 91:2314-2318.

Kuno Y: The significance of the pericardium. J Physiol 1915-1916; 50:1-36

Lai NC, Graham JB, Bhargava V, Shabetai R. Mechanisms of venous return and ventricular filling in elasmobranch fishes. Am J Physiol 1996; 270:H1766-1771

Laks MM, Garner D, Swan HJC: Volumes and compliances measured simultaneously in the right and left ventricles of the dog. Circ Res 1967; 20: 565-569

Lauson HD, Bloomfield RA, Cournand A: The influence of the respiration on the circulation in man with special reference to rressures in the right auricle, right ventricle, femoral artery and periperal veinsl Am J Med 1946; 1:315-336.

Lee MC, Fung YC, Shabetai R, Lewinter MM. Biaxial mechanical properties of human pericardium and canine comparisons. Am J Physiol 1987; 253:H75-H82

Lee MC, Lewinter MM, Freeman G, Shabetai R, and Fung YC. Biaxial mechanical properties of the pericardium in normal and volume overload dogs. *Am J Physiol* 1985; 249:H222-H230.

LeWinter MM and Pavelec R. Influence of the pericardium on left ventricular end–diastolic pressure-segment relations during early and late stages of experimental chronic volume overload in dogs. Circ Res 1982; 50: 501-509.

Ludbrook PA, Byrne JD, McKnight RC. Influence of right ventricular hemodynamics on left ventricular diastolic pressure-volume relations in man. Circulation 1979; 59:21-31.

Mangano DT. The effect of the pericardium on ventricular systolic function in man Circulation 1980; 61:352-357.

Mann D, Lew W, Ban-Hayashi E, Shabetai R, Waldman L et al. In vivo mechanical behavior of canine pericardium. Am J Physiol 1986; 251 (Heart Circ physiol 20): H349-H356.

McGregor M. Pulsus paradoxus. N Engl. J Med 1979; 301: 480-482.

Mirsky I, Rankin JS. The effects of geometry, elasticity and external pressures on the diastolic pressure-volume and stiffness-stress relations. How important is the pericardium? Circ Res 1979; 44: 601-611

Morgan BC,Guntheroth WC, Dillard DH. The relationship of pericardial to pleural pressure during quiet respiration and cardiac tamponade. Circ Res 1965; 16: 493-498.

Morris-Thurgood JA, Turner MS, Nightingale AK, Masani N, Mumford C et al.; Pacing in heart failure: improved ventricular interaction in diastole rather than systolic resynchronization. Europace 2000; 2: 271-275.

Moulopoulos SD, Sarcas A, Stamatelopoulos S, Arealis E: Left ventricular performance during bypass or distension of the right ventricle. Circ Res 1965; 17:484-491

Oh JK, Hatle LK, Mulvagh SL, Tajik AJ. Transient constrictive pericarditis: diagnosis by two-dimensional Doppler echocardiography. Mayo Clin Proc 1993; 68:1158-1164.

Patel AA, Hatle L, Mimish L. Pulmonary stenosis and severe biventricular dysfunction: improvement following percutaneous valvuloplasty J Heart Valve Dis 1999; 8: 305-306.

Saavedra WF, Tunin RS, Paolocci N, Mishima T, Suzuki G, Emala CW, Chaudhry PA, Anagnostopoulos P, Gupta RC, Sabbah HN, Kass DA. Reverse remodeling and enhanced adrenergic reserve from passive external support in experimental dilated heart failure. J Am Coll Cardiol 2002; 39:2069-2076.

Santamore WP, Constantinescu MS, Bogen D, Johnston WE. Nonuniform distribution of normal pericardial fluid. Basic Res Cardiol 1990; 85:541-549

Santamore WP, Lynch PR, Meier G, Heckman L Bove AA: Myocardial interaction between the ventricles. J Appl Physiol 1976; 41 (3):362-368

Scharf SM, Brown R Saunders N, Green LH, Ingram RH Jr. Changes in canine left ventricular size and configuration with positive end-expiratory pressure. Circ Res 1979; 44: 672-678.

Scott RW, Garvin CF. Cor pulmonale: Observations in fifty autopsy cases. Am Heart J 1941; 22:56-63

Shabetai R, Abel DC, Graham JB, Bhargava V, Keyes RS, et al. Function of the pericardium and pericardioperitoneal canal in elasmobranch fishes. Am J Physiol 1985; 248 (Heart Circ Physiol 17): H198-H207

Shaver JA, Reddy PS, Curtiss EI, Ziady GM, Reddy SC. Noninvasive/invasive correlates of exaggerated ventricular interdependence in cardiac tamponade. J Cardiol 2001; 37 Suppl 1: 71-76.

Shirato K, Shabetai R, Bhargava V, Franklin D, Ross J Jr. Alteration of the left ventricular diastolic pressure-segment length relation produced by the pericardium. Effects of cardiac distension and afterload reduction in conscious dogs. Circulation 1978; 57:1191-1198.

Shuler RH, Ensor C, Gunning RE, Moss WG, Johnson V. The differential effects of respiration on the left and right ventricles Am J Physiol 1942; 137:620-627.

Slinker BK, Ditchey RV, Bell SP, LeWinter MM. Right heart pressure does not equal pericardial pressure in the potassium chloride- arrested canine heart in situ. Circulation 1987; 76: 357-362.

Smiseth OA, Frais MA, Kingma I, Smith ER, Tyberg JV. Assessment of pericardial constraint in dogs. Circulation 1985; 71: 158-164

Smiseth OA, Kingma I, Refsum H, Smith ER, Tyberg JV. The pericardial hypothesis: a mechanism of acute shifts of the left ventricular diastolic pressure-volume relation. Clinical Physiol 1985; 5: 403-415

Smiseth OA, Refsum H, Junemann M, Sievers RE, Lipton MJ, et al. Ventricular diastolic pressure-volume shifts during acute ischemic left ventricular failure in dogs. J Am Coll Cardiol 1984; 3: 966-977.

Smiseth OA, Refsum H, Tyberg JV. Pericardial pressure assessed by right atrial pressure: a basis for calculation of left ventricular transmural pressure. Am Heart J 1984; 108:603-605

Smiseth OA, Scott-Douglas NW, Thompson CR, Smith ER, Tyberg JV. Non-uniformity of pericardial surface pressure in dogs. Circulation; 1987; 75:1229-1236.

Spodick DH: Medical history of the pericardium. The hairy hearts of hoary heroes. Am J Cardiol 1970; 26:447-454

Spotnitz HM, Kaiser GA. The effect of the pericardium on pressure-volume relations in the canine left ventricle. J Surg Res 1971; 11:375-380.

Starling EH, Linacre: Lecture on Law of the Heart. Cambridge, 1915. New York, Longmans, 1918

Starr I, Jeffers WA, Meade RH Jr.. The absence of conspicuous increments of venous pressure after severe damage to the right ventricle of the dog, with a discussion of the relation between clinical congestive failure and heart disease. Am Heart J 1943; 26: 291-301.

Stokland 0, Miller MM, Lekven J, Ilebekk A: The significance of the intact pericardium for cardiac performance in the dog. Circ Res 1980; 47:27-32

Stray-Gundersen J, Musch TI, Haidet GC, Swain DP, Ordway GA, et al. The effect of pericardiectomy on maximal oxygen consumption and maximal cardiac output in untrained dogs. *Circ Res* 1986;58:523-530.

Sudak FN. Intrapericardial and intracardiac pressures and the events of the cardiac cycle in *Mustelus canis* (Mitchill) Comp Biochem Physiol. 1965 14: 689-705.

Summer WR, Permutt S, Sagawa K, Shoukas AA, Bromberger-Barnea B. Effects of spontaneous respiration on canine left ventricular function. Circ Res 1979; 45: 719-728.

Taylor RR, Covell JW, Sonnenblick EH, Ross J Jr: Dependence of ventricular distensibility on filling of the opposite ventricle. Am J Physiol 1967; 213:711-718

Traboulsi M, Scott-Douglas NW, Smith ER, Tyberg JV. The right and left ventricular intracavitary and transmural pressure-strain relationshiiips. Am Heart J 1992; 123: 1279-1287.

Tyberg JV, Smith ER. Ventricular diastole and the role of the pericardium. Herz,1990;15: 354-361

Tyberg JV, Misbach GA, Glantz SA, Moores WY, Parmley WW. A mechanism for shifts in the diastolic left ventricular pressure-volume curve: The role of the pericardium. Euro J Cardiol 1978; 7 (suppl) 163-175

Wiggers CJ: Cardiac output, stroke volume, and stroke work, in Luisada A.A. (Ed): Cardiovascular Functions. New York, McGraw Hill, 1962, pp 81-91

Williams CBJ: The prognosis and treatment of organic diseases of the heart. Lond J Med 1850; 2:460-473

Chapter 3

PERICARDIAL EFFUSION

1.   HISTORICAL BACKGROUND

Even with copious effusion the onset and course may be so insidious that no suspicion of the true nature of the disease is aroused.
Probably no serious disease is so frequently overlooked by the practitioner. Postmortem experience shows how often pericarditis is not recognized or goes on to resolution and adhesion without attracting notice. (Osler 1892)

*Am I not right to infer that when this serosity exceeds six or seven ounces, a dropsy of the membrane exists? (*Corvisart 1812)

Corvisart, a contemporary of Laennec, was Napoleon's favourite physician. He drained pericardial effusion by surgical pericardiotomy.

The first published account of using echocardiography to detect pericardial effusion (*Edler1955)* launched the field of echocardiography that was to explode over the next half-century and become the prime modality for its detection and quantification, ending Osler's complaint about how hard it was to make the diagnosis. In this country, echocardiography was developed for this purpose, principally by Feigenbaum and co-workers *(Feigenbaum 1970; Feigenbaum, Waldhausen, Hyde 1966; Feigenbaum, Zaky, Waldhausen 1966 & 1967).* Notable contributions were made by other investigators, including Teichholz (1978), Popp (1976*),* and D'Cruz *(D'Cruz, Cohen, Prabhu 1975).* At that time the standard technique was M mode, but soon thereafter two-dimensional studies became the accepted modality, supplemented as appropriate by M mode.

2.   AETIOLOGY

The echocardiograms of 4,061 patients seen in an echocardiography laboratory were screened for pericardial effusion, enabling the investigators to study the aetiology of stable, asymptomatic pericardial effusion in 176 patients (*Kudo, Yamasaki, Doi 2002*). The aetiologies they found are listed in Table 1 and are considered representative.

Table 1. Aetiology of pericardial effusion in the study of Kudo, Yamasaki, Doi 2002

Dilated cardiomyopathy	11
Hypertensive heart disease	13
Old myocardial infarction	19
Valvular heart disease	11
Post-pericardiotomy syndrome	45
Malignant neoplasia	47
Connective tissue disease	13
Hypothyroidism	10
Chronic renal disease	7

3.   DIAGNOSIS

Physical examination is so insensitive and non-specific as to be worthless. Far be it from me to denigrate the value of a good history and physical examination, but I venture to suggest that few of my readers know of Ewart's sign (*Ewart 1896*) of pericardial effusion. Physicians of the 19th and early 20th centuries were doubtless a lot more proficient in the use of this sign than are we. Physicians used to percuss the thorax to elicit cardiac dullness beyond the cardiac apex, to establish the presence of pericardial effusion. Pericardial effusion, large enough to cause dullness in the fifth right intercostal space (as well as the left), was demonstrated by injecting fluid into the pericardium until a dull percussion note could be elicited. The volume needed was 25 to 30 ounces (*Rotch 1878*). Cardiac percussion is one of the lost clinical arts, but in any case was inaccurate for the diagnosis of pericardial effusion. False positives arise from left pleural effusion or thickening, or disease of the left lower lobe or lingula, whereas emphysema could be the cause of a false negative. Pericardial effusion is a condition in which the clinician should not even attempt to diagnose by clinical examination, but should proceed at once to laboratory tests. In echocardiography we have a highly reliable tool for the diagnosis of pericardial effusion. Now that this means has long been in hand, when the diagnosis is missed, it is not because of difficulty, but failure of the physician to think of it. One reason for this failure is the extraordinary number of diseases that may involve the pericardium. The number of systemic disorders that commonly involve the pericardium is, fortunately, much smaller (Table 1). Confronted with a patient with one of these disorders, one should always consider the possibility of pericarditis with possible effusion. When evaluating patients with a systemic disorder who manifest unexplained cardiovascular abnormalities, one should remember that pericardial disease may be the cause. The diagnosis thus becomes a matter of knowing when to suspect it. The physician who has a high index of suspicion that a pericardial effusion may be present need only obtain an echocardiogram to confirm or refute the diagnosis.

3.1   Presentations

Pericardial effusion may present in a variety of ways. Small pericardial effusions may fail to cause symptoms, clinical abnormalities, change in even serial chest roentgenograms or electrocardiographic abnormalities. Even large effusions may, if they develop slowly enough, cause few if any symptoms or physical findings. In this case, the heart appears large on the chest roentgenogram, but a confident differentiation from generalized cardiac enlargement is often not possible. Frequently the electrocardiogram does not show the features of acute pericarditis. It may be normal or show non-specific T wave changes or low voltage, neither of which, and not even the combination, is diagnostic of pericardial effusion. On the other hand, if a clinical clue has led the physician to suspect a disease in which the pericardium is likely to be involved and therefore orders an echocardiogram, the pericardial effusion will be recognized at once.

4.   SYNDROMES OF PERICARDIAL EFFUSION

The particular syndrome of pericardial effusion that manifests depends on the volume of the effusion, its rate of accumulation, the aetiology, the thickness of the pericardium, the presence or absence of co-existing cardiac disease and the nature of the fluid. Rapid accumulation of fluid in the pericardium causes acute tamponade, because the pericardium cannot be stretched fast enough to accommodate it without a severe increase in pericardial pressure. On the other hand, when the effusion accumulates more slowly, cardiac tamponade may be subclinical, mild, moderate or severe.

At the other extreme is the syndrome of massive chronic pericardial effusion of unknown cause, associated sometimes for many years with only subclinical tamponade (*Sagrista-Sauleda, Angel, Permanyer-Miralda 1999*).

Chronic effusive pericarditis was first described by Bedford *(1964),* who considered it an autoimmune phenomenon because of its frequent association with what was then called congestive cardiomyopathy. The pericardial pressure, although elevated, is usually less than the pressure in either atrium, thereby satisfying the definition of minimal tamponade (*Shaver, Reddy, Curtiss 2001*). The transmural pressure, however, is less than normal. A case studied in our laboratory in 1977 is illustrated in Figure 1. Long-term follow up has shown that these patients may eventually develop unexpected overt tamponade. Nevertheless, in my opinion, it is safe to manage conservatively patients who reliably attend the office or clinic for as long as the effusion persists and never display clinical tamponade. Sagrista-Sauleda et al., however, recommend a more active approach. They reported that, in a substantial proportion of cases, pericardiocentesis is not followed by recurrence. Based on their experience of 28 cases followed for up to 20 years (mean 7 years), they advise pericardiocentesis be done and, if the effusion recurs, be repeated, and that pericardiectomy be undertaken in those patients who develop further recurrence.

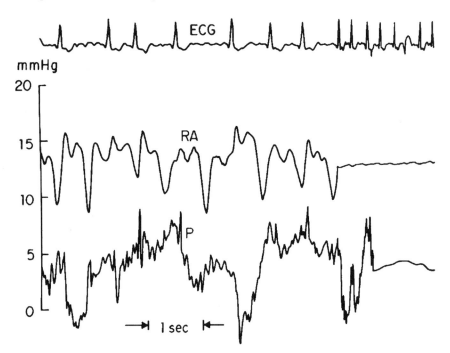

Figure 1. Chronic effusive pericarditis in idiopathic congestive cardiomyopathy. 1400 ml. of fluid was aspirated. From above down, ECG showing atrial fibrillation, greatly elevated right atrial pressure (RA) and slightly elevated pericardial pressure (P). Mean pressures are recorded at the end of the figure.

Some causes of pericardial effusion are known to have a proclivity to develop tamponade. These include tuberculosis, pericardial effusion related to chronic hemodialysis, remote mediastinal radiation, and neoplasm, but tamponade can occur in pericardial effusion of any aetiology. The tendency to develop tamponade may change in response to changing management of the primary cause. Thus, dialysis associated with pericardial effusion used to be one of the commoner causes of tamponade, but with changes that have been made in dialysis membranes, has become a very infrequent occurrence. AIDS is now a leading cause of pericardial effusion, but these effusions usually are small and tend not to create overt tamponade (*Heidenreich, Eisenberg, Kee 1995)*. The combination of a small- to medium-sized pericardial effusion with a thickened non-compliant pericardium is associated with tuberculous pericarditis and with prior mediastinal radiation. Again, this syndrome is becoming less common in response to more accurate targeting and improved shielding. Perforation of the heart or an intrapericardial vessel is now one of the commonest causes of cardiac tamponade.

5.   FACTORS THAT MODIFY THE PATHOPHYSIOLOGY

If the pericardium is thickened by scarring, neoplastic infiltration, tubercular or pyogenic infection, it resists stretching to an even greater degree than does the normal pericardium. The initial relative flat part of its pressure volume curve is absent; therefore, tamponade develops with lesser volumes of effusion than in patients whose pericardium was normal before effusion occurred.

Many of the models used to characterise the pathophysiology of pericardial effusion assume a normal underlying heart. This assumption includes practically all animal models and many clinical models as well. Information has been acquired from creating experimental cardiac tamponade in animals and from studies of young individuals with acute effusive idiopathic pericarditis. The information so gleaned has furnished the basis for our understanding of the pathophysiology of pericardial effusion and tamponade. On the other hand, the physician can never lose sight of the fact that significant pericardial effusion, with or without tamponade, can occur in patients with serious underlying heart disease that may greatly modify the hemodynamics. Likewise, the fluid balance greatly influences the hemodynamic impact of pericardial effusion, as is seen in patients receiving hemodialysis or ultrafiltration. Thick purulent pericardial effusion is more apt than serous effusion to cause adverse hemodynamic sequelae.

6.   EFFUSION IN ACUTE PERICARDITIS

Classical medicine and pathology draw a distinction between fibrinous, so-called "dry" pericarditis and pericardial effusion. This distinction arose because, prior to the advent of echocardiography, the means to detect a small accumulation of pericardial fluid in this condition were not then available. That acute pericarditis often caused a small effusion was well known to Sir William Osler who, like most great physicians of his day, was a competent pathologist who performed his own autopsies.

He wrote "*Acute Plastic Pericarditis – This, the most common form, occurs usually as a secondary process, and is distinguished by the small amount of fluid exudation, which does not, as in the next variety, give special characters to the disease... Slight fluid exudation is invariably present, entangled in the meshes of fibrin, but there may be very thick fibrinous layers without much serous effusion.*" *(Osler 1892)*

7.   CLINICAL APPROACH TO THE PATIENT WITH PERICARDIAL EFFUSION

Several steps should be taken when approaching a patient with suspected pericardial effusion. The first is to establish whether pericardial effusion is or is not present. Second, the aetiology must be established (see Table 1). Third, it must be decided whether the effusion is causing hemodynamic embarrassment. The fourth step, which should be limited to special clinical circumstances, is to determine the nature of the fluid. Finally, a very important step is to determine whether treatment is warranted.

7.1   Diagnosing the presence of pericardial fluid

Success in diagnosing pericardial effusion depends first upon a correct assessment, based on the patient's illness, of the probability of pericardial effusion. The next step is to seek clinical and laboratory evidence of pericardial disease. These two steps should lead to the appropriate decision regarding the need for echocardiography.

7.2   Evidence of pericardial disease

Perhaps the most helpful clue to pericardial effusion is detection of other evidence of pericardial abnormality. The leading contenders are a pericardial friction rub and the characteristic electrocardiographic findings of acute pericarditis. Electrocardiographic evidence of pericardial effusion *per se* is less helpful, because of its lack of specificity and sensitivity, which were documented in a study of 122 patients (*Unverferth, Williams, Fulkerson* 1979). They emphasized the multiplicity of causes of low voltage and also found no correlation between QRS amplitude and effusion size, but did find that an unexplained decrease in amplitude from that measured on a prior electrocardiogram indicated probable cardiac tamponade. Their observation that, after pericardiocentesis for tamponade, QRS voltage increased, as illustrated in Figure 2, was consistent with their deduction that low voltage is a sign of increased pericardial pressure.

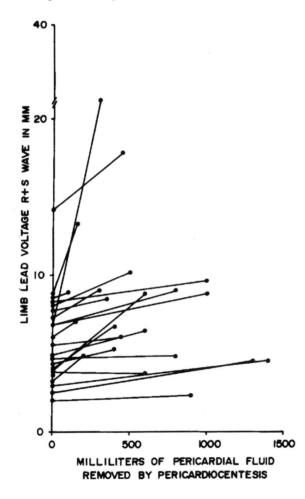

Figure 2. Electrocardiographic voltage in the limb leads plotted against aliquots of pericardial aspirate. A similar relation was found in the precordial leads. (From Unverferth, Williams, Fulkerson 1979, with permission)

A more recent study (*Bruch, Schmermund, Dagres 2001*) proves that Unverferth was correct, and also showed that low voltage is a feature of cardiac tamponade but not pericardial effusion itself. These two studies undermine several popular theories concerning the mechanism of low voltage associated with pericardial effusion, because they do not include pericardial pressure. By showing that QRS voltage increases to a comparable degree following anti-inflammatory treatment, they also cast new light on mechanisms that cause reduced QRS voltage in tamponade. The combination of low voltage and features of acute pericarditis is sufficiently suggestive of cardiac tamponade so that, faced with this syndrome, the physician is obligated to carry out suitable tests to rule out or include cardiac tamponade.

It has been shown that depression of the PR segment and, less commonly, elevation of the ST segment may be present when pericardial effusion is caused by an inflammatory or auto immune response such as the post-pericardiotomy syndrome, but is absent in pericardial effusion of other aetiology, such as heart failure (Kudo, Yamasaki, Doi, 2002). In cases where the aetiology was not known before the electrocardiogram that disclosed PR depression or ST elevation was performed, consideration of anti-inflammatory or immunosuppressive therapy is appropriate.

A clue to pericardial effusion may be the chest pain of acute pericarditis. This pain is somewhat variable in nature, sometimes imitating myocardial ischemia, but at other times it is pleuritic. It tends to be relieved by sitting up, and a characteristic radiation site is the trapezius ridge. Echocardiography is therefore indicated in patients with chest pain compatible with acute pericarditis. In pericardial effusion of other aetiology in which acute inflammation may well be absent, pericardial effusion is often entirely painless.

Clues to pericardial effusion may not be found even on diligent clinical examination, but still may be found on laboratory examination. Thus widespread ST segment elevation, especially when associated with PR segment depression, proves that acute pericarditis, in which there may be an associated effusion, is present. It is not uncommon for pericardial effusion to be first suspected by unexplained radiographic cardiomegaly, especially when the lungs are not congested.

7.3   Nature of the pericardial fluid

Clinicians use the term pericardial effusion for any abnormal quantity of pericardial fluid and it thus embraces the range from a simple transudate (hydropericardium) to inflammatory exudates that may or may not be purulent, and intrapericardial hemorrhage. More strictly, an effusion is fluid secreted from the visceral pericardium. Unfortunately, the distinction between a transudate and an exudate is often blurred, for example, the protein content may approach 4 g/dl, the value classically assigned to define exudative fluid. Analysis of pericardial fluid is covered in Chapter 5. Here, suffice it to say that a routine bacteriological analysis, often including polymerase chain reaction, and chemical analysis should be performed from any sample of pericardial fluid that has been obtained, and that numerous additional tests are frequently appropriate in specific clinical circumstances. It is wise to err on the side of including tests that may turn out not to be useful, because of the obvious need to avoid a second pericardiocentesis. Information concerning the nature of the pericardial fluid, especially when there is evidence of tamponade or infection, can be crucial for diagnosing the cause of effusion. Sanguinous fluid, in the case of pericardial fluid, is less ominous than in the case of pleural effusion, where so often it denotes that the effusion is malignant (*Chiu, Atar, Siegel, 2001).* In this study, the leading cause of bloody pericardial effusion was idiopathic pericarditis, but other causes included complications of myocardial infarction, tuberculosis, and uremia. Often, malignant pericardial effusion was serous.

7.4   Aetiologic Diagnosis

7.4.1   Pericardial Infection

Pericardial effusion may complicate virtually any infectious pericarditis, be it acute or chronic, but the number of infections especially apt to inflame the pericardium is limited. Among these are viral infections, especially echovirus and Coxsackie. For bacterial pericarditis, one needs to consider septicemia, intrathoracic infections, including fungal acquired in the course of cardiac operation, pneumonia, empyema, myocardial abscess complicating infective endocarditis, infected chest wounds, and subdiaphragmatic abscess. In any of these infections, pericardial friction rub, chest pain or change in the radiological size or configuration of the heart furnishes a clue that pericarditis, and hence a pericardial effusion, may be present. In the last situation, caution is necessary when comparing portable with standard radiograms. When assessing cardiac and pericardial problems, the physician should insist on standard anterior-posterior and lateral views and should not accept as adequate a portable radiogram, except when the patient cannot tolerate the routine procedure.

Diagnostic difficulties include distinguishing between pericardial friction rub, pleural rub, and mediastinal crunch. This difficulty is common when assessing patients soon after cardiac surgery in whom pericardial effusion is common and may be highly significant, but in whom these auscultatory phenomena are very frequent, whether or not they have pericardial effusion. In many infections in which pericardial effusion is present, the organism grows in the pericardial fluid, but a non-infectious pericardial effusion may occur in patients with systemic infection. Notable examples are meningeal septicaemia with sterile pericardial effusion. Tuberculosis, often drug resistant, is an important cause of pericarditis in many parts of the world, and threatens to become more frequent in the United States. Tuberculous pericarditis should be suspected when there are findings compatible with tuberculosis, a recent conversion to positive of the tuberculin skin test, history of contact with tubercular individuals, or predisposing conditions such as diabetes. See also Chapter 9.

Table 1. Classification of some of the more common causes of infectious pericarditis.

VIRAL DISEASES	BACTERIAL INFECTIONS
Coxsackie A&B	*Staphylococcus*
Echovirus	*Streptococcus*
Influenza virus	*Meningococcus*
Retrovirus, AIDS	*Francisella tularensis*
Opportunistic infections	*Pneumococcus*
Adenovirus	Rickettsial infections
Infectious mononucleosis	*Typhus*
Mumps, herpes zoster	*Q fever*
Chicken pox	*Boutonneuse fever*
Mycobacterial infections	Other infections
Tuberculosis	*Actinomyces*
Protozoal infections	*Nocardia*
Toxoplasmosis	Psittacosis-lymphogranuloma
Entamoeba histolytica	venereum group
Trypanosoma cruzi	
Fungal infections	
Histoplasma	
Coccidioides	
Blastomyces	
Aspergillus	

Modified from Fowler and Manitsas, 1973. Reprinted by permission.

7.4.2   Metabolic disorders

At one time, uremia may have been the most frequent metabolic disorder associated with pericardial disease. Pericarditis frequently complicates the terminal stages of chronic renal disease, and pericardial effusion supervenes in a considerable proportion. This association was well known to Bright (1789-1858), the English physician credited with the first description of acute and chronic nephritis (*Bright 1836*). He was a graduate of Edinburgh University Faculty of Medicine and was a contemporary of Addison and Hodgkin at Guy's Hospital, London. His portrait is reproduced in Figure 3. The blood urea nitrogen level usually exceeds 100 mg/dl before pericarditis supervenes. The rub of this kind of pericarditis is very coarse and often palpable. The electrocardiogram often does not provide evidence of acute pericarditis, presumably because the epicardium is spared.

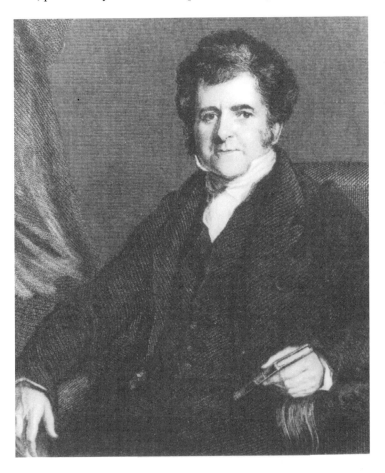

Figure 3. Richard Bright (1789-1858) who described pericardial disease in nephritis. (Reproduced from TJ Pettigrew: Medical Portrait Gallery, London, with permission)

Of greater importance in the current era is pericarditis that may develop during the course of hemodialysis. In 1981, when the first edition of this book was published, dialysis-related cardiac tamponade was, along with hepatitis, a major scourge of the dialysis unit. Cardiac tamponade is now uncommon in patients undergoing chronic hemodialysis. It is believed that responsible agents, able to pass through the membranes of earlier dialysis machines, are filtered out by the membranes of modern machines.

Pericardial effusion may appear rapidly and with little warning, and must be considered in the differential diagnosis whenever the combination of hypotension, raised central venous pressure and increased heart size (all frequent occurrences in dialysis patients) are not readily explained by volume overload. Many patients undergoing chronic hemodialysis have severe heart disease secondary to the combination of hypertension, anemia, arteriosclerosis and the shunt required for haemodialysis or ultrafiltration. The signs of cardiac tamponade are sometimes mistaken for those of fluid retention due to heart failure or renal insufficiency and inadequate dialysis. Echocardiography must be performed whenever pericardial effusion is suspected under such circumstances. In some cases, clues to pericardial involvement, such as pericardial friction rub, typical pain or ECG changes make the diagnosis more straightforward. Treatment is considered in Chapter 9. Suffice it to say here that increased intensity of dialysis may resolve the pericardial effusion in many patients, but at the opposite extreme, other patients need volume expansion (see Chapter 4).

Myxoedema is another metabolic disease in which pericardial effusion is not uncommon. In the earlier literature, the stated prevalence of pericardial effusion in hypothyroidism, although quite variable, was much higher than the five percent encountered now (*Kabadi and Kumar 1990*). The authors attribute the change to the doubtful accuracy of the diagnosis in the past and to the current high frequency of routine testing of thyroid function practiced in modern medicine. The effusion is usually of little hemodynamic significance, but tamponade may occur. I believe that it is sound clinical practice to obtain an echocardiogram in all patients who have myxoedema with cardiac symptoms or cardiomegaly, but echocardiography in patients with hypothyroidism found on routine testing of patients without evidence of myxoedema is not cost effective.

7.4.3   Specific heart muscle disease

Specific cardiomyopathies, such as amyloidosis (*Navarro, Rivera, Ortuno 1992*) or sarcoidosis (*Angomachalelis, Hourzamanis, Salem, 1994*) may be accompanied by pericardiopathy with effusion. Although, on occasion the pericardial effusion may come to dominate the clinical picture, for example with cardiac tamponade, much more often it is an incidental finding, and diastolic dysfunction, when present, is usually predominantly of myocardial, not pericardial origin

7.4.4   Heart failure

In the literature published before effective treatment of heart failure was possible, heart failure was given as a common cause of pericardial effusion and, indeed in the pathology literature, as the most common cause. As late as 1994, the prevalence is given as 14 percent (*Maisch 1994*). This figure, while much lower than the earlier ones, is still too high, judging from experience in reading echocardiograms for heart failure clinics.

7.4.5   Collagen Vascular Diseases

Pericardial involvement, often with effusion, may complicate practically all of the collagen vascular diseases, but is of special importance in lupus erythematosus and rheumatoid arthritis. In these two conditions, the likelihood of pericardial effusion is so high, that any hint of its possible presence calls for echocardiography, as rheumatologists, judging by their referrals, know well. One quarter to one half of patients with disseminated lupus develop pericardial disease at some stage of the disease. The prevalence is even higher in autopsy series.

7.4.6   Myocardial Infarction

Pericardial effusion may be a feature of different stages of myocardial infarction. During the early stages of acute myocardial infarction, serial echocardiograms frequently disclose pericardial effusion in the absence of any evidence of pericarditis. These effusions are most often small and of no clinical importance (*Galve, Garcia-Del-Castillo, Evangelista 1986*). Patients who develop a pericardial effusion early after a myocardial infarction have a worse prognosis than those who do not. The reason is that early pericardial effusion is an indication that the infarction was large. The effusion itself is almost always hemodynamically innocuous, and therefore is not the cause of the worse prognosis. While intuition may suggest that the clinician should be particularly alert for pericardial effusion in patients who have received throbolytic therapy, in fact, effusion is less likely in these patients because the infarctions are smaller (*Correale, Maggioni, Romano 1993*).

Pericardial effusion may appear after several days, weeks, or even months after acute myocardial infarction (Dressler's syndrome). The first evidence is pericardial pain, and often also pleuritic pain, in the absence of signs of recurrent ischemia. Fever, elevated erythrocyte sedimentation rate, and leucocytosis are usually found. The chest radiogram frequently shows, in addition to increased size of the cardio-pericardial silhouette, a pleural effusion (*Dressler 1959*).

7.4.7   Other thoracic catastrophes

Aortic aneurysm, dissecting hematoma and intramural clot may cause the vessel to rupture with massive hemorrhage into the pericardium. Myocardial aneurysm or infarction may also rupture into the pericardium. Making the diagnosis is usually a matter of considering the possibility of intrapericardial bleeding in the appropriate clinical circumstances.

7.4.8   Trauma

It is important to suspect bleeding or effusion into the pericardial space in patients who have sustained a chest injury. A sharp injury that has penetrated the heart or a great vessel causes acute tamponade, indicating the need for urgent echocardiography. Blunt injuries also cause pericardial effusion, often bloody. These effusions may appear soon after the offending trauma, but may be delayed for several weeks or months (*Parmley, Manion, Mattingly 1958*). Patients who have sustained a severe contusion such as from a baseball blow to the chest or a steering wheel injury are at great risk of developing either an early or late pericardial effusion. This complication must always be considered when the clinical course is unsatisfactory or deteriorates for unexplained reasons.

The pericardial injury may occur during invasive diagnostic or therapeutic cardiac intervention. Disappearance of cardiac pulsation on the image on the fluoroscopic monitor, a drop in blood pressure and increase in venous pressure should immediately alert the operator to this emergency and the need for pericardiocentesis, preceded whenever possible by echocardiography. Cardiopulmonary resuscitation is a known, if uncommon, cause of pericardial hemorrhage.

7.4.9   Neoplastic disease and radiation therapy

Many neoplasms may affect the heart or pericardium causing effusion. Especially important are mammary and bronchogenic carcinoma, and the lymphomas. Pericardial effusion should be suspected when patients with neoplasm develop evidence of cardiovascular disease. The chest radiogram usually shows considerable enlargement of the cardio-pericardial silhouette, but cases with extensive invasion of the pericardium have effusive-constrictive pericarditis in which the silhouette may or may not be enlarged, depending on the severity of the constrictive element. Radiotherapy, particularly for Hodgkin's, may cause pericardial effusion and, subsequently, constriction (*Benoff and Schweitzer, 1995*).

7.4.10   Pregnancy

Pericardial effusion is common in normal pregnancy. The prevalence increases with each succeeding trimester. Effusion is more common in primagravidas and in those who gain excessive weight. These effusions are innocuous (*Abdulijabbar, Marzouki, Zawawi 1991*).

7.4.11   Miscellaneous diseases associated with pericardial effusion

Pericardial effusion may occur in a number of seemingly unrelated syndromes, but the mechanism and pathophysiology are often obscure. The list is far too long to be useful for this chapter, but some of the more useful and interesting ones can be singled out, such as Reiter's syndrome (*Csonka and Oates 1957)*, cardiac transplantation when it may mark the incidence and severity of acute rejection (*Ciliberto, Anjos, Gronda 1995)*, inflammatory bowel disease (especially ulcerative colitis) (*Dubowitz and Gorard 2001*), and Whipple's disease (*Pastor and Geerken* 1973). Pericardial effusion is also more common in patients with anorexia nervosa than in a demographically matched population (*Frolich, von Gontard, Lehmkuhl 2001*), and in patients who have had a Fontan operation to palliate a congenital cardiac malformation *(Zahn, Houde, Benson 1992)*.

7.5   Clinical significance of pericardial effusion

Pericardiopathy with effusion may be the primary illness, or appear secondarily in the course of almost any disease. There are, however, particular diseases and clinical situations in which the physician must be on the lookout for pericardial effusion. Chief among these number chest trauma, neoplasm and its treatment by radiation, infections, especially viral and tubercular, the collagen vascular diseases, especially rheumatoid arthritis and lupus erythematosus, prior myocardial infarction, and renal disease treated by dialysis or ultrafiltration.

Pericardial effusion may mimic the features of the causative disease. For example, just as hydralazine or procainamide-induced pericardial effusion may be mistaken for congestive heart failure, or ruptured myocardial infarction with tamponade be mistaken for cardiogenic shock without a mechanical cause, so too may pericardial effusion during dialysis be mistaken for nephrogenic derangement of fluid balance, or for heart failure.

8.   IMAGING

8.1   Echocardiography

8.1.1   M mode

Echocardiography is virtually a hundred percent specific and sensitive for the detect4ion of pericardial effusion. It should be recalled that, in the early days of echocardiography, when only the M mode modality was available, the operator was deprived of the means provided by two-dimensional images to guide the beam; therefore the study depended highly on the operator's knowledge and skill. The acoustic impedances of pericardial fluid and myocardium are similar, and the pericardial lung interface reflects the strongest echoes. Advantage of these two considerations was (and still is) taken by using appropriate attenuation and damping.

8.1.1.1   Technique

The direction and position of the M mode beam is critical. When the gain is set high, the sonolucent space between the pericardium and epicardium is obliterated by multiple echoes. The attenuation and damping controls are progressively increased until the posterior pericardium alone is visualized. In patients without pericardial effusion, this structure appears as a thin line exhibiting cardiac motion, and when attenuation and damping are appropriately decreased, the myocardial structures appear, and the epicardial surface of the posterior wall of the left ventricle is contiguous with the pericardium, as seen in Figures 4 and 5. In the case of a pericardial effusion, the pericardium appears as a motionless, thin straight line when the controls have been adjusted to remove all other echoes. After the controls have been readjusted, the hyperactive epicardial surface of the heart appears and is separated from the motionless pericardium by an echo-free space.

After identifying the mitral valve, the transducer is angled laterally and inferiorly to avoid confusion with the vertebral column and mediastinal structures, the standard structures are identified next, and then the controls are adjusted for optimal visualization of the pericardium. False positive diagnosis is much less common when real time two-dimensional images are created, because sources of error are fewer and easier to recognize.

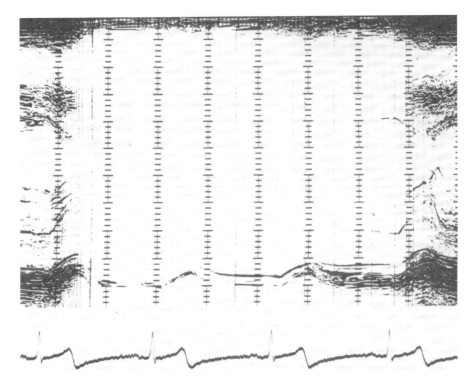

Figure 4. Echocardiogram demonstrating absence of pericardial effusion. The location of the pericardium is identified as a thin linear echo.

For inexperienced operators, the major pitfall is pleural effusion, but left pleural effusion can be recognized easily by its location posterior to the descending aorta. It is less well known that right pleural effusion may simulate pericardial effusion by creating an echo free space between the right atrium and the liver in the subcostal view (*D'Cruz 1984*). Sonlucent spaces adjacent to the heart may also be due to ascites or pericardial cyst (*D'Cruz and Constantine 1993*) or localized fat deposit, or an atypical diaphragmatic hernia (*D'Cruz and Kanura 2001*).

8.1.2 M mode and real time echocardiography

8.1.2.1 Quantification

While the quantity of pericardial fluid can be estimated fairly well by M mode (*Horowitz, Schultz, Stinson 1974*) or two dimensional and even three-dimensional echocardiography (*Vazquez de Prada, Jiang, Handschumacher*

1994), for most clinical purposes it suffices to classify effusion as trivial, small, moderate, large or massive.

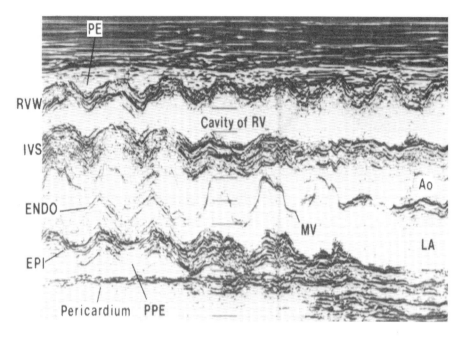

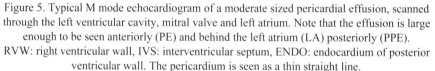

Figure 5. Typical M mode echocardiogram of a moderate sized pericardial effusion, scanned through the left ventricular cavity, mitral valve and left atrium. Note that the effusion is large enough to be seen anteriorly (PE) and behind the left atrium (LA) posteriorly (PPE).
RVW: right ventricular wall, IVS: interventricular septum, ENDO: endocardium of posterior ventricular wall. The pericardium is seen as a thin straight line.

A useful way to consider the size of an effusion is to estimate its width. An effusion extending less then one centimetre from the myocardial border is considered small and unsuitable for pericardiocentesis, except by a very experienced operator. Two centimetres is considered moderate and safe for pericardiocentesis. The size of the effusion is judged also by its appearance in the various image planes, as can be appreciated from Figure 6. Two-dimensional images clearly demonstrate the regional distribution of the effusion, important when selecting the site on the skin for performing peicardiocentesis.

The pericardium itself is less easily identified on two-dimensional images than by M mode. The pericardium creates the brightest images, so that when the gain is set too high, abnormally increased thickness suggesting constrictive pericarditis may be falsely diagnosed. CAT scans and transaesophageal echocardiograms are far superior in this regard. When pericardial fluid organizes, fibrin strands or coats may be visualized (*Alio-*

Bosch, Candell-Riera, Monge-Rangel 1991). An example is illustrated in Figure 7.

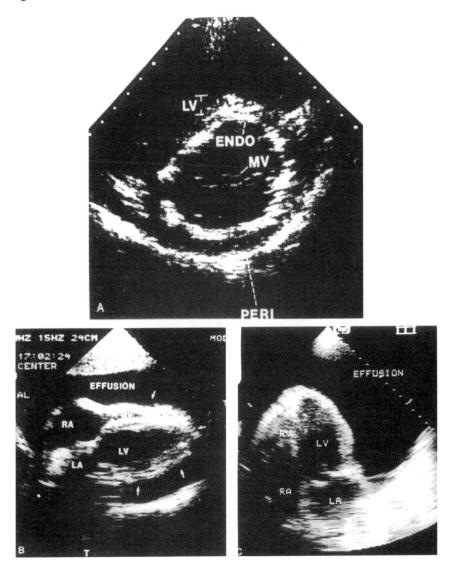

Figure 6. Two-dimensional echocardiograms of three patients with pericardial effusion. **A:** Short axis view at the mitral valve level of the left ventricle(LV). The effusion is moderate in size. ENDO: endocardium, MV: mitral valve, PERI: pericardium. Note echo-free space separating the heart from the pericardium. **B:** Large effusion (arrows) in the subcostal view. The effusion is seen anterior to the right ventricle (RV) and posterior to the left ventricle (LV) The right ventricle is severely compressed indicating tamponade. RA: right atrium, LA: left atrium. **C:** Massive circumferential effusion in the four chamber view. (From Shabetai 2000, with permission)

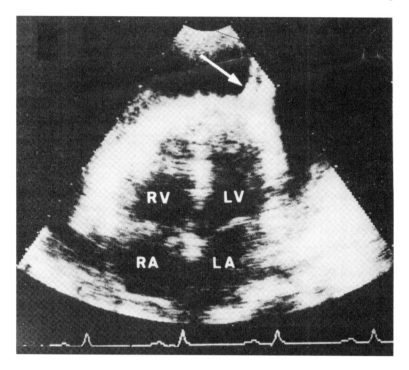

Figure 7. Apical four chamber view echocardiogram, showing large pericardial effusion and coat-like echoes within the pericardium (arrow). LV: left ventricle, RV: right ventricle (From Alio-Bosch, Candell-Riera, Monge-Rangel 1991, with permission)

Findings of this kind may be a precursor of constrictive pericarditis (*Sinha, Singh, Jaipuria 1996*)**.** A fascinating study is depicted in Figure 8, showing an echo-Doppler study of a postoperative patient who was receiving warfarin and suffered a large hemorrhagic effusion without clots. The low viscosity of the effusion permitted recognition of flow signals due to movement of the fluid related to changes in volume of the cardiac chambers throughout the cardiac cycle (*Gerber and Safford, 1999*). Spontaneous contrast was imaged in a case of septic pericardial effusion and pneumopericardium (*Martana, Marvric, Vukas 1992*).

M mode imaging may provide valuable additional information. Expertise is needed to evaluate real time images for cardiac tamponade because of the need to determine that chamber collapse is occurring during diastole. An M mode record that clearly identifies the phase of the cardiac cycle, for instance, by showing whether the aortic or mitral valve is open or closed, allows any observer to decide with confidence that the right ventricular dimension diminishes in diastole (see Chapter 4). Likewise, M mode can provide a static image of the inferior vena cava over several respiratory cycles, helpful in quantifying absence of raised central venous pressure and thus inspiratory decrease in its dimension, a finding indicative of tamponade.

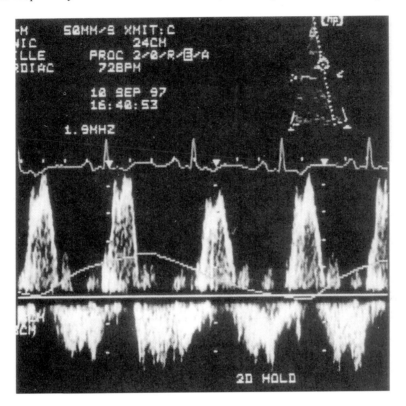

Figure 8. Pulsed-wave Doppler showing "flow" caused by movements of the pericardial fluid within the pericardial cavity. (From Gerber and Safford 1999, with permission)

8.1.2.2   Postoperative and loculated pericardial effusion

Echocardiography has been highly informative about both the high incidence of this sequel to cardiac surgery and establishing the presence of atypical effusions such as loculation in postoperative cases as well as in cases due to bacterial infection, bleeding and other factors favoring organization of the fluid. In a series of 780 patients studied by echocardiography before and eight days after cardiac surgery, pericardial effusion was detected in 64 percent, but was moderate or large in only 31 percent. The effusion was loculated in 60 percent of the cases. Less then 2 percent developed tamponade (*Pepi, Muratori, Barbier 1994*). In a similar study involving 510 patients, the incidence of tamponade was 2 percent (*Russo, O'Connor, Waxman 1993*). The presentation of cardiac tamponade in these patients may be atypical due to loculation causing selective chamber compression.

8.2   Other imaging modalities

8.2.1   Radiology

Because water and blood are similar in radiodensity, the plain chest x-ray is an inferior tool for diagnosing pericardial effusion. An outstanding recent review of what can be accomplished from the chest x-ray, however, is that by Woodring *(1998)*. In addition to reviewing well-known radiographic signs of pericardial effusion, less well-known newer signs are also described. Clinicians now rely much less on the chest radiogram for this purpose, its place having rightfully been usurped by the echocardiogram. In spite of these limitations, the chest radiogram may provide the first suggestion of pericardial effusion. When heart size has increased significantly between films without apparent cause, pericardial effusion should be suspected, especially when an acute increase in heart size is not accompanied by pulmonary congestion. The radiological signs described below may also furnish the first clue to the presence of pericardial effusion.

The transverse diameter of the heart is increased and the cardio-pericardial silhouette often assumes a globular or water bottle shape. The cardiophrenic angles often appear hyperacute, and the lung fields, in contradistinction to heart failure, appear normal. The obvious exception is the patient who has coexisting heart disease causing pulmonary congestion. Although the radiodensities of blood and pericardial fluid are similar, they are not identical. It is therefore sometimes possible to identify a double density, especially along the left heart border, as shown in Figure 9 (Tehranzadeh and Kelley 1979). Cardiomyopathy, with enlargement of all four chambers and functional tricuspid regurgitation, diverts blood destined to the lungs to the systemic veins, thereby protecting the lungs from flooding. In these patients, the heart is enlarged and the lung fields are not congested, a combination difficult or impossible to tell from pericardial effusion.

The signs of pericardial effusion detectable on the posterior anterior projection include widening of the carinal angle in the absence of signs of left atrial enlargement, and the differential density sign. An ectopic location of the epicardial fat pad and a postero-inferior bulge are detected on the lateral projection. A wide carinal angle is seen in about 20 percent of medium-sized effusions, but less frequently in small effusions. The differential density sign, described several years ago by Tehranzadeh and Kelley **(1979),** is insensitive, but is fairly specific (*Woodring 1998*).

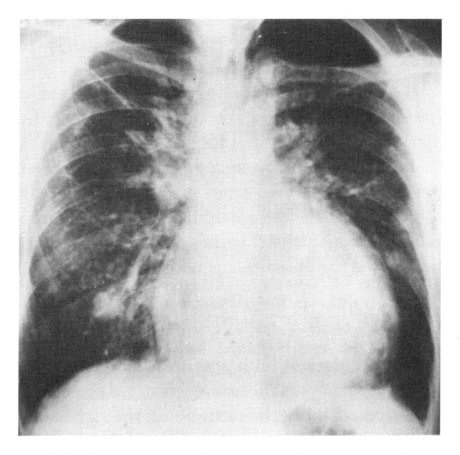

Figure 9. The differential density sign. Chest radiogram of a 70 year-old woman with a large pericardial effusion by echocardiography. The heart appears large and the lung fields are normal. Note also the differential density along the left heart border. (From Tehranzadeh and Kelley 1979, with permission)

Kremens (1955) and Torrance (1955) were the first to draw attention to what is now called the epicardial fat pad sign (Figure 10). They pointed out that the epicardial fat pad allowed the silhouette of the two layers of the pericardium to appear separate from the heart on plain chest radiograms. When visible in the normal heart radiogram, the pericardium measures one to two mm thick *(Woodring 1998)* and a thickness exceeding 2 mm suggests pericardial effusion. Pericardial effusion separates the layers of the pericardium. The consequent widening of the pericardial shadow creates the appearance of inward displacement of the epicardial fat. This sign is present in about half the cases of moderate or large effusion. Rarely, the fat pad sign is due to extrapericardial disease, for example, teratoma (*Demos, Cardella, Moncada 1983*).

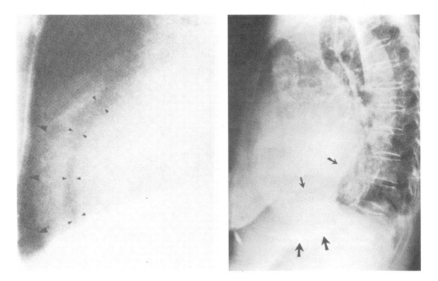

Figure10. Displaced epicardial fat pad sign of pericardial effusion

The posteroinferior bulge sign (*Holmes 1920*), according to Woodring, is the best sign of pericardial effusion, and is present in the vast majority of cases. The explanation is that pericardial fluid usually accumulates along the diaphragmatic surface of the heart and in the posteroinferior pericardial recess (*Woodring 1998*), as shown in Figure 11.

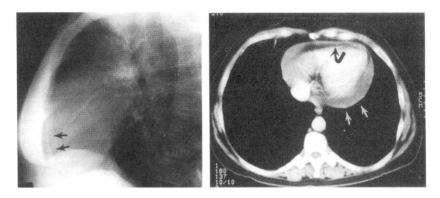

Figure11. Postero-inferior bulge sign of pericardial effusion. **Left:** Lateral chest radiogram showing prominent postero-inferior bulge due to small pericardial effusion. The postero-anterior projection showed only mild cardiomegaly. **Right:** Thoracic CT showing postero-inferior accumulation of pericardial effusion (white arrows) as well as anterior effusion present in front of the epicardial fat. (From Woodring 1998, with permission)

Mediastinal masses may simulate pericardial effusion (*Schlesinger and Fernbach,1986*). Mediastinal lipoma furnishes a good example. Figure 12 depicts a striking case. The chest x-ray of an asymptomatic young woman was mistaken for pericardial effusion until further studies were done. After removal of the lipoma, the x-ray was normal. A virtually identical case was presented to me when visting Torino, Italy.

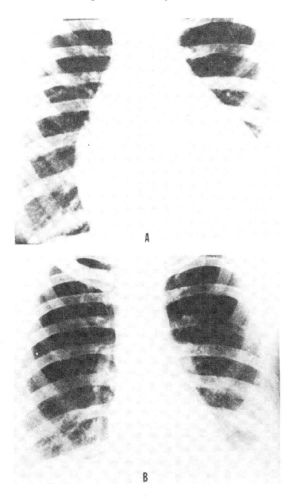

Figure12. Mediastinal lipoma simulating pericardial effusion. **A**: preoperative, **B**: after excision. (From Hipona and Paredes, 1976, with permission)

8.2.2   Cardiac fluoroscopy

Diagnostic cardiac fluoroscopy is seldom performed now, so will not be discussed in detail. When the heart of a patient with pericardial effusion is examined under the fluoroscope, cardiac pulsations are greatly diminished. Total absence of cardiac pulsation is highly suggestive of cardiac tamponade. In severe dilated cardiomyopathy, the enlarged silhouette with diminished pulsations may mimic pericardial effusion. Fluoroscopy is a good way to see epicardial fat lines in multiple projections. Failure to find a projection that brings the fat line to the edge of the cardio-pericardial silhouette constitutes reliable evidence of pericardial effusion.

8.2.3   Computer assisted tomography and magnetic resonance imaging

Although pericardial effusion is easily identified and localized on a computer assisted tomogram or magnetic resonance image, it is seldom indeed that either of these procedures is performed just to diagnose or evaluate pericardial effusion. Pericardial effusion, however, is not uncommon as an incidental finding, seen on studies done for other reasons. Both techniques exceed echocardiography in their ability to characterize the nature of the pericardial fluid (Figure 13).

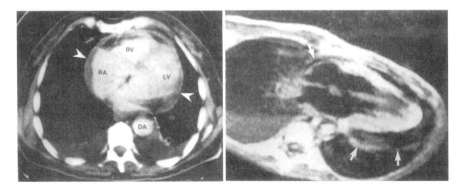

Figure 13 Pericardial effusion **Left:** contrast enhanced computerized tomogram; RA: right atrium, RV: right ventricle, LV: left ventricle, DA: descending aorta (arrow heads point to the effusion). **Right:** magnetic resonance image. The pericardium (arrows) is displaced from the epicardium by a large low-density effusion. Right pleural effusion is also seen. (From Maksimovic and Goldner 2000, with permission)

8.2.4   Early imaging techniques

The need to image the pericardium was apparent long before the modern imaging modalities we now take for granted had been developed. Pericardial effusion could be visualized on angiocardiography as a density less dense than the contrast-filled cardiac chambers, and immobile. Durant (*1961*) was the first to use negative contrast to outline the pericardium. In the past, I used it frequently, but have long since abandoned it; I describe it here solely for its interest. CO_2 was injected into the right atrium and a radiogram was taken with the patient in the left decubitus position. The pericardial image separated the air density of the gas from that of the lung, and a pericardial effusion was imaged as a wide water-density separating the two, as illustrated by Figure 14.

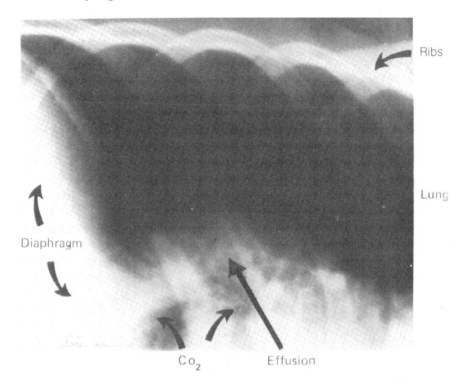

Figure14. Pericardial effusion demonstrated on a cross-table x-ray using CO_2 injected into the right atrium.

Another technique commonly employed to image pericardial effusion used to be to inject CO_2 into the pericardial cavity at the time of pericardiocentesis, as illustrated by Figure 15. Pericardial effusion is sometimes discovered accidentally during abdominal ultrasound examination or cardiac scintigraphy.

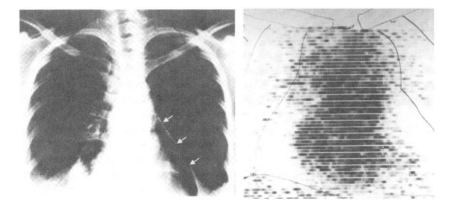

Figure15. ***Left:*** Pneumopericardium induced during pericardiocentesis to show gas-fluid interface and outline of the pericardium ***Right:*** Superimposed blood pool scan using human serum albumen and the chest radiogram. The cardiac scan is separated by a large space relatively clear of radioactive counts from the lungs and liver in which counts are present. Arrows indicate pericardium.

9.   CHYL0PERICARDIUM AND CHOLESTEROL PERICARDITIS

Chylopericardium is an effusion of chyle, the fluid normally present in the lacteals and thoracic duct. Chylopericardium is divided into idiopathic or primary, and secondary. Both forms are uncommon, but of the two, the secondary is much more common (*Svedjeholm, Jansson, Olin 1997).* The milky opaque appearance of the effusion is diagnostic. The exact constituents of the effusion depend upon the diet but, generally, the triglyceride (chylomicron) content is high. The ratio of triglyceride to cholesterol is characteristically less than one. Other characteristics of the fluid include a high content of protein, cholesterol, fat globules and lymphocytes.

In spite of the elevated cholesterol content, chylopericardium must be distinguished from cholesterol pericarditis (*vide infra*). In this entity, cholesterol crystals (absent in chylopericardium), foam cells, macrophages and giant cells are seen in the fluid. The fluid is translucent and its colour varies from case to case, but the classic description is that of a glittering gold paint.

9.1   Primary chylopericardium

Only a few cases have been reported in the literature; the number stood at 24 in the year 2000. It occurs in all age groups and may affect either sex (*Riquet, Gandjbakheh, Rabago 1993*). Occasionally, the source of the responsible leak has been identified by lymphangiography, sometimes combined with computerised tomography. Intraoperative opacification of the thoracic duct has also been used. Chylopericardium may occur in patients with idiopathic chylothorax.

9.1.1   Clinical Presentation

Fatigue and dyspnea are common, but the spectrum ranges from asymptomatic to cardiac tamponade. Some cases were diagnosed after unexplained cardiomegaly was detected on a chest radiogram. In addition to the standard means of diagnosing and evaluating pericardial effusion, chylopericardium may be disclosed by precordial imaging with labelled erythrocytes and oral administration of 1311-triolein (*Gallant, Hunziker, Gibson, 1977*).

9.2   Secondary chylopericardium

This type of chylopericardium results from injury of the thoracic duct. The commoner causes of the injury are trauma and thoracic surgery. Others include radiotherapy, infection (especially tuberculous), subclavian vein thrombosis and mediastinal neoplasm (especially lymphoma). Acute pancreatitis is a rare cause of chylopericardium (*Arendt, Bastian, Lins 1996*). Chylothorax is a rare complication of cardiac surgery (*Valentine and Raffin 1992*), much of the pertinent literature consisting of single case reports. Chylothorax, with or without chylopericardium, is commoner than isolated chylopericardium. Most often it affects children and young adults. Neoplasm and thoracic surgical operation, damaging or obstructing the thoracic duct, are leading causes. Extrinsic venous thrombosis may raise venous pressure to levels that result in lymphatic leaks (*Kurekci, Kaye, Koehhler 1998*). Disruption of the thoracic duct anywhere along its course may cause chylothorax; thus, injury of its intra-abdominal portion engenders chylous ascites that may pass through the diaphragm to cause chylopericardium.

9.2.1   Diagnosis of secondary chylopericardium

Symptoms are often non-specific or absent; therefore, diagnosis usually depends on finding milky opalescent pericardial fluid with the same contents described for primary chylopericardium. The lymphocytes are predominantly T type and the number varies from a few hundred to several thousand per ml. The electrolyte concentration is that of the plasma. Sudan 111 stains identify the fat globules. Contrast-enhanced tomography may identify the lesion responsible for disrupting or blocking the thoracic duct.

9.2.2   Treatment

Treatment of asymptomatic cases is seldom warranted when the effusion can be controlled by adhering to a diet high in medium chain triglycerides. The effusion may not recur after several weeks of this treatment (*Nguyen, Shum-Tim, Dobell 1995*).

Although the majority of cases have few or no symptoms, cardiac tamponade has been described as a complication of chylopericardium requiring pericardiocentesis or pericardiotomy (*Campbell, Benson, Williams* 2001). Ligation of the thoracic duct is often required in cases of combined chylothorax and chylopericardium, but usually pericardial drainage alone suffices in simple chylopericardium that fails to respond to dietary treatment. Refractory chylopericardium may require a pericardio-peritoneal shunt for long-term drainage (*Griffin and Fountain, 1989*).

9.3   Cholesterol pericarditis

This rare condition is a complication of chronic pericardial effusion or scarring. Commoner causes are tuberculous and rheumatoid pericarditis and myxoedema (*Fernandes, Vieira, Arteaga 2001*). In most myxoedematous effusions, however, the cholesterol content is elevated, but crystals are absent. In acute pericardial effusion, cholesterol is dissolved in the pericardial fluid, but in chronic effusion the normal ability to dissolve cholesterol may be impaired, resulting in the deposition of irritating cholesterol crystals. The concentration of cholesterol in the effusion exceeds that in the blood, often attaining values in excess of 500 mg/dl.

9.3.1   Treatment

Pericardiocentesis seldom suffices because the effusion tends to recur and the procedure does not address the pericardial scarring and injury inflicted by cholesterol crystals. Optimal treatment is radical pericardiectomy and treatment of the underlying cause.

References

Abdulijabbar HS, Marzouki KM, Zawawi TH, Khan AS. Pericardial effusion in normal pregnant women. Acta Obstet Gynecol Scand 1991; 70:291-294.

Alio-Bosch J, Candell-Riera J, Monge-Rangel L, Soler-Soler J. Intrapericardial echocardiographic images and cardiac constriction. Am Heart J. 1991; 121:207-208.

Angomachalelis N, Hourzamanis A, Salem N, Vakalis D, Serasli E, et al. Pericardial effusion concomitant with specific heart muscle disease in systemic sarcoidosis. Postgrad Med J. 1994; 70 Suppl 1:S8-S12

Arendt T, Bastian A, Lins M, Klause N, Schmidt WE, et al. Chylous cardiac tamponade in acute pancreatitis. Dig Dis Sci 1996; 41:1972-1974.

Bedford DE. Chronic effusive pericarditis. Br Heart J 1964; 26:499-512.

Benoff LJ, Schweitzer P: Radiation therapy-induced cardiac injury. *Am Heart J* 1995; 129:1193-1196.

Bright R. Tabular view of the morbid appearances in 100 cases connected with albuminous urine: with observations. Guys Hosp Rep 1836; 1: 380-400.

Bruch C, Schmermund A, Dagres N, Bartel T, Campari G, et al. Changes in QRS voltage in cardiac tamponade and pericardial effusion: reversibility after pericardiocentesis and after anti-inflammatory drug treatment. J Am Coll Cardiol 2001; 38: 219-226.

Campbell RM, Benson LN, Williams WW, Adatia I. Chylopericardium after cardiac operations in children. Ann Thorac Surg 2001; 72:193-196.

Chiu J, Atar S, Siegel RJ. Comparison of serous and bloody pericardial effusion as an ominous prognostic sign. Am J Cardiol 2001; 87:924-926

Ciliberto GR, Anjos MC, Gronda E, Bonacina E, Danzi G, et al. Significance of pericardial effusion after heart transplantation. *Am J Cardiol* 1995; 76:297-300.

Correale E, Maggioni AP, Romano S, Ricciardiello V, Battista R, et al. Comparison of frequency, diagnostic and prognostic significance of pericardial involvement in acute myocardial infarction treated with and without thrombolytics. Gruppo Italiano per lo Studio della Sopravvivenza nell'Infarto Miocardico (GISSI). Am J Cardiol. 1993; 71:1377-1381.

Corvisart JN. Of hydro-pericardium; in an essay on the organic diseases and lesions of the heart and great vessels: Philadelphia 1812. pp 66-174.

Csonka GW, Oates JK. Pericarditis and electrocardiographic changes in Reiter's syndrome. Br Med J 1957; 1:866-869.

D'Cruz IA. Echocardiographic simulation of pericardial fluid accumulation by right pleural effusion. Chest. 1984; 86:451-453.

D'Cruz IA, Cohen HC, Prabhu R, Glick G. Diagnosis of cardiac tamponade by echocardiography. Circulation 1975; 52: 460-465.

D'Cruz IA, Constantine A. Problems and pitfalls in the echocardiographic assessment of pericardial effusion. Echocardiography 1993; 10:151-166.

D'Cruz IA, Kanura N. Echocardiography of serous effusions adjacent to the heart. Echocardiography 2001; 18:445-456.

Demos TC, Cardella RG, Moncada R, Reynes CJ, Love L, et al. Epicardial fat sign due to extrapericardial disease. AJR 1983; 141:289-291.

Dressler W. The post-myocardial infarction syndrome. Arch Intern Med 1959; 103:28-42.

Dubowitz M, Gorard DA.Cardiomyopathy and pericardial tamponade in ulcerative colitis. Eur J Gastroenterol Hepatol 2001; 13:1255-1258.

Durant TM. Negative (gas) contrast angiocardiography. Am Heart J 1961; 61:1-4.

Edler I. Diagnostic use of ultrasound in heart disease. Acta Med Scand 1955; Suppl 308: 32-36.

Ewart W. Practical aids in the diagnosis of pericardial effusion in connection with the question as to surgical treatment. Br Med J 1896; 1: 717-721.

Feigenbaum H. Echocardiographic diagnosis of pericardial effusion Am J Cardiol 1970; 26:475-479.

Feigenbaum H, Waldhausen JA, Hyde LP. Ultrasound diagnosis of pericardial effusion. Ann Intern Med 1966; 65: 443-552.

Feigenbaum H, Zaky A, Waldhausen JA. Use of ultrasound in the diagnosis of pericardial effusion. Ann Intern Med 1966; 65:443-452.

Feigenbaum H, Zaky A, Waldhausen JA: Use of reflected ultrasound in detecting pericardial effusion. Am J Cardiol 1967; 19:84-90.

Fernandes F, Vieira GS, Arteaga E, Ianni BM, Pego-Fernandes P, Mady C. Cholesterol pericarditis. A specific but rare cause of pericardial disease. Arq Bras Cardiol 2001; 76:391-394

Fowler NO, Manitsas GT. Infectious pericarditis. Prog Cardiovasc Dis 1973; 16:323-336.

Frolich J, von Gontard A, Lehmkuhl G, Pfeiffer E, Lehmkuhl U. Pericardial effusions in anorexia nervosa. Eur Child Adolesc Psychiatry. 2001; 10:54-57.

Gallant TE, Hunziker RJ, Gibson TC. Primary chylopericardium: the role of lymphangiography. AJR Am J Roentgenol 1977; 129:1043-1045

Galve E, Garcia-Del-Castillo H, Evangelista A, Batlle J, Permanyer-Miralda G, et al. Pericardial effusion in the course of myocardial infarction incidence, natural history, and clinical relevance. Circulation 1986; 73:294-299.

Gerber TC, Safford RE. Intrapericardial Doppler flow signals in cardiac tamponade. Clin Cardiol. 1999; 22:231-232.

Griffin S, Fountain W. Pericardio-peritoneal shunt for malignant pericardial effusion. J Thorac Cardiovasc Surg 1989; 98:1153-1154

Heidenreich PA, Eisenberg MJ, Kee LL, Somelofski CA, Hollander H, et al. Pericardial effusion in AIDS: Incidence and survival. *Circulation* 1995; 92:3229-3234

Hipona FA, Paredes S. The radiology of pericardial disease. In Spodick DH (ed): Pericardial Diseases. Philadelphia, FA Davis, 1976, p112.

Holmes GW. The radiographic findings in pericarditis with effusion. Am J Roentgenol 1920; 7:7-15.

Horowitz MS, Schultz CS, Stinson EB, Harrison DC, Popp RL. Sensitivity and specificity of echocardiographic diagnosis of pericardial effusion. Circulation 1974; 50:239-247.

Kabadi UM, Kumar SP. Pericardial effusion in primary hypothyroidism. Am Heart J. 1990; 120:1393-1395.

Kremens V. Demonstration of the pericardial shadow on the routine chest roentgenogram: a new roentgen findingpreliminary report. Radiology 1955; 64:72-80.

Kudo Y, Yamasaki F, Doi Y, Sugiura T. Clinical correlates of PR-segment depression in asymptomatic patients with pericardial effusion. J Am Coll Cardiol 2002; 39:2000-2004

Kurekci E, Kaye R, Koehler M. Chylothorax and chylopericardium: a complication of a central venous catheter. J Pediatr 1998; 132:1064-1066.

Maisch B. Pericardial diseases, with a focus on etiology, pathogenesis, pathophysiology, new diagnostic imaging methods, and treatment. Curr Opin Cardiol. 1994; 9:379-388.

Maksimovic R, Goldner B. Computed tomography and magnetic resonance imaging in pericardial disease. In Pericardiology: Comtemporary Answers to Continuing Challenges. PM Seferovic, DH Spodick, B Maisch (eds). Belgrade, Science, 2000.

Martana A, Marvric Z, Vukas D, Beg-Zec Z. Spontaneous contrast echoes in pericardial effusion: Sign of gas-producing infection. Am Heart J 1992; 124:521-523.

Navarro JF, Rivera M, Ortuno J. Cardiac tamponade as presentation of systemic amyloidosis. Int J Cardiol. 1992; 36:107-108.

Nguyen DM, Shum-Tim D, Dobell AR, Tchervenkov CI. The management of chylothorax/chylopericardium following pediatric cardiac surgery: a 10-year experience. J Card Surg 1995; 10:302-308.

Osler W. The Principles and Practice of Medicine. 1892, New York, Appleton and Co.

Parmley LF, Manion WC, Mattingly TW. Non-penetrating traumatic injury of the heart. Circulation 1958; 18:371-396.

Pastor BM, Geerken RG. Whipple's disease presenting as pleuropericarditis. Am J Med 1973; 55:827-831.

Pepi M, Muratori M, Barbier P, Doria E, Arena V, et al. Pericardial effusion after cardiac surgery: incidence, site, size, and haemodynamic consequences. Br Heart J 1994; 72:327-331.

Popp RL. Echocardiographic assessment of cardiovascular disease. Circulation 1976; 54: 538-552.

Riquet M, Gandjbakhch I, Rabago G, Jault F, Dupont JC, et al. Isolated chylopericardium. Review of the literature apropos of a case. Ann Chir 1993; 47:124-131.

Rotch TM. Boston Med and Surg J 1878: quoted in Major RH. Classic Description of Disease with biographical sketches of the authors, 3rd ed. Charles C Thomas, Springfield, 1948 pp 410-411

Russo AM, O'Connor WH, Waxman HL. Atypical presentations and echocardiographic findings in patients with cardiac tamponade occurring early and late after cardiac surgery. Chest 1993; 104:71-78.

Sagrista-Sauleda J, Angel J, Permanyer-Miralda G, Soler-Soler J. Long-term follow-up of idiopathic chronic pericardial effusion. N Engl J Med. 1999; 341:2054-2059.

Schlesinger AE, Fernbach SK. Pericardial effusion presenting as an anterior mediastinal mass Pediatr Radiol. 1986; 16:65-66.

Shabetai R. Etiology, Pathophysiology, Recognition and Treatment: in Cardiovascular Medicine (ed. 2). JT Willerson and JN Cohn editors. Churchill Livingstone, Philadelphia, 2000.

Shaver JA, Reddy PS, Curtiss EI, Ziady GM, Reddy SC. Noninvasive/invasive correlates of exaggerated ventricular interdependence in cardiac tamponade. J Cardiol. 2001; 37 Suppl 1:71-76.

Sinha PR, Singh BP, Jaipuria N, Rao KD, Shetty GG, et al. Intrapericardial echogenic images and development of constrictive pericarditis in patients with pericardial effusion. Am Heart J 1996; 132:1268-1272.

Svedjeholm R, Jansson K, Olin C. Primary idiopathic chylopericardium--a case report and review of the literature. Eur J Cardiothorac Surg 1997; 11:387-390

Tehranzadeh J, Kelley MJ. The differential density sign of pericardial effusion. Radiology 1979; 133:23-30.

Teichholz LE. Echocardiographic evaluation of pericardial diseases. Prog Cardiovasc Dis 1978; 21: 133-140.

Torrance DJ. Demonstration of subpericardial fat as an aid in the diagnosis of pericardial effusion or thickening Am J Roentgenol Rad Therapy Nuc Med 1955; 74:850-855.

Unverferth DV, Williams TE, Fulkerson PK. Electrocardiographic voltage in pericardial effusion. Chest. 1979; 75:157-160

Valentine VG, Raffin TA. The management of chylothorax. Chest 1992; 102:586-591

Vazquez de Prada JA, Jiang L, Handschumacher MD, Xie SW, Rivera JM, et al. Quantification of pericardial effusions by three-dimensional echocardiography. J Am Coll Cardiol 1994; 24:254-259.

Woodring JH. The lateral chest radiograph in the detection of pericardial effusion: A re-evaluation. KMA Journal 1998; 96:218-224.

Zahn EM, Houde C, Benson L, Freedom RM. Percutaneous pericardial catheter drainage in childhood. Am J Cardiol 1992; 70:678-680.

Chapter 4

CARDIAC TAMPONADE

1.   HISTORICAL BACKGROUND

"Although the fluid in the pericardium serves effectively for lubricating the surface of the heart and facilitating its movement, it sometimes happens that a profuse effusion oppresses and inundates the heart. The envelope becomes filled with hydrops of the heart; the walls of the heart are compressed and cannot dilate sufficiently to receive the blood; then the pulse becomes exceedingly small, until finally it becomes utterly suppressed by the great inundation of fluid whence succeed syncope and death itself."

"What is the final and efficient cause why the human pericardium is always attached to the diaphragm, when the same structure in the quadruped is free, and separated by a clear space from the diaphragm?" (Richard Lower 1669).

William Harvey, after publishing De Motu Cordis, served as the King's personal physician in the civil war and attended him on the battlefields. After the "Cavaliers" (Royalists) were defeated by the "Roundheads" (parliamentarians), Harvey moved from Caius College, Cambridge, where, before the war, he had done the research that led to his discovery of the circulation, to Oxford University where he gathered around him a remarkable group of talented researchers, including Boyle, Hooke, Mayow, Lower and Willis, to mention just a few of the better known. Lower (Figure 1) was an experimental cardiovascular and respiratory physiologist, in whose time Harvey's theory of the circulation was still hotly disputed. Lower's research helped to discredit Harvey's opponents and support Harvey's views; in this endeavour, his research on muscular contraction was of great importance. He pioneered blood transfusion and he noted and appreciated the importance of the change of color of the blood after it passed through the lungs. He conducted experiments that proved this was due to the addition to the blood of a substance from inhaled air. He also was interested in the formation and circulation of chyle. Relevant to the subject of this chapter, in his Tractatus de Corde, he describes, in a way difficult to surpass to this day, the pathophysiology of cardiac tamponade and constrictive pericarditis. This remarkable achievement, based on clinical and autopsy observations, was the outcome of deductive reasoning. In spite of these accomplishments, however, he sometimes resorted to speculation and Aristotelian thought, as can be seen from the second of the two quotations above.

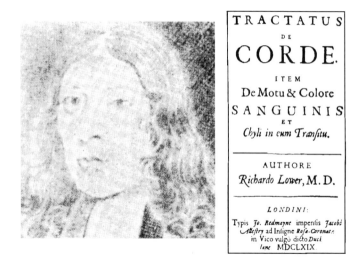

Figure 1. Left: Richard Lower who published a description of the physiology of cardiac tamponade. Right: Title page of the book, Tractatus de Corde, in which it was published.

2.   PATHOPHYSIOLOGY

Cardiac tamponade is the hemodynamic disturbance that results from the accumulation of fluid within the pericardial sac causing pericardial pressure to increase. For the purposes of this chapter, pericardial pressure will be considered as the conventionally measured liquid pressure, not as the contact pressure which assumes absence of pericardial fluid over the flatter cardiac surfaces and allows for significant regional variation of contact pressure (see Chapter 2). This choice is appropriate, because clinicians measure liquid pressure to assess cardiac tamponade and the results of treating it. When tamponade develops in a previously healthy subject, pericardial and therefore right and left ventricular diastolic pressures rise progressively and eventually become equal to each other.

The normal pericardial pressure measured in the standard manner, using an intrapericardial catheter connected to an external transducer, is very close to the pleural pressure measured in the same way, and is a few mm. lower than the left or right ventricular diastolic (and atrial) pressures throughout the respiratory cycle. Using this standard means to measure pericardial pressure, one can assume no significant variations in its magnitude in differing pericardial locations; therefore, to calculate transmural pressure, the same pericardial pressure is subtracted from the luminal pressure of any chamber. For example, in a normal subject, the left atrial or pulmonary wedge and the right atrial pressures may be 10 and 4 mmHg and the pericardial pressure minus 2 mmHg. The corresponding cardiac transmural pressures would then be 12 and 6 mmHg.

Assume that this subject develops tamponade. There is room for a small increase in pericardial pressure before it rises to the level of right ventricular diastolic pressure. This early increase in pericardial pressure has no clinical importance and cannot be detected without direct instrumentation of the pericardium and heart. From the physiological point of view, however, it defines latent or a *forme fruste* of tamponade, because respiratory variation in early diastolic filling of the ventricles is increased. In the example given above, pericardial pressure may rise from minus 2 to plus 3 mmHg, but remain 1 mmHg lower than the right atrial pressure of 4 mmHg (latent tamponade). When pericardial pressure has reached 10 mmHg., the three pressures are equal and mild clinical tamponade is present. As the pressures continue to climb, tamponade becomes increasingly severe. This spectrum of the severity of hemodynamic compromise depending on pericardial pressure is nicely illustrated in the diagram published by Reddy et al. (*1978*) and reproduced below (Figure 2), that depicts what happened to hemodynamics when a large pericardial effusion causing pericardial pressure to increase to 15 mmHg was aspirated. The magnitude of pulsus paradoxus fell progressively as pericardial fluid was removed. The point where pericardial pressure fell below the ventricular diastolic pressures during pericardiocentesis marks the end of the progressively improving hemodynamics seen during reduction of pericardial pressure from 15 to 5 mmHg. This 10 mmHg reduction in pericardial pressure progressively increased systemic blood pressure, cardiac output and stroke volume, and reduced the heart rate, but no further hemodynamic improvement occurred when pericardial pressure was lowered below the level of right ventricular diastolic pressure.

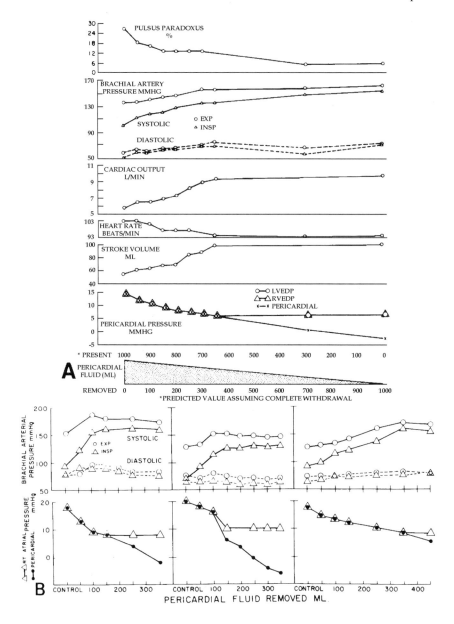

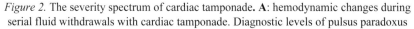

Figure 2. The severity spectrum of cardiac tamponade. **A**: hemodynamic changes during serial fluid withdrawals with cardiac tamponade. Diagnostic levels of pulsus paradoxus persist as long as left ventricular pressure equilibrates with pericardial pressure. **B**: Hemodynamic changes in 3 patients with cardiac tamponade during 50 ml aliquot aspiration of pericardial fluid. The most significant hemodynamic changes happen during the initial aspiration while right atrial and pericardial pressures remain equilibrated. After pericardial pressure falls below right atrial pressure, the latter remains constant. (From Reddy, Curtiss, O'Toole 1978, with permission)

To generalize: From the clinicians point of view, tamponade begins when pericardial pressure rises to the level of the right atrial pressure, but at that point is trivial, usually remains unrecognized and does not require pericardiocentesis. When pericardial pressure increases further as the volume and pressure of the effusion increase, right ventricular diastolic pressure rises with it and the two pressures therefore remain equal. An example is shown in Figure 3. Assuming no pre-existing heart disease that would have chronically elevated left ventricular diastolic pressure, continuing increase in the size of the effusion causes the pericardial pressure to rise to the level of the left atrial pressure The left and right ventricular diastolic pressures are then all equal to each other, but not excessively elevated, defining mild clinical cardiac tamponade that also may not merit aspiration. With increasing severity of tamponade, pericardial pressure and both ventricular diastolic pressures continue to rise. Figure 2 depicts the parallel decline in all three pressures during pericardiocentesis.

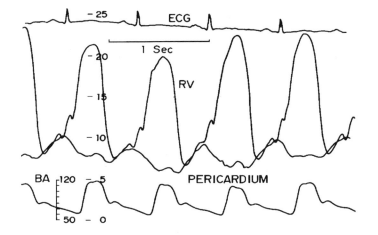

Figure 3. Mild cardiac tamponade. Right ventricular pressure, although only slightly elevated, is equal to pericardial pressure throughout diastole. Pulmonary hypertension, systemic hypotension and pulsus paradoxus are absent, defining early tamponade.

Severe tamponade may elevate pericardial pressure to 30 mmHg or more. Consequently, the atrial and ventricular diastolic pressures rise to the same level, and pulsus paradoxus with hypotension becomes evident. In the worst cases, hypotension and diminished perfusion progress to a point that simulates cardiogenic shock. The data illustrated in Figure 4 were obtained during cardiac catheterisation of a young man with tamponade secondary to viral pericarditis. It can be seen that central venous pressure is extremely high and lacks the *y* descent, and that inspiration causes central venous pressure to fall, causing an increase in systemic venous return.

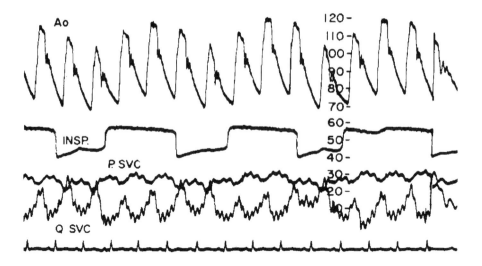

Figure 4. Severe, subacute tamponade. Tracings from above down, aortic pressure showing pulsus paradoxus, respirometer, superior vena caval pressure (P.SVC), blood flow velocity in the superior vena cava (Q.SVC), ECG, one second time marks *(Shabetai, Fowler, Fenton 1965).*

Exceptions to the rule of pressure equalization are found when heart disease coexists such that diastolic pressure in one ventricle greatly exceeds that in the other, and pericardial pressure has not achieved the diastolic pressure in the ventricle with the higher pressure. In the case of pathophysiology that increases right heart filling pressure, pericardial pressure rises to the level in the left, but not the right atrium, and therefore compression of the right atrium and right ventricular diastolic collapse are not observed.

2.1   Transmural pressure

In cardiac tamponade, atrial, ventricular diastolic and pericardial pressures are all equal, therefore the cardiac *transmural* pressures are near to zero; thus, distending pressure (preload) is greatly reduced. Although the clinical picture is the same as in heart failure, in cardiac tamponade the heart is unloaded, not overloaded. In contradistinction, when ventricular diastolic pressures increase due to chronic heart failure, the increase in pericardial pressure is far less; therefore, the slopes of absolute and transmural diastolic pressures are almost parallel and the heart is overloaded. The relationship of the two slopes in acute heart failure is intermediate between those of tamponade and chronic heart failure *(Fowler, Shabetai, Braunstein 1959).*

2.2   Cardiac volume

Cardiac tamponade reduces cardiac volume as was demonstrated long ago by left ventricular pressure-volume loop analysis in acute experimental tamponade in dogs (*Craig, Whalen, Behar 1968*) illustrated in Figure 5A. Changes induced by tamponade in pericardial and left ventricular and pericardial diameter are shown in Figure 5 (B and C) (*Pegram, Kardon, Bishop 1975*). Cardiac compression by pericardial fluid under pressure increases the thickness of the left ventricular wall normalized to end-diastolic radius, but does not change ventricular mass (pseudohypertrophy) (*Di Segni, Beker, Arbel 1990*).

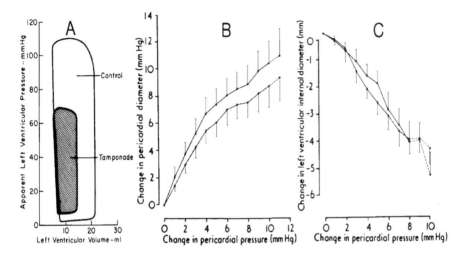

*Figure 5.***A**: Left ventricular pressure-volume loops before and after acute tamponade induced in a dog. Cardiac volumes, stroke volume and systolic pressure are drastically reduced and diastolic pressure has increased. (From Craig, Whalen, Behar 1968, with permission) **B**: Changes in pericardial diameter; and **C**: Left ventricular internal dimension during induction of experimental cardiac tamponade. Upper graph, end-diastole; Lower graph, end-systole. (From Pegram, Kardon, Bishop 1975, with permission.)

Opacifying both ventricles simultaneously in a canine model of acute cardiac tamponade (*Shabetai, Mangiardi, Bhargava, 1979*) demonstrated not only greatly reduced volumes of both ventricles, but also the altered geometry of the right ventricle with blunting and, in some cases, obliteration of the apex and bowing of the interventricular septum toward the left ventricle (Figure 6). Not shown in the figure, compression of the atria was clearly visualized. Biventriculography is too invasive to be useful in clinical practice, but provided relevant data on the pathophysiology of tamponade.

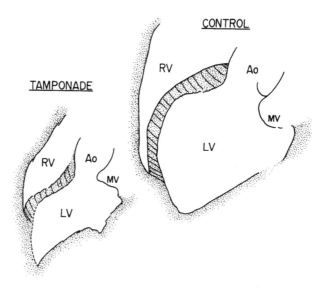

Figure 6. Diagram reconstructed from biventriculograms of dogs before and with acute experimental cardiac tamponade by simultaneously injecting opaque contrast medium into both ventricles. Tamponade has reduced the volume of both chambers and reversed the curvature of the septum, such that it is no longer toward the right ventricle but toward the left. Other shape and volume changes induced by tamponade are described in the text. (From Shabetai, Mangiardi, Bhargava, 1979, with permission.)

2.2.1   Right ventricle

For many years it was tacitly assumed that reduction of left ventricular volume by cardiac tamponade is caused by direct compression by pericardial fluid under increased pressure, but this is not the chief mechanism, because the thin-walled right ventricle and the atria are considerably more compressible than the thicker-walled left ventricle, so a major proportion of the reduction in left ventricular volume simply reflects reduced pulmonary venous return due to compression of the more susceptible thin-walled right heart chambers (series ventricular interdependence). Evidence supporting this hypothesis was obtained from canine studies made in both fresh post-mortem and *in situ* beating hearts (*Ditchey, Engler, LeWinter 1981*). Both sides of the post-mortem heart were filled with saline to physiological volumes, after which fluid was instilled into the pericardial space. The saline previously introduced into the two sides of the heart was displaced by the increased pericardial pressure into two graduated cylinders (Figure 7). In all experiments, as pericardial pressure and volume rose, the volume of fluid displaced from the right heart exceeded that displaced from the left, and higher pericardial pressures were required to displace a given volume of fluid from the left heart than from the right. This study proved that with the left and right sides of the heart at physiological volume, pericardial pressures commonly encountered in cardiac tamponade compress the right heart more severely than the left (Figure 7).

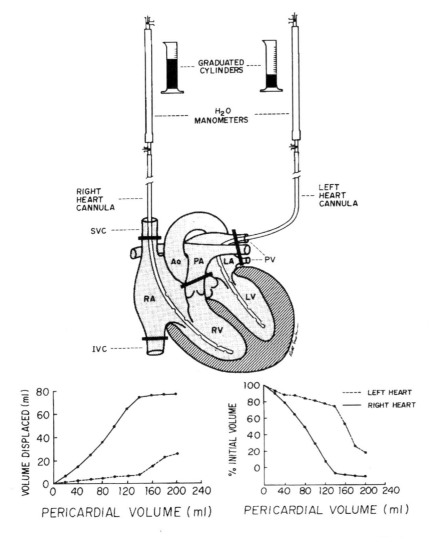

Figure 7. **Top**: Schematic representation of the post-mortem heart experiment. The intact pericardium and indwelling catheter for pressure measurement are not shown. SVC and IVC: venae cavae; RA and LA: right and left atria; LV and RV: left and right ventricles; PV: pulmonary veins. Heavy black lines indicate the positions of clamps and ligatures used to isolate the two sides of the heart within the pericardium. **Bottom:** Data from one of the 7 dogs showing more fluid displaced from the right heart than the left. This phenomenon was recorded in all 7 dogs. (From Ditchey, Engler, LeWinter 1981, with permission.)

Companion *in vivo* studies in dogs with intact circulation were done to confirm the importance of right ventricular compression in tamponade. Flow meters were placed around the ascending aorta and a branch pulmonary artery (Figure 8A). Abrupt cardiac tamponade was created by the sudden introduction into the pericardium of a quantity of warmed physiological saline sufficient to raise pericardial pressure promptly by several mmHg. The immediate effect was an instantaneous fall in pulmonary arterial stroke flow.

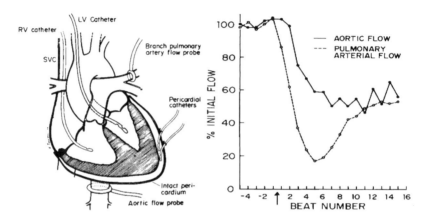

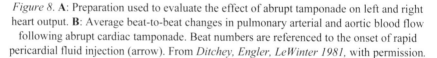

Figure 8. **A**: Preparation used to evaluate the effect of abrupt tamponade on left and right heart output. **B**: Average beat-to-beat changes in pulmonary arterial and aortic blood flow following abrupt cardiac tamponade. Beat numbers are referenced to the onset of rapid pericardial fluid injection (arrow). From *Ditchey, Engler, LeWinter 1981,* with permission.

At this moment, the left ventricle, subject to the same external compressive force, maintained its original stroke volume. Following its dramatic decline, pulmonary arterial stroke flow continued to fall over the next several cardiac cycles, as right ventricular pressure was progressively depleted. Coincidentally, left ventricular stroke volume fell as a result of reduced return of blood from the pulmonary circulation. The phase of falling pulmonary arterial blood flow was followed over the next several cardiac cycles by an increase due to transfer of blood from the pulmonary venous bed to the systemic. Eventually, pulmonary arterial and aortic flows achieved an equilibrium well below the control level. This study suggests that the initial event in acute tamponade is an acute reduction in right ventricular volume that subsequently reduces left ventricular volume and stroke output. This reduction in turn effectively moves blood from the pulmonary venous to the systemic venous bed, partially restoring cardiac output (Figure 8B). Both studies showed that the right heart is much more susceptible than the left heart to compression by pericardial fluid under increased pressure. Severe reduction of right heart pressure and volume thus make a major contribution to the hemodynamic deterioration characteristic of tamponade.

In experimental animals, the effect of tamponade on right ventricular geometry can also be dramatically shown by right or biventriculography *(Shabetai, Mangiardi, Bhargava 1979)*. The diastolic volume of both ventricles is greatly reduced (Figure 6). Severe generalized reduction of systolic volume is also seen. In addition to generalized compression, selective narrowing of the right ventricular outflow tract is a striking feature, and is consistent with observations from Schiller's laboratory made two years previously using M mode echocardiography, and now routinely used in the evaluation of two-dimensional echocardiography for cardiac tamponade *(Schiller and Botvinick 1977)*.

Except in agonal cases, left ventricular global systolic function remains normal, or is hyperdynamic in response to increased sympathetic tone *(Pegram, Kardon, Bishop 1975)*. Impaired cardiac output and work are secondary to impaired ventricular filling, not to depression of contractility. Decreased systolic pump function resulting from operating at a lower preload is compensated by increased adrenergic and sympathetic activity. Impairment of systolic performance by severe cardiac tamponade can, nonetheless, be quite impressive, as illustrated in Figure 9, showing no significant change in end-systolic volume with marked reduction of stroke volume, end-diastolic volume and mean circumferential shortening rate.

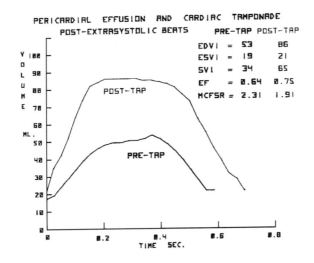

Figure 9. Left ventricular volume-time curves in a patient with severe cardiac tamponade before (lower curve) and after pericardiocentesis. During tamponade, left ventricular volume is reduced and the chamber fills more slowly. End-systolic volume is not significantly different under the two conditions.

A somewhat different conclusion was reached after a meticulous study of cardiac tamponade in chronically instrumented conscious dogs, breathing spontaneously but deeply, and under sympathetic blockade with propanolol (*Savitt, Tyson, Elbeery, 1993*). The authors proposed that, during inspiration, the transmural pressure on the left side of the interventricular septum is lower than on the right at end-diastole. This reversal of transseptal pressure would diminish the arc length of the septum, and these changes would abolish the contribution that the septum makes to right ventricular systole during inspiration. They also proposed that this inspiratory impairment of systolic function in tamponade is an important mechanism of pulsus paradoxus.

Left ventricular function, evaluated from pressure-volume curves in a canine model of acute tamponade, also proved that reduced stroke volume is not caused by impaired contractility (*Johnston, Vinten-Johansen, Klopfenstein 1990*). Three levels of cardiac tamponade were induced at differing cardiac volumes produced by transient bicaval occlusion (Figure 10). Contractility indices were calculated from the loops. This method has the advantage of being relatively independent of preload.

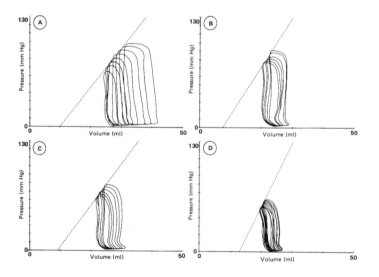

Figure 10. Left ventricular pressure-volume loops during bicaval occlusion at **A**: baseline; **B**: mild, **C**: moderate, **D**: severe tamponade. No significant change in E_{max} was observed. (Reproduced from Johnston, Vinten-Johansen, Klopfenstein, 1990, with permission)

2.2.2   Role of the atria

The study by Ditchey et al., cited in section 2.2.1, provided convincing evidence that reduced left ventricular stroke volume and diastolic volume is not a consequence of direct pressure exerted on the chamber by tamponade, but is a consequence of compression of the right heart lowering right ventricular stroke output and consequently left ventricular stroke input. That study, however, did not investigate which right heart chamber is the primary agent of impaired left ventricular function, an issue that was taken up by different investigators in a subsequent study (*Fowler and Gabel 1985*). They created a model of regional cardiac tamponade in dogs breathing spontaneously several days after surgical preparation, in which they divided the surface of the heart into separate compartments by means of sutures from the pericardium to the heart. They compared the effects of tamponade of the right ventricle plus both atria to the right ventricle alone, and tamponade of the left ventricle plus both atria to tamponade of the left ventricle alone. When the pericardial pressure surrounding either ventricle alone was raised to 20 mmHg, the change in left atrial pressure and cardiac output was slight. Tamponade of the right ventricle together with both atria, however, depressed aortic pressure and cardiac output more profoundly than tamponade of either ventricle alone. Comparable results were obtained when tamponade of the left ventricle alone was compared with tamponade of the left ventricle and both atria. The investigators' conclusion is summarized in the title of their paper, "The hemodynamic effects of cardiac tamponade: mainly the result of atrial, not ventricular, compression."

The authors modified these conclusions after performing a follow-up study using the same preparation (*Fowler and Gabel 1987*). They reasoned that compression of a single ventricle would not increase ventricular interaction to the same extent as compression of both ventricles and that, consequently, tamponade of a single ventricle would cause less hemodynamic derangement than tamponade of both ventricles. They therefore studied the comparative effects of compression of the great veins and both atria together, both ventricles together, and then all four chambers of the heart. This study showed that tamponade of both ventricles had a greater hemodynamic effect than tamponade of either ventricle alone, and that tamponade of all four chambers has the greatest hemodynamic effect. The findings with limited tamponade are congruent with reports of localized tamponade that may occur after cardiac surgery or be caused by compression by a tumour or haematoma, within or close to the pericardium. Tamponade, either limited to the atria, or involving all four cardiac chambers, caused a significant increase of superior and inferior vena caval pressure above right atrial pressure. This observation proved, once more, that narrowing of the caval-to-atrial junctions contributes to the hemodynamic derangements seen in cardiac tamponade. Interestingly, tamponade of both ventricles did not create a pressure gradient from the venae cavae to the right atrium.

This technically demanding study did not go on to distinguish between compression of the atria or the great veins or both, or attempt to elucidate the relative importance of left versus right atrial compression. Although in the past an attempt to measure pressure gradients from the venae cavae to the right atrium and pulmonary veins to the left atrium failed to find any such gradient (*Isaacs, Berglund, Sarnoff 1954*), it must be acknowledged that on-line measurement of very small pressure differences using analog-to-digital conversion, now considered essential, was not available in that era. The question remains open for further study. Supporting some contribution by compression of the great veins is the angiographic demonstration of caval compression in canine models of tamponade (*Spitz and Holmes 1972; Shabetai, Mangiardi, Bhargava 1979*), and clinical tamponade (*Miller, Feldman, Palacios 1982*).

2.2.3   Coronary circulation

Investigators have considered the possibility that tamponade may compress the epicardial coronary arteries and cause myocardial ischemia (*Jarmakani, McHale, Greenfield 1975*). These authors found that with severe tamponade, flow in the circumflex artery decreased by 51 percent and that the systolic component was retrograde. They went on to propose that left ventricular dysfunction was the outcome of the resulting ischemia. It had been demonstrated some years earlier, however, that reduction of coronary flow in tamponade does not cause myocardial ischemia because the reduced preload balances the decreased perfusion (*O'Rourke, Fischer, Escobar 1967*). More recent highly convincing evidence that myocardial contractility is not impaired in cardiac tamponade confirms that myocardial ischemia should not be included as a pathophysiological feature of cardiac tamponade.

3.   HEMODYNAMICS

We have seen that the instantaneous hemodynamic result that occurs with the onset of tamponade is reduced left ventricular filling due to reduced input from the compressed right ventricle. Soon thereafter a steady state is established, provided that fluid ceases to accumulate in the pericardium. This is the situation that confronts the clinician. There are important differences among cases, depending in the main on the speed with which the fluid has accumulated. These differences and their clinical impact will be described in later portions of this section. The essentials of the hemodynamic derangement, however, are the same in all cases and are subject to precise measurement by either invasive or non-invasive means. These hemodynamic alterations (pathophysiology) underlie all the clinical manifestations. I will therefore depart from tradition and describe these in detail before embarking on descriptions of the various clinical syndromes of cardiac tamponade. The principal non-invasive hemodynamic tool is echo-Doppler cardiography, but because much of what it reveals was validated by earlier investigators using cardiac catheterisation, and although increasing reliance is placed on echo-Doppler studies, I will discuss the findings obtained invasively before discussing hemodynamics measured non-invasively.

The pathological changes of cardiac tamponade provide the substrate for the hemodynamic alterations. When fluid enters the pericardium faster than it can be absorbed, pericardial pressure increases with multiple hemodynamic consequences. When the pericardium is stretched over a period of weeks or months, it becomes increasingly more compliant, as shown by the shape of its pressure-volume curves (Figure 11). With rapidly occurring pericardial effusion, the pericardium does not have time to creep and is then less compliant than the normal pericardium. The more acute the tamponade, the more rapidly does the pericardium become inextensible and lose its ability to stretch and accommodate an increase in cardiac volume or the volume of one side of the heart. Once pericardial strain is no longer possible, the total pericardial content is absolutely fixed. One ventricle therefore cannot expand without compressing the opposite ventricle, that is, parallel ventricular interaction is dramatically increased. In addition to this greatly enhanced ventricular interdependence, series ventricular interaction and atrio-ventricular interaction are also increased. When the pericardium has been stretched by pericardial effusion, it becomes much more compliant.

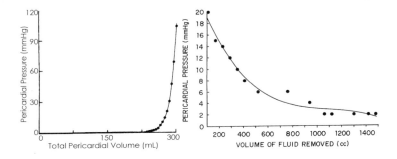

Figure 11 Pericardial pressure-volume curves: **Left**: From post-mortem study of a normal canine heart. The curve from the canine begins at the volume of the heart and illustrates the steep increase in pressure characteristic of normal pericardium. The shape of the curve of normal human pericardium is similar. **Right**: Plotted from data acquired during pericardiocentesis of a large effusion causing moderately severe tamponade. The curve acquired during pericardiocentesis is less steep, because the clinical effusion was not acute; the pericardium was therefore more distensible.

3.1   Ventricular suction

In normal physiology, the left ventricle fills by active suction only in the early rapid filling period (*Brecher 1958*), but in any condition that greatly impedes the filling of either ventricle, that ventricle may develop negative transmural pressure throughout diastole. Extreme cardiac tamponade is one such condition. Thus, in canine models of extreme tamponade (Figure 12) or massive exsanguination, both ventricles rely on suction for pan-diastolic filling. Negative ventricular transmural diastolic pressure can also be demonstrated by canine experiments in which the orifice of the mitral or tricuspid valve is severely restricted (*Fowler, Shabetai, Braunstein 1959*).

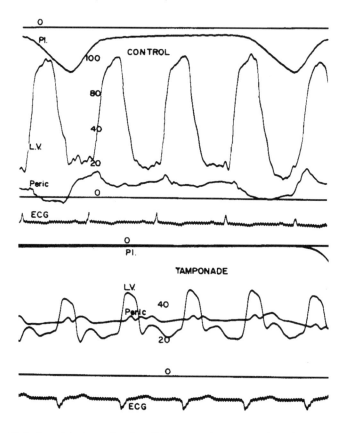

Figure 12. Left ventricular and pericardial pressure in an open-chest dog. With extreme tamponade, ventricular transmural pressure is negative. **Above**: Control. The zero line for pleural pressure is on top. **Below**: Extreme tamponade. From above down, zero for pleural pressure, pleural pressure (pl), left ventricular (LV) and pericardial (Peric) pressures, common zero line for left ventricular and pericardial pressures. Near end-stage tamponade causes severe hypotension and pan-diastolic negative transmural pressure. (From Fowler, Shabetai, Braunstein 1959, with permission).

In patients with severe tamponade we were able to demonstrate negative left ventricular diastolic pressure using a differential transformer, but it was of lesser magnitude than in the experimental model described above. An example is shown in Figure 13. Both left ventricular and left ventricular minus pericardial pressure were recorded. Left ventricular pressure was 115/16, and pericardial pressure 18 mmHg. Pulsus paradoxus was present.

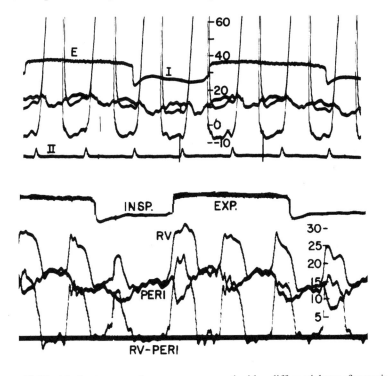

Figure 13. Ventricular transmural pressures measured with a differential transformer in a patient with severe tamponade. Left ventricular data are shown in the upper panel. **From above:** The recordings show left ventricular diastolic pressure (16 mmHg), pericardial pressure (18 mmHg), left ventricular minus pericardial pressure, the respiratory cycle and the electrocardiogram. **Lower panel:** Left ventricular transmural diastolic pressure is below atmospheric. Right ventricular data are shown in the lower panel. Transmural diastolic pressure is zero. **Tracings from above down**: Respirometer, right ventricular and pericardial pressures, right ventricular minus pericardial pressure.

3.2   Systemic congestion

The increased pericardial pressure lowers ventricular transmural pressure *vide infra,* but not absolute right atrial pressure. The resulting changes in the venous return curve at the onset of tamponade transfers blood from the central to the venous circulation. When steady state conditions are established, comparable changes in the pulmonary venous return curve together with reflex changes in inotropy and arteriolar resistance partially restore central blood volume, but systemic venous congestion persists. The increased systemic venous return raises atrial and ventricular diastolic pressures to the level of the pericardial pressure, reducing their transmural diastolic pressures to zero (*Shabetai, Fowler, Braunstein 1961*). Thus pressures in both atria, both ventricles in diastole, and the venae cavae are all equal to the pericardial pressure. This pressure equilibration is one of the chief hemodynamic hallmarks of cardiac tamponade (*Shabetai, Fowler, Guntheroth 1970*) and occurs because circumferential pericardial effusion compresses all four chambers equally.

3.3   Cardiac catheterisation

Cardiac catheterisation is by no means essential for the diagnosis of cardiac tamponade. Typical cases are readily diagnosed from the clinical features and characteristic echo-Doppler findings, but is needed in some atypical cases. When coexisting heart disease is found by echocardiography, further evaluation using invasive means, sometimes including coronary arteriography, may be needed. Right heart catheterisation during pericardiocentesis is useful for confirming the diagnosis and its severity, and assessing the hemodynamic result.

3.4   Atrial ventricular filling

3.4.1   Normal subjects

Tamponade alters the profile of venous return and the pattern of ventricular filling. Before considering the changes, I will briefly review the relevant normal physiology (Figure 14). The waveform of atrial pressure comprises the ascent of the *a* wave generated by atrial systole, the descent of the *a* (sometimes rather confusingly designated the *x* descent) marking atrial relaxation, the *c* wave caused by movement of the closed atrio-ventricular valves toward the atrium during isovolumic ventricular systole, the *x* or *x'* descent marking descent of the closed atrio-ventricular valves during isovolumic relaxation, the *v* wave that results from increased atrial pressure when the atria are filling passively from the veins and, finally, the *y* descent that occurs when the atrioventricular valves open and equalize atrial and ventricular pressures while the ventricles are actively relaxing and aspirating blood from the great veins and atria. Normal atrial filling is thus bimodal with one peak accompanying the *x* descent and ventricular ejection, and the other during the y descent and early rapid ventricular filling. The a and c waves may merge, as they do in this example (*Uther, Peterson, Shabetai 1974*).

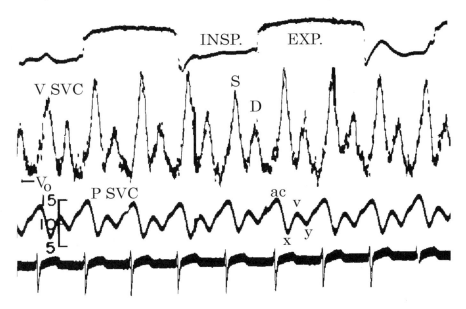

Figure 14. Blood flow velocity and pressure in the superior vena cava of a patient with mild congestive cardiac failure. V_o indicates zero flow. V SVC and P SVC are velocity and pressure respectively in the superior vena cava. The predominant peak (S) is systolic and corresponds with the x descent of pressure. The second and smaller peak (D) corresponds with the y trough.

3.4.2   Patients with tamponade

The normal contour of right atrial pressure during diastole is profoundly altered by tamponade (Figure 15). Venous return is absent during diastole (y descent) and is confined to the period of time that the x descent is inscribed, which is the ejection period of ventricular systole. In mild tamponade, the y descent is attenuated; in more severe tamponade it is absent altogether (*deCristofaro and Liu 1969*). In tamponade, systemic venous return is thus unimodal (Figure 15). The explanation is that cardiac volume is minimal during ejection because ejection is much faster than venous return. The lesser cardiac volume slightly lowers pericardial pressure; therefore, tamponade is slightly less severe in systole than diastole, permitting the heart to fill. Early diastolic filling is inhibited by the severe external pressure restraint; therefore, the *y* descent is absent.

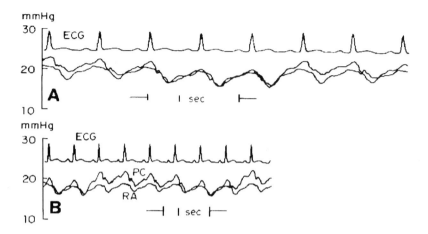

Figure 15 Cardiac catheterisation data from a patient with severe cardiac tamponade. **A:** Right atrial and pericardial pressures are elevated to 20 mmHg, the y descent is absent. Both are monophasic with an x descent. **B**: Right atrial and wedge pressures showing that these pressures also are equal and that left and right atrial pressure wave contours are similar. Compare the pressure contours with the normal shown in Figure 14.

3.4.3   The effects of respiration

It is important to appreciate that, in spite of tamponade, the normal drop in right heart pressure is preserved in spite of the elevated pericardial pressure. The reason for this is that when the subject inspires, a substantial proportion of the decline in intrathoracic pressure is still transmitted to the pericardium and thence to the right heart chambers. Therefore, just as in normal subjects, inspiration increases the pressure gradient from the extrathoracic great veins to the intrathoracic veins and right atrium, thereby increasing systemic venous return. Cardiac catheterisation therefore shows lower caval and right atrial pressures during inspiration. Figure 16 illustrates a case of very severe tamponade in which the right ventricular diastolic and right atrial pressures and the caval and pericardial pressures (not shown) were elevated to 30 mmHg but still fell with inspiration.

When blood flow or velocity is also recorded, flow and its peak velocity increase with inspiration, as seen in Figures 4 and 16 (*Shabetai, Fowler, Fenton 1965*). Ideally, respirometer tracings that accurately record the onset of inspiration and expiration should be included in the data acquired. In practice, however, most laboratories are not equipped with a respirometer, but the respiratory cycle can be shown adequately by recording the pulmonary wedge pressure along with the right atrial pressure.

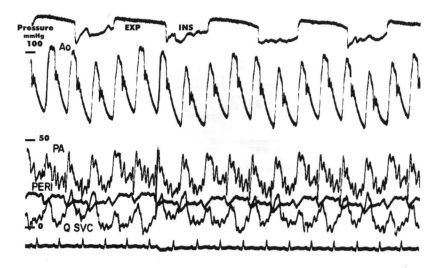

Figure 16 Severe cardiac tamponade due to idiopathic pericarditis. **Tracings from above down:** Respirometer, aortic pressure (Ao), pulmonary arterial pressure (PA), pericardial pressure (PERI), superior caval blood flow velocity (Q SVC). With inspiration, Q SVC increases and aortic systolic and pulse pressures decline. Pulmonary arterial pressure is 45 mmHg. Pericardial pressure is 20 mmHg and declines with inspiration.

3.4.4 Ventricular filling

The right ventricular diastolic pressure contour is also abnormal. The slight decline in early diastolic pressure and the plateau indicating diastasis present in normal subjects are absent. Instead, diastolic pressure increases slowly but progressively throughout diastole and the ventricles fill slowly (Figure 17). In a patient with tamponade, when a dip-and-plateau configuration of diastolic pressure is recorded by a catheter-tip manometer or a critically damped fluid-filled system an element of constriction is also present, so-called effusive-constrictive pericarditis, described in Chapter 6. Under-damped tracing may simulate the early diastolic dip. The pulmonary arterial diastolic pressure, like the atrial and ventricular diastolic pressures, becomes equal to the pericardial pressure (Figure 17, top). Indeed, in cardiac tamponade it is often difficult to distinguish the right ventricle from the pulmonary artery by inspection of the pressure recording; thus, pericardial pulmonary wedge and right atrial pressures equilibrate (Figure 15). In the case shown in Figure 17, left and right ventricular pulmonary arterial and pericardial pressures were all 17 mmHg in diastole. In the case shown in Figure 16, pulmonary arterial systolic pressure was 45 mmHg. The pulmonary hypertension of cardiac tamponade is commensurate with the elevation of right ventricular diastolic pressure. A pulmonary arterial systolic pressure significantly above 40 mmHg suggests other causes contributing to pulmonary hypertension. The cases illustrate the typical hemodynamics of constrictive pericarditis.

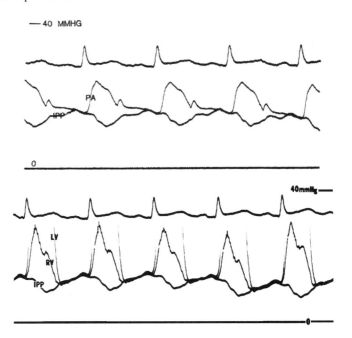

Figure 17. Top: Pericardial and pulmonary arterial pressure in clinical cardiac tamponade. Below: Micromanometer (high fidelity) pressure recording of right and left ventricular pressure with conventional pressure recording of pericardial pressure and the ECG. Left ventricular end diastolic, pericardial and pulmonary arterial end diastolic pressures are all 17 mmHg. (From Reddy PS, Hemodynamics of cardiac tamponade in man. In Pericardial Diseases. PS Reddy, DF Leon, JA Shaver (eds). Raven Press, New York, 1982, with permission)

3.4.5   Ventricular interaction

The remaining hemodynamic markers of cardiac tamponade are based on the strongly enhanced ventricular interaction (interdependence) brought about by the loss of pericardial compliance, the major manifestation being pulsus paradoxus. In the systemic circulation, pulsus paradoxus is manifested by an abnormally large drop in systolic and pulse pressures that commence at the onset of inspiration. Paradox of the pulmonary arterial pressure is in the opposite direction, such that the highest systolic pressure corresponds in time with the lowest aortic pressure. The mechanisms of pulsus paradoxus are described in Chapter 7. Suffice it here to single out ventricular interaction, which is the chief one. When inspiration increases right heart volume in a situation in which total heart volume cannot change, the right ventricle compresses the left, reducing its volume and distorting its shape. The consequence of this interaction is reduced left ventricular systolic performance and therefore stroke volume during inspiration.

3.5   Non-invasive hemodynamic assessment

The diagnosis and evaluation of cardiac tamponade does not usually necessitate cardiac catheterisation, but can usually be made with confidence from the clinical and echo-Doppler findings. Of course, a *sine qua non* is a pericardial effusion, but it must be emphasised again that, in acute cases, the effusion need not be large. Intrapericardial bleeding during interventional cardiac procedures has now overtaken neoplasm as the leading cause of tamponade in many institutions, and in these cases tamponade is often extreme, yet the effusion is so small that, under other circumstances, it would be considered too small to tap.

Once the presence of pericardial effusion has been established, the remainder of the examination is devoted to detecting hemodynamic embarrassment compatible with tamponade. The three main lines of such evidence are compression of cardiac chambers, usually the right atrium and ventricle, increased respiratory variation of left and right ventricular inflow and outflow, and plethora of the inferior vena cava. Exaggerated respiratory variation of blood flow velocities to and from the ventricle are such that with inspiration they increase on the right and decrease on the left, and are a direct manifestation of ventricular interdependence that has been greatly heightened by the tightly stretched and therefore non-compliant pericardium.

3.5.1   Normal respiratory variation of blood flow

In normal subjects, a number of mechanisms cause transtricuspid flow velocity to increase and transmitral to decrease with inspiration. The most important of these is the transit time required for the increased right ventricular output that accompanies inspiration to appear at the systemic circulation, where it does not arrive until the subsequent expiration. This normal respiratory variation in ventricular inflow velocity is most pronounced in the early filling wave and amounts to 10 percent or less when respiration is normal.

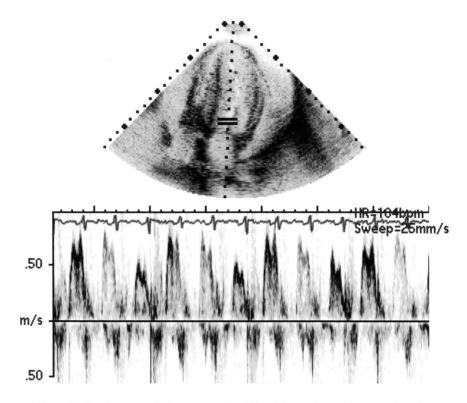

Figure 18. Respiratory variation in transmitral blood flow velocity in a case of cardiac tamponade. **Top**: Four chamber echocardiogram showing a large pericardial effusion severely compressing the right ventricle. **Bottom**: Spectral Doppler tracing showing the exaggerated respiratory variation. (Courtesy of Nelson Schiller, M.D., UCSF)

3.5.2   Respiratory variation of blood flow in tamponade

In cardiac tamponade, respiratory variation of early rapid left ventricular inflow is significantly increased and may exceed 40 percent (see Figure 18 above). Pericardial effusion without overt tamponade induces a smaller increase in respiratory variation of ventricular inflow. A landmark study combined echo-Doppler cardiography with meticulous invasive measurements of cardiovascular and pericardial pressure in patients with tamponade and those with effusion, but without classic tamponade (Figure 19) (*Appleton, Hatle, Popp 1988)*. Respiratory variation is measured conveniently for clinical purposes as change in peak velocity but, from the physiological point of view, it is important to realize that it is the respiratory variation of stroke input volume that is important *(Shabetai, Fowler, Fenton 1965)*. The reason for this greatly exaggerated respiratory variation on ventricular inflow in tamponade is that strongly enhanced ventricular interaction predominates over the normal mechanisms, such that any change in filling of one side of the heart has a dramatic effect on the volume of the contralateral side. In addition, reduced left ventricular filling delays opening of the mitral valve, and thus isovolumic relaxation time is lengthened. Impaired early rapid ventricular filling is associated with an increased rather than a decreased speed of myocardial relaxation due to the heightened sympathetic tone characteristic of tamponade *(Nishikawa, Roberts, Talcott 1994)*. The resulting tachycardia and increased rate of myocardial inactivation accelerate myocardial relaxation. The resulting small increase in the atrio-ventricular pressure difference, however, is usually insufficient to compensate for the reduced venous return that diminishes it. The time-velocity index of mitral inflow also declines, indicating reduced pulmonary venous return. Just as the magnitude of pulsus paradoxus increases with greater severity of tamponade, reflecting respiratory variation in stroke volume, so does respiratory variation of ventricular Doppler inflow parameters. In patients with mild or subclinical tamponade, augmented respiratory variation of left ventricular filling may be confined to the atrial component. Stroke output varies directly with stroke input and therefore aortic stroke volume and peak velocity decline with inspiration, while those of the pulmonary artery increase. When evaluation of respiratory variation in ventricular inflow and outflow is precluded by swinging motion of the heart within the pericardium, the variation can be seen in the descending aorta *(Ho, Eisenberg, Schiller 1994)*. The inspiratory fall in aortic time-velocity index is the equivalent of clinical pulsus paradoxus. Doppler interrogation of the pulmonary veins confirms that pulmonary venous return falls with inspiration.

3.5.3   Echo-Doppler signs of tamponade

In addition to the Doppler evidence of tamponade that depend on respiratory variation and ventricular interdependence, the two most important of these signs are right ventricular diastolic collapse *(Armstrong, Schilt, Helper 1982)*, and right atrial compression *(Gillam, Guyer, Gibson, 1983; Kronzon, Cohen, Winer 1983)*. The echocardiogram itself thus makes an important contribution to the likelihood that a pericardial effusion is or is not causing tamponade.

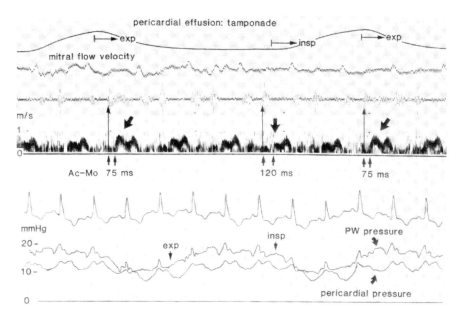

Figure19. Reciprocal respiratory variation of mitral and tricuspid inflow velocities in a patient with severe cardiac tamponade. **TOP PANEL:** Tracings from above down: respirometer, mitral inflow velocity, ECG. The three heavy arrows show sequentially, apnea, the onset of inspiration, and expiration. The small arrows mark isovolumic relaxation times. **LOWER PANEL**: Pulmonary wedge and pericardial pressures. Note that with inspiration, the pressure gradient from pulmonary wedge to pericardium (and thus presumably ventricular diastolic pressure) falls. (From *Appleton, Hatle, Popp 1988,* with permission.

Right ventricular diastolic collapse is an abnormal diastolic motion of the anterior wall of the right ventricle, as shown in Figure 20. The hemodynamic explanation of this phenomenon is a reversal of the ratio of pericardial to right ventricular diastolic pressure, thus causing right ventricular transmural pressure to become slightly negative. This is a reasonably sensitive and specific sign of tamponade, but it must be recalled that the underlying reversal of the normal ratios of pericardial pressures is prevented by right ventricular hypertrophy or elevated diastolic pressure, which therefore prevents the appearance of this otherwise useful sign of tamponade (*Plotnick, Rubin, Feliciano 1995*).

3.5.3.1   The effusion

The effusion does not have to be large in order to cause tamponade; its size depends upon how rapidly it has accumulated. Tamponade can be hyperacute, virtually instantaneous, for instance, following trauma or rupture of the heart or aorta, or puncture of a coronary artery. In such cases, a remarkably small blood collection can quickly produce extreme tamponade.

3.5.4 Echocardiographic signs of tamponade

In addition to the Doppler signs of alterations in hemodynamics dependent on respiration and a feature of heightened ventricular interaction, a number of abnormalities on the echocardiogram itself also provide strong evidence upon which to decide whether or not an effusion is causing clinically significant tamponade. Of these, the most important are right ventricular diastolic collapse (*Armstrong, Schilt, Helper 1982*) and compression of the right atrium (*Gillam, Guyer, Gibson 1983*). Right ventricular collapse is an abnormal posterior motion of the anterior wall of the right ventricle caused by a transient increase in pericardial pressure that causes it to exceed right ventricular pressure slightly in early diastole. This abnormality of regional right ventricular wall motion in diastole is well seen in the subcostal imaging plane (Figure 20). Its timing in diastole can be appreciated by experienced echocardiographers, but is more easily recognized on M mode images in which the open position of the mitral valve and closed position of the aortic valve unequivocally document the phase of the cardiac cycle (Figure 20).

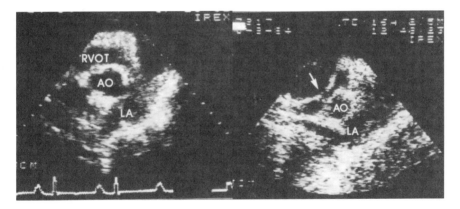

Figur20. Right ventricular diastolic collapse. **Left**: Subcostal view. **Right**: M mode. (From Klopfenstein, Schuchard, Wann 1985, with permission.)

In a study using a chronically instrumented canine model of cardiac tamponade, right ventricular diastolic collapse began at a lower pericardial pressure, cardiac output and blood pressure when the animals were rendered hypovolemic (*Klopfenstein, Cogswell, Bernath 1985*). This observation has been borne out many times in clinical evaluation of tamponade. Hypervolemia had the opposite effect. These phenomena are commonly seen in clinical practice; right ventricular diastolic collapse must therefore always be interpreted within its clinical context, especially the volume status, and other imaging findings. For instance, its presence in spite of a low central venous pressure may be because the patient is hypovolemic (see also low pressure cardiac tamponade) or it may be absent in a patient who does have tamponade because the right ventricular diastolic pressure is very high, or the chamber is greatly hypertrophied (*Leimgruber, Klopfenstein, Wann 1983*).

A canine study of the effects of coexisting left ventricular dysfunction showed that ventricular diastolic collapse occurs at a lower pericardial pressure than when ventricular function is normal. The left ventricle was damaged by intracoronary injection of non-radioactive microspheres. Left ventricular dysfunction shifted the pericardial pressure-volume curve upwards and to the left, causing compression of the right heart at smaller pericardial volumes than were required before left ventricular dysfunction had been produced (*Hoit, Gabel, Fowler 1990*). The authors speculated from their data that echocardiographic signs of tamponade may be found in patients who have left ventricular dysfunction even when the effusion is quite small. The results obtained by Klopfenstein, Cogswell, Bernath (1985) and Hoit, Gabel, Fowler (1990) should serve to emphasize the importance of clinical correlation with echocardiographic signs of tamponade. Right ventricular diastolic collapse is more specific and sensitive than pulsus paradoxus in detecting cardiac tamponade, and appears earlier in its course.

The onset of right ventricular diastolic collapse, earlier in the course than pulsus paradoxus, was established by studies using a conscious dog model in which the investigators recorded combined echocardiographic and invasive hemodynamic data at increasing pericardial pressure induced by intrapericardial administration of saline (*Klopfenstein, Schuchard, Wann 1985; Leimgruber, Klopfenstein, Wann 1983; Singh, Wann, Klopfenstein 1986*). The investigators correlated the appearance of right ventricular diastolic collapse with the severity of the resulting hemodynamic derangement, as shown in Figure 21. Data were recorded every two minutes while pericardial volume was continuously increased at a rate of 10 ml/min. When this echocardiographic abnormality first appeared, definite but not yet severe reductions in blood pressure and stroke volume and heart rate were present, allowing the investigators to conclude that, although pulsus paradoxus had not by then appeared, significant but compensated cardiac tamponade was present. Administration of more intrapericardial fluid induced pulsus paradoxus and severe reductions of stroke volume, cardiac output, blood pressure and increased tachycardia, defining decompensated cardiac tamponade (Figure 21). While right ventricular diastolic collapse is more sensitive than pulsus paradoxus as a detector of increased pericardial pressure when blood volume is normal, they are equally sensitive in hypovolemic states. It has been stated that low pressure cardiac tamponade increases the sensitivity of right ventricular diastolic collapse (*Labib, Udelson, Pandian 1989*), but a comparison with pulsus paradoxus was not included in that publication. Easier to recognize and probably more important than these right heart regional wall motion abnormalities is compression of the whole right ventricle (*Schiller and Botvinick 1977*).

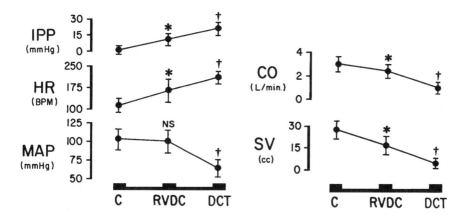

Figure 21 Correlation of right ventricular diastolic collapse with hemodynamics in experimental cardiac tamponade. Details are described in the text. IPP: intrapericardial pressure. C: control. RVDC: right ventricular diastolic collapse. DCT: decompensated tamponade. (From Leimgruber, Klopfenstein, Wann 1983, with permission.)

Right atrial compression (Figure 22) is highly sensitive for cardiac tamponade, but less specific than right ventricular diastolic collapse. Although it is generally considered as an aid to the diagnosis of tamponade, it is also important in the pathogenesis of its hemodynamic consequences. Its specificity is increased without decreasing its sensitivity when it lasts longer than one third of the cardiac cycle. Atrial compression is greatest in diastole and in inspiration, when right heart volume and therefore pericardial stretch are maximal. These factors are responsible for the transient reversal of the ratio of pericardial to atrial pressure and for its timing in the respiratory and cardiac cycles (*Kronzon, Cohen, Winer 1983*). Kronzon suggested that atrial compression plays a significant role in reducing cardiac output and blood pressure, a view strongly supported by experimental studies (*Fowler and Gabel 1985*).

Transoesophageal echocardiography in critically ill, hypotensive patients may reveal that the cause is compression of the heart, not ventricular dysfunction, and therefore determines the appropriate therapy (*Heidenreich, Stainback, Redberg 1995*). Compression of right heart chambers can occur in patients with large, often bilateral pleural effusion, with (*Traylor, Chan, Wong 2002*) or without (*Venkatesh, Tomlinson, O'Sullivan 1995*) other signs of tamponade. Based on experience with patients who had extensive pleural effusion but an insignificant pericardial effusion, investigators have compared intrapericardial with intrapleural effusion of saline in canine models (*Vaska, Wann, Sagar 1992; Klopfenstein and Wann 1994*). The increase in pleural pressure induced a parallel increase in pericardial pressure and right ventricular diastolic collapse but, in spite of this, the hemodynamic signs of tamponade were milder. In patients like these, it is well to remove pleural fluid before proceeding to pericardiocentesis *(Kaplan, Epstein, Schwartz 1995)*. Another unusual cause of cardiac tamponade is a large intrathoracic pancreatic pseudocyst *(Nagy, Olah, Raez 2000)*. The paper is in Hungarian, but the abstract is in English.

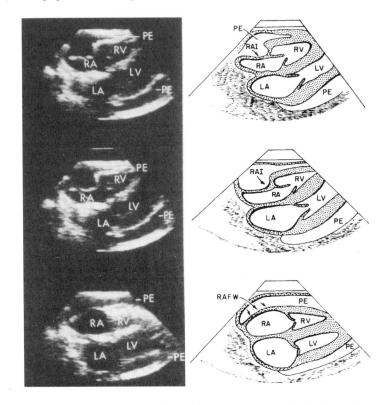

Figure 22. Right atrial compression. Subcostal long axis cross-sectional echocardiogram from a patient with right atrial compression. Inversion is initiated at end-diastole (top) and continues through early diastole (middle). By end-systole (bottom) the right atrial free wall appears normal. (From Gillam, Guyer,Gibson, 1983, with permission.)

3.5.4.1   Compression of left heart chambers

Echocardiographic evidence of compression of the right-sided cardiac chambers is common and highly specific and is sensitive in tamponade of moderate or greater severity. It is important to know that, under certain circumstances, for instance after cardiac surgery, compression of the left atrium or left ventricle, or both, may be seen on the echocardiogram (Figure 23). In a study of 18 postoperative patients, the investigators found only 3 with collapse of either the right atrium or the right ventricle, but 15 with left ventricular diastolic collapse associated with posterior loculation of the effusion (*Chuttani, Pandian, Mohanty 1991*). In a subsequent study from this laboratory, the incidence of left ventricular diastolic collapse in posterior loculated effusion was seen in 89 percent *(Chuttani, Tischler, Pandian 1994)*. In a similar study, the incidence of postoperative tamponade was 2 percent of all cases of tamponade. Clinical, hemodynamic and echocardiographic findings were atypical in the 10 patients identified. Specifically, left ventricular diastolic collapse, either alone or in combination with collapse of other chambers, was frequent. In this context, it is appropriate to consider that the Doppler findings of cardiac tamponade were more sensitive and more specific than chamber collapse in a study of 159 patients with moderate to large pericardial effusion, of whom 38 were suspected on clinical grounds to have tamponade (*Merce, Sagrista-Sauleda, Permanyer-Miralda 1999*).

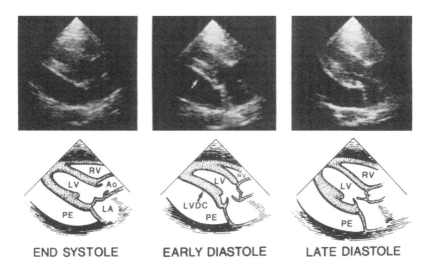

Figure 23. Left ventricular compression in a case of atypical tamponade following cardiac surgery. (From Chuttani, Tischler, Pandian, 1994, with permission)

3.5.5   Abnormal motion of the whole heart

Electrical alternans, with or without mechanical alternans (*Ratib and Perrenoud 1984; Gabor, Winsberg, Bloom, 1971*), may be a feature of cardiac tamponade in cases with a large effusion, usually with associated tamponade under increased pressure. It is said to be particularly associated with effusion due to malignant tumours (*Gaffney, Keller, Peshok 1984*). It has been reasoned that the cardiac displacement is so great that the heart cannot return to its original position before the next cardiac cycle commences. The heart would then begin its next depolarisation in an altered position. The subsequent depolarisation would cause much less displacement, enabling the heart to return to its original position (*Feigenbaum 1994*).

A large pericardial effusion frees the heart from the constraints imposed by the lungs and mediastinum, allowing it to rotate about its attachments to its vascular pedicle. The heart, because of torque generated by ventricular ejection, swings within the effusion at a frequency that depends on the heart rate (*Rigney and Goldberger 1989; Sacks and Widman 1993*). A striking example was evaluated in our laboratory (Figure 24). Rigney and Goldberger's models were developed by applying non-linear dynamics (Chaos theory). They predicted from their two models that the heart would swing every other heart beat when the heart rate is between 105 and 106 or 88 and 119. At slower or faster rates the swinging would happen with every cardiac cycle. The derived critical rates at which swinging occurs agree with clinical reports.

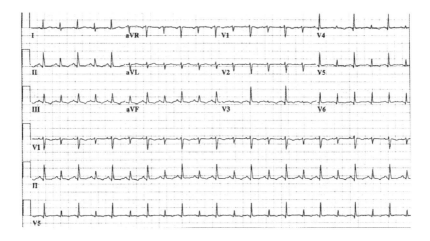

Figure 24. A striking example of electrical alternans in a case of tamponade. Often, this finding is more subtle.

The swinging heart is a very dramatic finding when viewed in real time. The vastly differing positions of the heart within the mediastinum can be seen on the still frames shown in Figure 25, even though they lack the drama of the moving pictures.

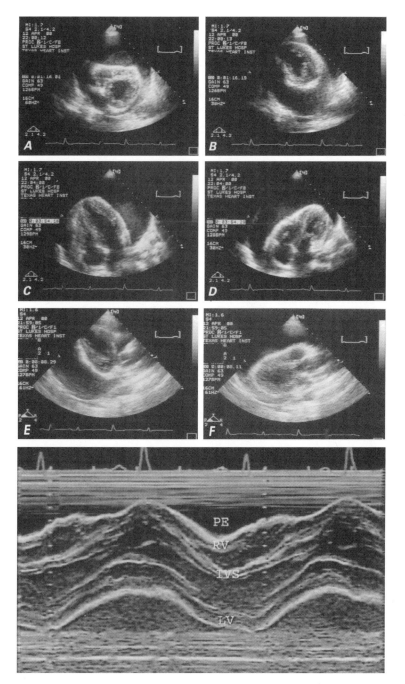

Figure 25. Still frames and M mode echocardiogram from a study that showed the heart swinging in real time. The patient had cardiac tamponade and the electrocardiogram showed electrical alternation. (From *Lau, Civitello, Hernandez, 2002,* with permission).

3.6   Summary

From the early days of echocardiography, this imaging modality has been of inestimable value in the diagnosis and evaluation of pericardial effusion and has contributed significantly to the recognition of cardiac tamponade. The last two decades have witnessed major advances in the ability of echocardiography to advance our understanding and management of this often life-threatening condition. Of vital importance have been the introduction of Doppler imaging, the development of high-resolution real-time images and the ability of echo-Doppler cardiography to provide critical hemodynamic as well as anatomical data. In this last connection, elegant studies coordinating findings obtained by cardiac catheterisation with the imaging findings have been invaluable. All this is not to say that echo-Doppler has usurped clinical evaluation. The numerous examples of situations in which the echo-Doppler study may fail to rule in or rule out cardiac tamponade attest to the need to correlate the findings on imaging with the clinical picture.

4.   BEDSIDE AND CLINICAL ASPECTS OF CARDIAC TAMPONADE

4.1   Aetiology

All injuries of the pericardium may cause pericardial effusion, and any effusion may lead to cardiac tamponade. The number of systemic disorders that may injure the pericardium is legion but, as always in clinical medicine, it is appropriate to consider first the common aetiologies. Only after these have been ruled out, or clinical clues in individual cases suggest an unusual cause is it necessary to probe for unusual causes. The aetiology of cardiac tamponade seen by clinicians depends very much on the population they serve and the type of practice in which they are engaged, so these factors influence their approach to the diagnosis, and rightly so. The order in which aetiologic categories are listed here must therefore be arbitrary. A catalogue of all known causes of tamponade is more a concern for the epidemiologist than the practitioner.

4.1.1   Idiopathic and viral pericarditis

These two categories are here considered as one, as frequently it is difficult to distinguish between them and, because management is the same, the effort often is not made. Viral and idiopathic pericarditis are often dry and fibrinous, but pericardial effusion may occur, as in other inflammations of the pericardium. In general, the effusion is of more diagnostic than therapeutic importance, but it can become very large, progressively distending the pericardium until finally it becomes inextensible and the pressure rises to levels that mandate urgent pericardiocentesis.

The offending virus is commonly Coxsackie or echo, but any viral infection may cause pericarditis with tamponade.

4.1.2   Other infections

Non-viral infections are important causes of tamponade. Tubercular pericarditis should be singled out because of its propensity to cause tamponade, both in the acute phase in which a large effusion may supervene, or in the subacute phase in which tamponade is a component of effusive constrictive pericarditis. Purulent pericarditis is a life-threatening disease even when tamponade is absent and more so when it is complicated by tamponade. Pericardial infection with any living organism is a potential cause of tamponade.

4.1.3   Trauma

Trauma (immediate, recent or remote) is an important cause of tamponade. Mention has been made already of the high and rising incidence of tamponade complicating interventional cardiac procedures. Steering wheel injuries and baseball blows may be followed by early or late tamponade. Some of the largest effusions with severe tamponade that I have encountered occurred weeks or months after cardiac operation.

4.1.4   Neoplasia

While just about any neoplasm could be responsible for tamponade, by far the more common are carcinoma of the lung or breast, and lymphoma. Primary tumours of the pericardium are more apt to cause constriction than tamponade. Clearly, the greatest variety of tumours is seen on oncology services and in cancer hospitals.

4.1.5   Other causes

The most important metabolic cases are myxedema, although it is among
the less common causes overall, and patients undergoing dialysis, although
the numbers have declined sharply in recent decades. Numerous systemic
disorders involve the pericardium, with or without effusion, and in turn the
effusion may or may not be a tamponading one.

4.2   Clinical syndromes of tamponade

Claude S. Beck, who pioneered surgical intervention for ischemic heart
disease and who was the first to describe open chest resuscitation for cardiac
arrest, described what he designated as two triads of cardiac compression.
The components of the acute triad were falling arterial pressure, rising
venous pressure and a small, quiet heart. We now appreciate that this triad is
relevant only to the most acute cases of tamponade, for instance, those that
follow immediately upon trauma, or are a consequence of rupture of an
aneurysm of the aorta or the heart. They do not apply to most patients seen
in the practice of internal medicine, in which the effusion is not caused by
haemorrhage, is subacute or chronic, and large. Systolic and pulse arterial
blood pressures are mostly within a normal range. An enlarged cardio-
pericardial silhouette and pulsus paradoxus are commonly present
(*Guberman, Fowler, Engel 1981*). The components of Beck's second triad,
high venous pressure, ascites and small, quiet heart do not apply to chronic
tamponade, but to constrictive pericarditis and will not be considered here.

The history and past history are very helpful in making the diagnosis.
When a patient presents with hemodynamic compromise, the presence or
history of any of the conditions mentioned under aetiology of cardiac
tamponade should enter the differential diagnosis, unless a cardiac cause is
apparent.

4.2.1   Hyper-acute tamponade

Cardiac stab or bullet wounds, ruptured aneurysm of an intrapericardial
artery or the heart itself, perforation of the left atrium or its appendage
during trans-septal catheterisation, perforation or tear of a coronary artery
during angioplasty or stent deployment, in which high level anti-platelet
therapy increases the danger, are important causes of this catastrophic
syndrome that carries a startlingly high mortality. A case is described below
and illustrated in Figure 26.

After a stent had been deployed in the right coronary artery, the patient
became drowsy and showed air hunger. An emergency echocardiogram

showed severe cardiac compression and pericardial opacity only 1 cm from the heart at its widest point. Nevertheless, echo-guided pericardiocentesis via the apical route was undertaken, and blood was aspirated after agitated saline was injected, to ascertain that the needle tip was in the pericardium, not the heart. A balloon was deployed to seal the leak and protamine was administered. These measures resolved the hemodynamic crisis and the patient went on to make a complete recovery. He was fortunate indeed, considering the high mortality of this complication.

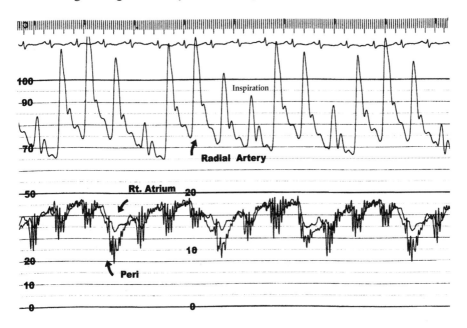

Figure 26. Acute cardiac tamponade during coronary angioplasty. The radial arterial tracing shows tachycardia and extreme pulsus paradoxus. The right atrial and pericardial pressures are equally elevated, but the amount of effusion was very small. Note deeper y descent in the pericardial pressure, compared with right atrial. Heavy time markings = 1 second.

4.2.2   Cardiac tamponade in medical patients

Among the patients I have seen personally, the majority were suffering from one of seven conditions: bronchogenic carcinoma, mammary carcinoma, lymphoma, renal failure (often on dialysis), tuberculosis, idiopathic pericarditis and postpericardial injury syndrome, most often following cardiac operation. In these circumstances it is most unusual to find either of Beck's triads of cardiac compression. Usually the cardiac silhouette is moderately enlarged, sometimes greatly, and the patients do not have hypotension. Furthermore, the heart sounds, a widely held opinion notwithstanding, are usually of normal intensity and quality. Moreover, unlike patients with severe acute tamponade, these patients are seldom in extremis, have little or no alteration in cerebral function, and dyspnoea is seldom extreme. They may complain of a degree of dyspnoea, often associated with a feeling of fullness or tightness in the chest. When there is accompanying acute pericarditis, they complain specifically of chest pain. Symptoms of the underlying causative disease may be prominent, for instance, dyspnoea is often aggravated by impaired pulmonary function in patients with bronchogenic carcinoma and those with pulmonary tuberculosis. Patients with tuberculosis or lymphoma often report severe constitutional symptoms.

The patient's symptoms and past history are very helpful in making the diagnosis. When a patient presents with hemodynamic compromise, and the presence or history of any of the conditions mentioned under aetiology, cardiac tamponade should enter the differential diagnosis, unless a cardiac cause is apparent.

Examination is easier than in the more acute cases because the heart rate is slower, respiration less laboured and the patient's condition does not preclude cooperation with the examiner. The jugular pressure is elevated, often extremely so, and its pulse contour can be evaluated more easily. The waveform lacks the y descent, but the x descent is prominent. These two nadirs of the jugular pulse can be distinguished on clinical examination. The x is synchronous with the palpated contra-lateral carotid pulse, whereas the y is seen between successive carotid pulsations. When the jugular pressure elevation is not extreme, it is often possible to see that its level drops during inspiration. Palpation of the pulses discloses pulsus paradoxus. The severity of the pulsus can be gauged by taking the blood pressure and finding the difference in systolic pressure at which Karatkoff sounds are audible only during expiration as against when they can be heard throughout the respiratory cycle. Details of the technique are given in Chapter 7.

The literature often states that orthopnea is not a feature of cardiac tamponade because, for a given elevation of pulmonary and systemic venous pressure, the compromised right ventricle is less able to flood the lungs, as it does in left heart failure or mitral stenosis. Besides, we have already seen that tamponade shifts an appreciable portion of pulmonary blood volume to the systemic circulation. I have often observed that patients with severe tamponade are unable to lie down because they are short of breath when they attempt to do so. This phenomenon was recognized many years ago (Figure 27)

In severe cases, the blood urea nitrogen level is frequently elevated because of greatly reduced renal blood flow. In spite of the greatly elevated atrial pressure, atrial naturetic peptide concentration remains normal, because transmural pressure is low. Other abnormal laboratory findings are related to the underlying disease, not to tamponade *per se*. If the clinical evaluation has not eliminated cardiac tamponade, the next step is echocardiography.

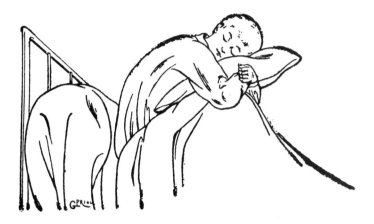

Figure 27. The pillow sign of acute pericardial effusion from *Blechmann, quoted by Bedford 1964.*

4.2.3   Low pressure tamponade

This treacherous form of cardiac tamponade is found in patients with severe hypovolemia in which, as discussed previously, tamponade occurs at much lower pericardial, and therefore also central venous pressure than in euvolemic patients (Figure 28). In trauma cases, massive haemorrhage from multiple extra-cardiac sources is the usual reason for tamponade without greatly elevated jugular pressure. In other cases, low venous pressure has resulted from high dosage of diuretic, often given in the mistaken belief that the patient had heart failure, and in which tamponade had not been considered until later. Central blood volume may have been depleted by starvation, dialysis or excessive fluid loss. Left, rather than right, ventricular diastolic collapse in a patient with low pressure tamponade has been reported (*Dwivedi, Saran, Narain 1998*). Abnormal respiratory variation of ventricular inflow velocities is helpful in the diagnosis (*Hayes, Freeman, Gersh 1990*).

Many of the patients whom I have observed were early in the stage of development of effusion due to malignant neoplasm. Others had severe blood loss outside the pericardium. One of the case reports in the literature described an elderly dehydrated man who developed low-pressure tamponade from tuberculous pericarditis (*Antman, Cargill, Grossman 1979*). Dialysis is an important cause of low-pressure tamponade.

The modest elevation of jugular pressure may be missed on clinical examination, but pulsus paradoxus (Figure 28), right ventricular diastolic collapse and right atrial compression are present. Often pallor, peripheral cyanosis, cool extremities and other signs suggesting depressed cardiac output can also be observed.

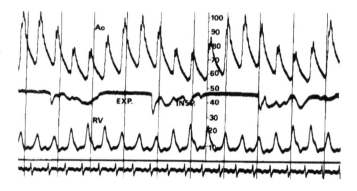

Figure 28. Low pressure cardiac tamponade. The right ventricular diastolic pressure was only 10 mmHg, but otherwise the characteristic findings of tamponade were present, including pulsus paradoxus, out of phase between the right ventricle (RV) and aorta (Ao), and absent dip and plateau of RV diastolic pressure.

4.3   Atypical tamponade

Tamponade is often atypical when it is a complication of cardiac surgery (*Bommer, Follette, Pollock 1995*), when it is often localized *(Russo, O'Connor, Waxman 1993)*, and in which concurrent heart disease may further complicate the hemodynamics. Localized tamponade may be found in patients with extensive pericardial adhesion. Air in the pericardium is a rare cause of tamponade, and a pericardial cyst in association with an otherwise innocuous pericardial effusion may cause tamponade. Pericardial effusion is frequently found when looked for prospectively, before and after cardiac surgery. The majority are small and do not increase in size *(Pepi, Muratori, Barbier 1994)*. In Pepi's study, 430 of 803 post-cardiac operative patients had an effusion, but only 1.9 percent of them had cardiac tamponade.

4.3.1   Effusive-constrictive pericarditis

Pericardial effusion may develop along with constrictive pericarditis. Neoplasm, radiation and tuberculosis are among the more prominent causes.

The hemodynamic and therefore also the clinical features differ from those of uncomplicated cardiac tamponade. The hemodynamic outcome, after successful pericardiocentesis, also differs. This syndrome is more appropriately discussed in the context of constrictive pericarditis (see Chapter 6).

4.4   Differentiation from superior vena caval syndrome

Distinguishing between cardiac tamponade and obstruction of the superior vena cava by a tumour or other mass is usually straightforward and generally is made without cardiac catheterisation. Nevertheless, I am occasionally requested to evaluate a case of "tamponade" when the true problem is mechanical obstruction of the superior vena cava. In this condition, the neck veins are extremely distended, but since they are cut off from the right atrium, they do not pulsate. Furthermore, a network of collateral veins is often visible around the clavicle and the offending mass is readily identified by chest roentgenography. Most of the patients had bronchogenic carcinoma, in itself a good reason to suspect cardiac tamponade and, adding to the confusion, many had pulsus paradoxus from laboured breathing. Some had a pericardial effusion. These features explain why such cases may be mistaken for cardiac tamponade. This error is easily avoided by proper evaluation of the jugular pulse. The data recorded from a patient with obstruction of the superior vena cava, who did come to cardiac catheterisation, are shown in Figure 29.

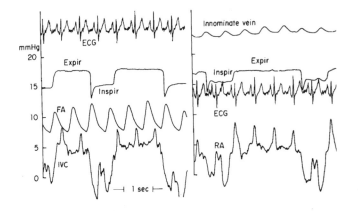

Figure 29. Superior vena caval syndrome. On the left panel observe that, save for excessive respiratory variation, the inferior vena caval pressure is normal. On the right panel, observe innominate pressure of 23 mmHg and pressure in the right atrium equal to that in the inferior cava. In the record from the innominate vein, respiratory variation is absent and the pressure is severely damped.

5.   TREATMENT OF TAMPONADE

Standard treatment is evacuation of the tamponading fluid, accomplished usually by pericardiocentesis, but sometimes by surgical operation. The former has the advantages that it is performed without the services of an operating room and surgical team, does not require general anaesthesia, and the patient is spared postoperative discomfort. Another major advantage of pericardiocentesis is that it provides an excellent opportunity to refine the diagnosis, assess the hemodynamics, and to detect underlying cardiac abnormalities. A good example was provided by a case of post-traumatic pericardial effusion with severe tamponade in which elevated right atrial pressure with abnormal waveform led to right ventriculography, which revealed severe tricuspid regurgitation. At a subsequent operation, traumatic rupture of the chordae was seen. In the present era, it should be added, all these features would be detected by echo-Doppler cardiography.

In some circumstances, surgical exploration and evacuation of fluid is preferred. Examples include tamponade with only a small effusion and in cases in which biopsy is required. When a large pericardial effusion recurs after multiple pericardiocenteses, drainage by surgical means is appropriate. The decision of whether to employ pericardiectomy or subcostal pericardiotomy often depends on the clinican's preference, availability of facilities at the time of an emergency, local experience and expertise and institutional policy. Technical details of pericardiocentesis and various means of obtaining pericardial and, where indicated, epicardial biopsy are discussed in Chapters 3 and 5.

5.1   Pharmacological palliation

Administration of drugs should never be considered definitive therapy, and volume expansion seldom suffices. Adrenergic tone is heightened; therefore, any amelioration following the infusion of an inotrope depends largely on its vasodilating properties. Thus it increases cardiac output and lowers right atrial and pericardial pressures, as well as decreasing end-systolic volume (*Fowler and Holmes 1969*). A subsequent study from Fowler's laboratory showed that nitroprusside infusion lowers the elevated systemic vascular resistance and right atrial pressure, but fails to increase cardiac output. Transfusion alone raises right atrial pressure, but does not increase cardiac output. They showed that the combination is highly effective in raising cardiac output without increasing right atrial pressure (*Fowler, Gabel, Holmes 1978*). These measures afford some temporary relief in severe cases awaiting pericardiocentesis or pericardiectomy. They should not be considered as definitive treatment.

References

:

Antman EM, Cargill V, Grossman W. Low-pressure cardiac tamponade. Ann Intern Med 1979; 91:403-406.

Appleton CP, Hatle LK, Popp RL. Cardiac tamponade and pericardial effusion: respiratory variation in transvalvular flow velocities studied by Doppler echocardiography. J Am Coll Cardiol 1988; 11:1020-1030

Armstrong WF, Schilt BF, Helper DJ, Dillon JC, Feigenbaum H. Diastolic collapse of the right ventricle with cardiac tamponade: an echocardiographic study. Circulation 1982; 65:1491-1496.

Bedford DE. Chronic effusive pericarditis. Br Heart J 1964; 26:499-512

Bommer WJ, Follette D, Pollock M, Arena F, Bognar M, et al. Tamponade in patients undergoing cardiac surgery: a clinical-echocardiographic diagnosis. Am Heart J 1995; 130:1216-1223.

Brecher GA: Critical review of recent work on ventricular diastolic suction. Circ Res 1958; 6:554-566

Chuttani K, Pandian NG, Mohanty PK, Rosenfield K, Schwartz SL, et al. Left ventricular diastolic collapse. An echocardiographic sign of regional cardiac tamponade. Circulation 1991; 83:1999-2006.

Chuttani K, Tischler MD, Pandian NG, Lee RT, Mohanty PK. Diagnosis of cardiac tamponade after cardiac surgery: relative value of clinical, echocardiographic, and hemodynamic signs. Am Heart J 1994; 127:913-918

Craig RJ, Whalen RE, Behar VS, McIntosh HD: Pressure and volume changes of the left ventricle in acute pericardial tamponade. Am J Cardiol 1968; 22:65-74

DeCristofaro D, Liu CK. The haemodynamics of cardiac tamponade and blood volume overload in dogs. Cardiovasc Res 1969; 3:292-298

Di Segni E, Beker B, Arbel Y, Bakst A, Dean H, et al. Assessment of pseudohypertrophy as a measure of left-ventricular compression in patients with cardiac tamponade. Cardiology 1990; 66: 508-511.

Ditchey R, Engler RL, LeWinter MM, Pavelec R, Bhargava V, et al. The role of the right heart in acute cardiac tamponade in dogs. Circ Res 1981; 48:701-710.

Dwivedi SK, Saran R, Narain VS. Left ventricular diastolic collapse in low-pressure cardiac tamponade. Clin Cardiol 1998; 21:224-226.

Feigenbaum H. Echocardiography (5th Ed) 1994, Febiger, Philadelphia. pp 556-588

Fowler NO, Gabel M. The hemodynamic effects of tamponade: mainly the result of atrial, not ventricular, compression. Circulation 1985; 71: 154-157.

Fowler NO, Gabel M. Regional cardiac tamponade: a hemodynamic study. J Am Coll Cardiol 1987; 10:164-169.

Fowler NO, Gabel M, Holmes JC. Hemodynamic effects of nitroprusside and hydralazine in experimental cardiac tamponade. Circulation 1978; 57:563-567.

Fowler NO, Holmes JC. Hemodynamic effects of isoproterenol and norepinephrine in acute cardiac tamponade. J Clin Invest 1969; 48:502-507.

Fowler NO, Shabetai R, Braunstein JR. Transmural ventricular pressures in experimental cardiac tamponade. Circ Res 1959; 7:733-739.

Gabor GE, Winsberg F, Bloom HS. Electrical and mechanical alternation in pericardial effusion. Chest 1971; 59:341-344.

Gaffney FA, Keller AM, Peshock RM, Lin JC, Firth BG. Pathophysiology mechanisms of cardiac tamponade and pulsus alternans shown by echocardiography. Am J Cardiol

1984; 53:1662-1666

Gillam LD, Guyer DE, Gibson TC, King ME, Marshall J, et al. Hydrodynamic compression of the right atrium: a new echocardiographic sign of cardiac tamponade. *Circulation* 1983; 68:294-301

Guberman BA, Fowler NO, Engel PJ, Gueron M, Allen JM: Cardiac tamponade in medical patients. *Circulation* 1981; 64:633-640.

Hayes SN, Freeman WK, Gersh BJ. Low pressure cardiac tamponade: diagnosis facilitated by Doppler echocardiography. Br Heart J 1990; 63:136-140

Heidenreich PA, Stainback RF, Redberg RF, Schiller NB, Cohen NH, et al. Transesophageal echocardiography predicts mortality in critically ill patients with unexplained hypotension. J Am Coll Cardiol 1995; 26:152-158.

Hoit BD, Gabel M, Fowler NO. Cardiac tamponade in left ventricular dysfunction. Circulation 1990; 82:1370-1376.

Isaacs JP, Berglund E, Sarnoff SJ. Ventricular function (III): The pathologic physiology of acute cardiac tamponade studied by means of ventricular function curves. Am Heart J 1954; 48:66-76.

Jarmakani JM, McHale PA, Greenfield JC Jr. The effect of cardiac tamponade on coronary haemodynamics in the awake dog. Cardiovasc Res 1975; 9:112-117.

Johnston WE, Vinten-Johansen J, Klopfenstein HS, Santamore WP, Little WC. Effect of acute cardiac tamponade on left ventricular pressure-volume relations in anaesthetised dogs. Cardiovasc Res 1990; 24:633-640

Kaplan LM, Epstein SK, Schwartz SL, Cao QL, Pandian NG. Clinical, echocardiographic, and hemodynamic evidence of cardiac tamponade caused by large pleural effusions. Am J Respir Crit Care Med 1995; 151:904-908.

Klopfenstein HS, Cogswell TL, Bernath GA, Wann LS, Tipton RK, et al. Alterations in intravascular volume affect the relation between right ventricular diastolic collapse and the hemodynamic severity of cardiac tamponade. J Am Coll Cardiol 1985; 6:1057-1063.

Klopfenstein HS, Schuchard GH Wann LS, Palmer TE, Hartz AJ, et al. The relative merits of pulsus paradoxus and right ventricular diastolic collapse in the early detection of cardiac tamponade: an experimental echocardiographic study. Circulation 1985; 71:829-833.

Klopfenstein HS, Wann LS. Can pleural effusions cause tamponade-like effects? Echocardiography 1994; 11:489-492.

Kronzon I, Cohen ML, Winer HE. Diastolic atrial compression: a sensitive echocardiographic sign of cardiac tamponade. J Am Coll Cardiol 1983; 2: 770-775.

Labib SB, Udelson JE, Pandian NG. Echocardiography in low pressure cardiac tamponade Am J Cardiol 1989; 63:1156-1157

Lau TK, Civitello AB, Hemandez A, Coulter SA. Cardiac tamponade and electrical alternans. Tex Heart Inst J 2002; 29:66-

Leimgruber PP, Klopfenstein HS, Wann LS, Brooks HL: The hemodynamic derangement associated with right ventricular diastolic collapse in cardiac tamponade: An experimental echocardiographic study. *Circulation* 1983; 68:612-620.

Lower R: Tractatus de Corde, Item de Motu, et Colare Sanguinis et Chyli in Sum Transiti, London, J. Allestry, 1669, quoted by Boyd LJ and Elias H, in Contributions to diseases of the heart and pericardium. 1. Historical introduction. Bull NY Med Coll 18:1-37, 1955.

Merce J, Sagrista-Sauleda J, Permanyer-Miralda G, Evangelista A, Soler-Soler J. Correlation between clinical and Doppler echocardiographic findings in patients with moderate and large pericardial effusion: implications for the diagnosis of cardiac tamponade. Am Heart J 1999; 138:759-764.

Miller SW, Feldman L, Palacios I, Dinsmore RE, Newell J, et al. Compression of the superior vena cava and right atrium in cardiac tamponade. Am J Cardiol 1982; 50:1287-1292.

Nagy SA, Olah A, Raez I, Gartner B. Cardiac tamponade caused by Intrathoracic pancreatic pseudocyst. Magy Seb 2000; 53:216-219

Nishikawa Y, Roberts JP, Talcott MR, Dysko RC, Tan P, Klopfenstein HS. Accelerated myocardial relaxation in conscious dogs during acute cardiac tamponade. Am J Physiol 1994; 266:H1935-1943

O'Rourke RA, Fischer DP, Escobar EE, Bishop VS, Rapaport E. Effect of acute pericardial tamponade on coronary blood flow. Am J Physiol 1967; 212:549-552

Pegram BL, Kardon MB, Bishop VS. Changes in left ventricular internal diameter with increasing pericardial pressure. Cardiovasc Res 1975; 9:707-714.

Pepi M, Muratori M, Barbier P, Doria E, Arena V, et al. Pericardial effusion after cardiac surgery: incidence, site, size, and hemodynamic consequences. Br Heart J 1994; 72:327-331

Plotnick GD, Rubin DC, Feliciano Z, Ziskind AA. Pulmonary hypertension decreases the predictive accuracy of echocardiographic clues for cardiac tamponade. Chest 1995; 107:919-924.

Ratib O, Perrenoud JJ. Demonstration of electrical and mechanical alternans in malignant pericardial effusion with 2-D echocardiography. J Clin Ultrasound 1984; 12:501-504.

Reddy PS, Curtiss EI, O'Toole JD, Shaver JA: Cardiac tamponade: Hemodynamic observations in man. Circulation 1978; 58:265-272.

Rigney DR, Goldberger AL. Nonlinear mechanics of the heart's swinging during pericardial effusion. Am J Physiol 1989; 257:H1292-1305.

Russo AM, O'Connor WH, Waxman HL. Atypical presentations and echocardiographic findings in patients with cardiac tamponade occurring early and late after cardiac surgery. Chest. 1993; 104:71-78.

Sacks E, Widman LE. Nonlinear heart model predicts range of heart rates for 2:1 swinging in pericardial effusion Am J Physiol 1993; 264:H1716-1722

Savitt MA, Tyson GS, Elbeery JR, Owen CH, Davis JW, et al. Physiology of cardiac tamponade and paradoxical pulse in conscious dogs. Am J Physiol 1993; 265:H1996-2008.

Schiller NB, Botvinick EH. Right ventricular compression as a sign of cardiac tamponade. An analysis of echocardiographic ventricular dimensions and their clinical implications. Circulation 1977; 56:774-779.

Shabetai R, Fowler NO, Braunstein JR, Gueron M: Transmural ventricular pressures and pulsus paradoxus in experimental cardiac tamponade. Dis Chest 1961; 39:557-568.

Shabetai R, Fowler NO, Guntheroth WG: The hemodynamics of cardiac tamponade and constrictive pericarditis. Am J Cardiol 1970; 26:480-489.

Shabetai R, Mangiardi L, Bhargava V, Ross J Jr., Higgins CB. The pericardium and cardiac function. Prog Cardiovasc Dis 1979; 22: 107-154.

Singh S, Wann LS, Klopfenstein HS, Hartz A, Brooks HL. Usefulness of right ventricular diastolic collapse in diagnosing cardiac tamponade and comparison to pulsus paradoxus. Am J Cardiol 1986; 57:652-656.

Spitz HB, Holmes JC. Right atrial contour in cardiac tamponade. Radiology 1972; 103:69-75.

Traylor JJ, Chan K, Wong I, Roxas JN, Chandraratna PA. Large pleural effusions producing signs of cardiac tamponade resolved by thoracentesis. Am J Cardiol 2002; 89:106-108 ·

Uther JB, Peterson KL, Shabetai R, Braunwald E. Measurement of force-velocity-length relationships in man using an electromagnetic flowmeter catheter. Adv Cardiol 1974; 12:198-209

Vaska K, Wann LS, Sagar K, Klopfenstein HS. Pleural effusion as a cause of right ventricular diastolic collapse. Circulation 1992; 86:609-617.

Venkatesh G, Tomlinson CW, O'Sullivan T, McKelvie RS. Right ventricular diastolic collapse without hemodynamic compromise in a patient with large, bilateral pleural effusions. J Am Soc Echocardiogr 1995; 8:551-553

Chapter 5

PERICARDIOCENTESIS
Pericardioscopy and pericardiotomy

It had been sometimes observed that great relief was given by the withdrawal of one or two ounces, and that this had been followed by the absorption of the rest of the fluid.

Mr. Hulke* hoped he should not be intruding on a subject of special interest to the physician if he made one or two remarks on the case that had been so admirably treated by Dr. West. He considered it more advisable to dissect down carefully to the pericardium before any incision was made, and if a trocar or cannula were employed, he advised very careful use of them, and that the trocar be frequently withdrawn, to form an opinion of the parts reached. He had himself, after medical consultation, a case which was believed to be one of pericardial effusion, once inserted a trocar and cannula somewhat boldly, and the withdrawal of the trocar had been followed by a jet of blood, which gave him great anxiety, but happily relieved the patient. (West 1883)

---

*In Britain, the title "Mr." is customary for surgeons who are Fellows of the Royal College of Surgeons. The title "Dr." is used by internists who are Members or Fellows of the Royal College of Physicians.

1.   HISTORICAL BACKGROUND

The interesting history of pericardiocentesis has been comprehensively reviewed elsewhere (*Kilpatrick and Chapman 1965*). In 1653, Riolanus suggested that pericardial fluid may compress the heart, and proposed that trephining the sternum might be a means to reduce this pressure. Senac is also said to have conceived the idea of pericardiocentesis. These ideas, however, did not bear fruit for another century. Around the turn of the 19th century, Desault and Larrey attempted to evacuate pericardial fluid by direct incision, perhaps following the method suggested by Romero, requiring an intercostal incision through which the pericardium could be palpated and cut if pericardial fluid were present.

The accounts we have of Romero's description are second hand, as the originals have been lost. The attempts by Desault and Larrey failed; Merat performed the operation successfully. Corvisart thought that entering the pericardium was too dangerous for general use, but when this operation was essential, he favoured a direct approach.

Kilpatrick and Chapman credit Franz Schuh (1804-1865), a Viennese physician (Figure 1) who worked closely with Skoda, the famous thoracic surgeon, with the first needle pericardiocentesis. Schuh suggested pericardiocentesis in 1839 and, a year later, carried out the procedure on a 24 year old woman suffering from extreme dyspnoea. The pericardiocentesis was carried out using a trocar introduced through the third intercostal space at the left sternal margin. The tap was dry and the trocar was therefore reintroduced in the fourth intercostal space, from which sizeable quantities of blood-stained fluid were aspirated. The patient immediately felt better. After death five months later, a mediastinal neoplasm was found. The trocar was a modification of one designed by Skoda for thoracocentesis. Indirect pericardiotomy using Schuh's trocar and cannula or modifications passed gradually into general use.

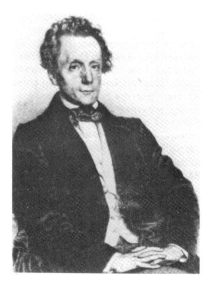

Figure 1. Franz Schuh (1804-1865) who in 1840 introduced blind pericardiocentesis. (From Kilpatrick and Chapman 1965, with permission)

West's cases, in which the tap was later followed by open drainage, was successful. The procedure was usually carried out without complications, presumably because only large pericardial effusions could be diagnosed, and therefore were safe to tap. Kilpatrick and Chapman mention another interesting case, in which the operator aspirated about 300 ml of blood from the heart before realizing that the trocar had penetrated beyond the pericardium.. The patient is said to have benefited from the mishap. One speculates that he must have been severely congested. The same source credits Sir Clifford Allbutt with introducing the English practice of pericardiocentesis in the 19th century; Roberts, among others, popularised the procedure in the United States at about the same time.

2. DECLINING RATES OF MORBIDITY AND MORTALITY

The last several decades have witnessed a steady decline in the morbidity and mortality of pericardiocentesis. The rather large number of citations in the first (1981) edition of this book, quoting a high incidence of death or serious complications, is not relevant to current practice. Several reasons account for this improved outcome. Around the middle of the last century, pericardiocentesis was treated as a bedside procedure requiring minimal aseptic precautions and frequently was performed by junior staff, usually without any means to monitor the cardiac silhouette or the position of the needle. A single channel electrocardiograph was generally the only monitor, and often even that was omitted. The needles and their bevels were unnecessarily long, adding to the risk of laceration.

Now, the procedure is performed in a suitable environment and is performed and supervised by trained personnel following strict aseptic precautions. Fluoroscopic guidance, except in extreme emergencies, became standard about thirty years ago, and about the same time, replacing the needle with a much less traumatic catheter immediately after the tip of the needle was securely within the pericardium was introduced and rapidly gained wide acceptance. In a review of 352 pericardiocentesis procedures using the subxiphoid approach and fluoroscopic guidance with substitution of the puncture needle by a straight polyethylene catheter with multiple side holes, and after successful puncture had been confirmed by injecting radio-opaque contrast medium, no deaths directly attributable to the procedure were reported. Cardiac perforation occurred in 23 instances, but bleeding was trivial, except in two postoperative patients receiving an anticoagulant. (*Duvernoy, Borowiec, Helmius,* 1992).

The steadily improving quality of echocardiographic images facilitated assessment of the size, distribution and nature of the effusion. Even when the standard practice was subxiphoid pericardiocentesis and fluoroscopic guidance, these advances increased the safety and success of pericardiocentesis. More recently, echocardiograhic guidance was introduced and soon thereafter became the method preferred by many operators. Because echocardiographic guidance enabled the operator, not only to determine where the effusion was most accessible, but also helped provide information on the proper trajectory for the needle, it contributed further to the safety and success of pericardiocentesis (*Tsang, Oh, Seward 1999*).

3.   INDICATIONS

3.1   Pericardiocentesis or pericardiotomy

A number of clinical situations require that pericardial fluid be removed, either by pericardiocentesis or pericardiotomy, usually as completely as possible; but sometimes only small samples for subsequent analysis need be procured. By far the most important indications are therapeutic. Dominant in this category are relief of cardiac tamponade and removal of infected, especially purulent pericardial effusion. A less common and less absolute indication is treatment of massive persistent or recurring pericardial effusion. Paradoxically, pericardiocentesis performed to establish the aetiology of pericarditis, pericardial effusion or a systemic disorder has a much lower diagnostic yield than does pericardiocentesis performed as therapy. A good example of this paradox is that the presence and source of malignant cells is often disclosed by cytological examination of pericardial fluid removed to treat cardiac tamponade. While this finding may only confirm a hitherto established diagnosis, it is sometimes new, revealing the cause for a pericardial effusion for the first time. Not all pericardial effusions in patients with extrapericardial malignancy are due to invasion of the pericardium. Malignant cells in the fluid prove that the effusion is malignant, but failure to find them does not rule out malignant effusion.

The literature does not include large multicenter trials; furthermore, I do not foresee that such a trial will become available. Trials involving some hundreds of patients and conducted by single large European centres, however, do provide helpful information that should be considered in individual practice in the U.S. where, generally, the structure of medical practice is not conducive to a large medical centre's ability to require that members of the staff follow a standard protocol.

Acute pericarditis and cardiac tamponade of uncertain aetiology at the time of initial hospitalisation for evaluation have been designated as primary pericardial disease and have been reviewed by the authors (*Soler-Soler, Permanyer-Miralda, Sagrista-Sauleda 1990*) since their original publication (*Permanyer-Miralda, Sagrista-Sauleda, Soler-Soler, 1985*) in which they reported the results of treating 231 consecutive patients. They designated pericardiocentesis, performed solely to learn the aetiology of pericardial effusion, diagnostic pericardiocentesis. The indications for what they called diagnostic pericardiocentesis were clinical activity and pericardial effusion persisting after one week, or suspicion of purulent pericarditis. The series also included 44 patients in whom they performed pericardiocentesis for therapy for cardiac tamponade. Similarly, they divided pericardial biopsy into diagnostic or therapeutic categories.

The results of this study show that neither pericardiocentesis nor pericardial biopsy and only standard histological examination without immunostaining have a high likelihood of finding the cause of either acute pericarditis or pericardial effusion. As has been noted already, therapeutic pericardiocentesis is considerably more likely than diagnostic pericardiocentesis to reveal the cause of pericardiopathy. Overall, the diagnostic yield of pericardiocentesis was only 19 percent. It was as low as 6 percent when carried out simply for diagnostic purposes, but even for therapeutic indications the diagnostic yield increased only to 29 percent. Pericardial biopsy, with an overall diagnostic yield of 5 percent fared even worse than pericardiocentesis. The difference in results comparing diagnostic versus therapeutic biopsy, however, was greater; therapeutic biopsy revealed the cause in 54 percent of cases. These results make it abundantly clear that when pericardial fluid or pericardial tissue is obtained for the sole purpose of discovering the aetiology of pericardial disease, the answer most likely will not be forthcoming; when performed as therapy for tamponade or purulent infection, one can anticipate that the procedure will disclose the aetiology in half of the patients.

The results of this study are not encouraging, but it was nonetheless a most important contribution, because we now know what it is reasonable to expect from these procedures. It has shown that neither is justified as a purely diagnostic endeavour, but that when either or both are performed as treatment of tamponade or purulent pericarditis, a diagnostic bonus may be forthcoming. Individual practitioners are mostly free from the constraints of a preset protocol, and it must be remembered that the one-week and three-week periods after the initial evaluation for removing fluid or obtaining biopsy were set for the purpose of designing a protocol and not as guidelines for practice, where each case must be judged individually.

3.2   Pericardioscopy

A more recent development has been the advent of rigid and flexible pericardioscopy that makes it possible to obtain epicardial biopsies (*Maisch, Bethge, Drude, 1994*). In patients with perimyocarditis, pathological lesions are more likely to be found on the epicardium than in pericardial tissue or on endomyocardial biopsy. With the use of a pericardioscope, biopsy ceases to be a blind procedure, because the bioptome can be directed to pathological or suspicious-looking areas (*Maisch and Ristic, 2002*). A series of 141 patients underwent examination with a rigid pericardioscope or mediastinoscope for the aetiological diagnosis of pericardial effusion (*Nugue, Millaire, Porte, 1996*). The patients were followed for two years. Receiver-operating curve analysis found that pericardioscopy was superior to both pericardiocentesis and open pericardial biopsy in finding the reason for pericardial effusion. The areas under the curves were 0.78 for pericardiocentesis, 0.89 for subxiphoid pericardiotomy, and 0.98 for pericardioscopy. Pericardioscopy was especially useful for neoplastic pericardial disease that would have been missed in 5 of 24 patients had not pericardioscopy been performed. The procedure requires a small subxiphoid incision and excision of the xiphoid process, and is usually performed under general anaesthesia.

The flexible pericardioscope is a less invasive instrument and does not call for general anaesthesia, or require an incision and excision of the xiphoid process.

The instrument must have an outer diameter less than 4 mm, but still be large enough to accommodate a bioptome of 2 mm outer diameter with which to perform biopsy of visualized targets. It also must be flexible in two directions and must provide sharp images. Not surprisingly, it is expensive and not easily commercially available. For all these reasons, pericardioscopy has not found a place in the general practice of cardiology. Most of the work with it has been done in Europe, especially France for the rigid instrument, and Germany and Yugoslavia for the flexible instrument. At this time, pericardioscopy is not a technique for use in most medical centres, but it would be desirable to develop centres in the U.S. at which there is a special expertise in myocardial and pericardial disease, to which large numbers of patients would be referred.

Pericardioscopy was first introduced in the U.S., not in Europe where it has been developed and practiced on a larger scale. Kondos, Rich, and Levitsky (1986) studied five patients. The instrument they used was a modified bronchoscope with associated camera and television. It was introduced using the same technique described above for the rigid pericardioscope. Bronchoscopes are designed for visualizing structures through air, not liquid. The pericardial effusion was therefore evacuated as completely as possible before carrying out the examinations.

In a recent study of 32 patients, the macroscopic appearance of lesions seen with the flexible pericardioscope was not very helpful, but the biopsies taken from them were informative (*Seferovic, Ristic, Maksimovic* 2000). These investigators compared blind biopsy with targeted biopsy. The number of samples taken was either 3 to 6 or 18 to 20. There was no difference in the results when the lower and higher numbers of samples were compared, but targeted biopsy increased the diagnostic yield from 43 percent to 86 percent.

A promising new application of pericardioscopy is the ability to obtain a greater number of samples. In addition, the fact that they are aimed at visualised lesions will provide more material for immunohistological studies, detecting viral infection by molecular techniques, and detecting pericardial malignancy by immunofluorescence.

4. TECHNIQUES FOR PERICARDIOCENTESIS

Variability in the details of how to perform pericardiocentesis is common and need not be discouraged. Individual operators have their preferences for equipment, site of puncture, where to perform the procedure, what sedative and local anaesthetic to use and for fluoroscopic or echocardiographic guidance. Pericardiocentesis is usually performed by cardiologists, surgeons (especially cardiac surgeons), emergency room physicians and, less commonly, interventional radiologists, all of whom are likely to have somewhat different preferences. Cardiologists who spend a lot of time in cardiac catheterisation laboratories often prefer fluoroscopic guidance, whereas intensive care cardiologists often opt for echocardiographic guidance. There is a lot to be said for having physicians work in the environment to which they are accustomed. These individual and local preferences should be kept in mind in relation to the descriptions that follow that are not meant to be more than general guidelines. Although fluoroscopic guidance has a longer history, I will first discuss pericardiocentesis using echocardiographic guidance, because of its increasing popularity (*Tsang and Seward 2001*).

4.1 Pericardiocentesis using echocardiographic guidance

The cardiovascular physicians at Mayo Clinic have maintained a great interest in pericardial disease for many years and have published a number of landmark papers on its diagnosis, physiology and treatment. Among these are numerous publications dealing with pericardiocentesis under echocardiographic guidance (*Tsang, Freeman, Sinak 1998*). The large number of procedures performed by this group, together with the large data base they have meticulously kept, approaches "evidence-based" data, something that is often lacking in diseases of the pericardium. The data are, however, retrospective. With this method, the effusion is imaged, and hemodynamic data can be easily acquired non-invasively (Figure 2).

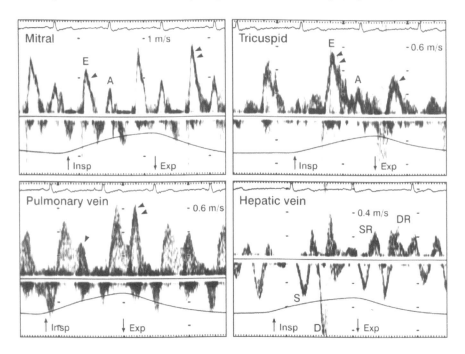

Figure 2. Doppler data in cardiac tamponade, showing increased respiratory variation in blood flow, and flow reversal in an hepatic vein Top left: left ventricular filling profile. Top right: right ventricular filling profile. Bottom left: inspiratory decrease in pulmonary venous flow. Bottom right: expiratory increase in hepatic flow reversal. (From Tsang, Oh, Seward, 1999, with permission)

The Mayo authors (*Tsang, Oh, Seward 1999*) and others (*Pandian, Brockway, Simonetti, 1988*) have employed this method in even more difficult clinical situations such as loculated effusion and acute tamponade complicating an invasive cardiac intervention. They believe that echocardiography is superior to fluoroscopy for monitoring pericardiocentesis, citing numerous advantages over subxiphoid puncture with fluoroscopic guidance. The advantages include ready availability and access to echocardiography in many sites, and the ability to find quickly where the effusion is largest and closest to the skin (*Tsang, Freeman,*

Barnes, 1998). With this information, the operator selects the most suitable point for the puncture and also visualises the optimal track, the required depth and the location of nearby vital structures to be avoided. The effusion is often maximal and most superficial in the region of the cardiac apex, not in the subxiphoid region. Puncture from this site is therefore easier and less traumatic. Agitated saline replaces iodine-based contrast agents used to verify proper placement of the needle (Figure 3). A probe mounted on the needle can be used to visualize it during pericardiocentesis (*Maggiolini, Bozzano, Russo, 2001*), but is considered unnecessary by many echocardiographers. Using echocardiography to guide the procedure, all that is needed for the puncture itself is a relatively short (5 to 8.5 cm long) "intracath" type of needle, gauge 18, or, for suspected thick effusion, 16. Once the needle tip enters the pericardium, the needle and sheath are advanced a further few mm, after which the needle is withdrawn. This technique greatly reduces the risk of laceration.

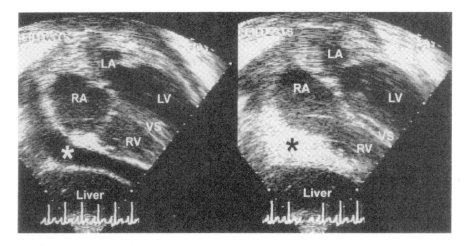

Figure 3. Echocardiographically-monitored pericardiocentesis. Agitated saline injection opacifies the effusion, confirming the appropriate position of the needle. **Left**: before injection. **Right**: after injection. * = pericardial cavity. (From Tsang, Freeman, Sinak, 1998, with permission)

4.2   Pericardiocentesis using the subxiphoid approach

The subcostal or subxiphoid route to the pericardium has been practiced for many years, either blindly or in conjunction with cardiac fluoroscopy. Marfan, better known for the syndrome that bears his name, introduced this means of reaching the pericardium in 1911 (*Marfan 1911*). It is still used quite extensively, in spite of the increasing popularity of echocardiographic guidance, in which the apical approach is much more frequently selected. Obesity or ascites present greater obstacle when the subxiphoid route is chosen. The needle track is longer and more muscle must be penetrated.

4.2.1   Technique

The skin is cleaned and prepared in the standard manner. After raising a skin bleb with a short 25-gauge needle, local anaesthesia is begun with 1-percent lidocaine and continued using a longer fine needle. Lidocaine is injected as the needle is advanced along the proposed pericardiocentesis track, described below. If the needle happens to penetrate the pericardium, a sample of the fluid should be removed and retained, after which the needle is removed.

To perform the definitive procedure, a small incision is made 3 to 5 mm to the left and below the tip of the xiphoid process and is widened and deepened with a small haemostat. The needle in the case of a slim patient need not be longer than the standard needle used for femoral puncture, and the bevel must be short. For the obese, the needle needs to be a few cm longer, but many lumbar puncture needles are too long and the use of a long needle invites inadvertent puncture of a vital structure. The needle is connected by a three-way stopcock to ports for pressure measurement and a 10 ml syringe for aspiration or administration of anaesthetic or contrast material. It is first directed in strictly posterior direction until it is deep in relation to the costal margin, after which the barrel of the syringe is pressed against the abdomen to direct the needle more anteriorly, while it is advanced in a cephalad direction, usually, but not necessarily, toward the left shoulder (Figure 4).

Intermittent gentle suction with the syringe is used while the needle is advanced. Often, a distinct pop or 'give' is felt when the needle pierces the pericardium. If clear or lightly blood stained fluid is obtained, the operator can be confident that the needle has entered the pericardial space, but if frankly bloody fluid is obtained, it is imperative to determine promptly and reliably whether it came from the pericardium or a cardiovascular structure. Several procedures are available for this important distinction. A turn of the stopcock allows instant display of the pressure. A ventricular pressure pulse can be recognized instantly and calls for withdrawal of the needle and careful hemodynamic monitoring. When an effusion is being tapped, but the patient does not have tamponade, pericardial pressure will be lower than atrial pressure, and the waveforms will differ. In the case of tamponade, pressures recorded from the pericardium or right atrium look the same. To make this critical distinction, a small amount of contrast agent is injected. If the needle is in the pericardial space, the contrast does not circulate, but collects in the most dependent portion. If the needle has penetrated a cardiac chamber, the contrast agent will be whisked away and disappear via the pulmonary arteries. Injection of contrast into the right ventricle to help to identify the anatomy has been suggested, but the publication has not gone beyond an abstract, so is not cited.

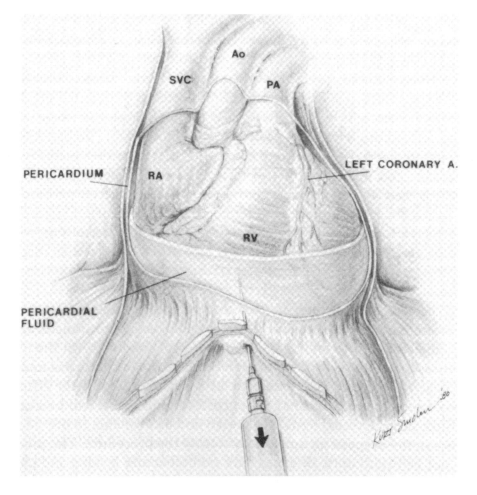

Figure 4. Subxiphoid approach to the pericardium

4.2.2   Electrogram as a monitor of the position of the needle

Another way to help to avoid myocardial puncture is to record the electrogram directly from the puncture needle (Figure 5). This technique is not applicable when the puncture is to be made with an intracath type of needle. Once the needle is under the skin, an insulated wire connects the needle to the V lead of an electrocardiograph. The resulting electrogram is displayed on the monitor along with a conventional limb lead. The ST segment of the electrocardiogram is isoelectric unless the needle contacts the epicardium. ST elevation is not prominent on a standard lead, but is dramatic on the electrogram, making it monophasic. Should this change be seen, the needle is withdrawn and a fresh attempt is made. The underlying theory is sound but, like the needle-mounted image probe suggested for echocardiographic guidance, in practice, most operators choose to avoid this extra encumbrance to the procedure. This type of monitoring should never be done if there is any doubt that all input circuits are isolated and that all the electrical grounds in the room are equipotential; otherwise there is danger to the patient of electrocution (*Stoner, Feldtman, Osborne 1978*).

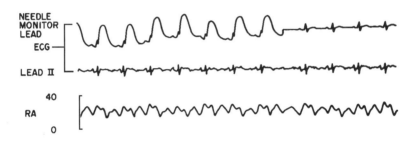

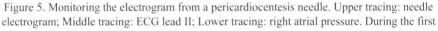

Figure 5. Monitoring the electrogram from a pericardiocentesis needle. Upper tracing: needle electrogram; Middle tracing: ECG lead II; Lower tracing: right atrial pressure. During the first 8 complexes, the needle touches the heart and the current of injury makes the complexes appear monophasic. Withdrawing the needle a few mm restores the ST segment to isoelectric. Right atrial pressure is 20 mmHg.

4.2.3   Blood or pericardial effusion

When bloody fluid first appears in the aspirating syringe, it may look suspiciously like whole blood. It is helpful to empty a few ml of the fluid onto a clean white sponge. A similar volume of blood can be emptied elsewhere on the sponge. The stain, even from very bloody effusion, is paler than that made by whole blood. If doubt persists, comparing the haematocrit of the pericardial aspirate with that of the blood provides a ready answer. In some situations, the source of whole blood may indeed be pericardial, for example in cases of trauma or rupture of the heart or an intrapericardial vessel. Clinical judgement should prevent the error of abandoning the pericardiocentesis when blood is aspirated when the needle is intrapericardial.

Another method that has been proposed is to inject indocyanine green into the pericardiocentesis needle and perform an indicator dilution curve with an ear oximeter (*Stone and Martin 1972*). If a curve is registered, the needle is intracardiac; if not, an intravenous injection is needed to ascertain that the system is working, before concluding that the needle is in the pericardium. This method is far-fetched and somewhat cumbersome and is seldom, if ever, used now. Chronic haemorrhagic pericardial fluid does not clot because of intrinsic fibrinolytic pericardial activity. This finding is often mentioned as a means to tell an intrapericardial from an intracardiac source of the blood (*Cheng 1973*). In acute pericardial bleeding, fibrinolysis does not take place; therefore the blood may clot. In pericardial fluid, pCO_2 is higher, and pO_2 and pH are lower than in arterial or venous blood. Although this method, using gas analysis, was suggested in the past (*Mann, Millen, Glauser, 1978*) and works; it is not often used any more.

4.2.4   Substitution of needle by catheter and hemodynamic evaluation

Once the needle tip is securely intrapericardial, a small sample of the fluid should be taken. If the case is one of tamponade, the sample volume should be no more than is necessary for laboratory examination, so as not to lower pericardial pressure before hemodynamics have been measured. Thereafter, the needle is replaced with a thin-walled catheter using the standard Seldinger method. The J-tipped guide-wire should be positioned at the level of the pulmonary artery in the posterior pericardium, which is the desired location for the catheter tip or pigtail. At this point, pericardial, right atrial, and pulmonary wedge pressures are recorded simultaneously at equal sensitivity, along with the systemic arterial pressure and the electrocardiogram. Cardiac output should then be determined. Aspiration of pericardial fluid, with collection of further samples of fluid for analysis if needed, proceeds until pericardial pressure is subatmospheric, at least during inspiration. At that point, hemodynamic evaluation is repeated. Finally, the catheter is attached to a vacuum bottle for continued drainage of fluid for several hours or days. Methods for preventing obstruction of the catheter have already been discussed. If the fluid becomes significantly bloodier during the procedure, it is desirable to check the patient's haematocrit and observe the clinical and hemodynamic status carefully.

4.2.4.1   Maintaining catheter patency

After completing pericardiocentesis using either guidance method, the catheter should remain in place until it drains less than 25-50 ml. daily, which often needs several days. If the catheter is allowed to drain continually, the lumen is apt to become plugged by fibrin. Drainage should therefore be intermittent.. Following each aspiration, or drainage, the catheter should be flushed with heparinised saline, after which it is filled with a fibrinolytic agent and sealed..

4.2.5   Relative merits of different approaches

The advantages of echocardiographic guidance and the consequent more frequent use of the apical site for puncture have been discussed above. The cardiac catheterisation laboratory is in many ways the ideal place for performing percardiocentesis, because hemodynamic data acquired there are, in general, more complete and more accurate. Also, if a cardiac lesion is discovered on fluoroscopy or echocardiography, it is likely that an interventional cardiologist can deal with it at the same time. Performing pericardiocentesis in the cardiac catheterisation laboratory by no means commits the operator to either fluoroscopic guidance or use of the traditional subxiphoid route. My preference is for pericardiocentesis in the catheterisation laboratory with echocardiographic monitoring and puncture from the site most accessible to the fluid.Laboratory study of pericardial fluid

4.2.6   Laboratory study of pericardial fluid

A good rule is to measure pericardial pressure and send fluid to the clinical laboratory virtually every time pericardiocentesis is done. At a minimum, the numbers of the contained blood cells, the content of proteins, lactic acid dehydrogenase and the specific gravity must be ascertained. The fluid should always be stained and cultured for the presence of organisms. The extent of investigation varies with the clinical assessment of likely aetiology. Tuberculosis is often a consideration. Anaerobes and fungi are sought in immunosuppressed patients and in those who have received prolonged treatment with potent antibiotics. Expert cytological evaluation, which is discussed under neoplastic diseases in Chapter 9, is critical. Adenosine deaminase is elevated in patients with tubercular infection of the pericardium; therefore, its activity in pericardial fluid and, when present, pleural fluid, should be measured routinely (*Burgess, Reuter, Taljaard 2002*). Polymerase chain reaction should be done if infection is under consideration, or to establish viral aetiology.

4.2.7   Alternative approaches

Occasionally the echocardiogram reveals that the effusion is not maximal or most superficial either para-apically or substernally. Alternatively, these areas may be infected, or made inaccessible by a dressing. The puncture can then be done parasternally, on either side. The internal mammary vessels are avoided by moving slightly lateral to the sternal edge. On the other hand, too lateral an approach increases the risk of pneumothorax. The safest location is the fourth intercostal space, which avoids the aortic arch and main pulmonary trunk, and half to one cm lateral to the sternal edge to avoid the pleura.

4.3 Pericardiotomy or pericardiocentesis?

When the first edition of this book was published, the mortality after pericardiocentesis, although decreasing, was still sufficient to give rise to the suggestion that subxiphoid pericardiotomy would be a safer and wiser option. In several places in his 1997 book on the pericardium, Spodick, well known for his work on pericardial disease, comes down strongly in favour of pericardiotomy (*Spodick 1997*). The sombre statement, *"It probably is not too much to add that any clinician who uses the blind method at all frequently can confidently expect, sooner or later, to tear an atrial or thin ventricular wall or to wound a coronary artery."* (*Kilpatrick and Chapman 1965*) no longer applies. Pericardiocentesis is no longer blind but is guided by echocardiography or fluoroscopy. Both procedures now are done with a similar low mortality. The incision needed for pericardiotomy is small, but after excision of the xiphoid process and downward retraction of the diaphragm, exposure of the pericardium is perfectly sufficient for drainage and removal of adequate tissue for microscopic examination.

Because of the poor sensitivity of pericardial biopsy when not performed in conjunction with a therapeutic procedure, it is usually done while performing pericardiotomy or sometimes pericardiectomy. Indeed the opportunity to add pericardial biopsy to pericardial drainage is cited as an argument against pericardiocentesis by clinicians who prefer surgical approaches to the pericardial fluid (*Allen, Faber, Warren 1999*). These authors performed subxiphoid pericardiotomy in 94 patients and pericardiocentesis in 23 considered too unstable for surgery. No mortality occurred in the surgical group, and only one complication, bleeding in a uremic patient with coagulopathy. The mortality from pericardiocentesis was 4 percent and the complication rate was 17 percent. Based on these findings, they advocated that pericardiocentesis be reserved for patients who are too unstable hemodynamically to undergo a surgical procedure. Most cardiologists, including myself, do not agree that a surgical approach to removing fluid from the pericardium should be the standard method.

Pericardioscopy in suitable cases is an attractive alternative, but is seldom a viable option in current U.S. practice. It can usually be performed under local anaesthesia with suitable sedation. As is the case after pericardiocentesis, pericardiotomy should be followed by drainage for several days. Here, I would point out that the popular term, pericardial window, is a misnomer. In reality, the operation induces fusion of the pericardium to the epicardium with obliteration of the pericardial space (*Sugimoto, Little, Ferguson, 1990).* The authors demonstrated the mechanism by echocardiography in 28 patients, in whom the operation was performed and followed until drainage became minimal. In 4 of the patients, they confirmed their findings at autopsy. Thus, it seems that there is little difference in the mode of action of pericardiotomy, instillation of sclerosing agents or prolonged catheter drainage. The procedure is not technically challenging and is as safe as pericardiocentesis. Trauma surgeons point out that pericardiotomy allows for inspection for associated cardiac injury (*Grewal, Ivatury, Divakar 1995*). Pericardioscopy can also be performed via laparoscopy (*Mann, Nguyen, Corbet 1994*)*.* Pericardiotomy can be performed using the thoracoscope (*Liu, Chang, Lin* 1994) instead of a laparoscope, but is more invasive and often requires general anaesthesia. Both these endoscopic techniques allow adequate biopsy of visualised lesions, but most surgeons prefer simple pericardiotomy without special instrumentation.

There is no "right answer" to the question of whether to drain the pericardium by pericardiocentesis or pericardiotomy, since both are safe and simple. The decision depends upon the clinical features of the case, the preferences of patient and doctor, the local expertise and customary approach.

5.   BALLOON PERICARDIOT0MY

Pericardiotomy can be achieved by pericardial catheterisation and creating a pericardial tear by means of balloon dilation. The first report described the procedure performed on eight patients with malignant pericardial effusion. (*Palacios, Tuzcu, Ziskind 1991*) and was followed by a larger series and the creation of a registry (*Ziskind, Pearce, Lemmon 1993*). This method has been used primarily for patients with malignant pericardial effusion because, with either pericardiocentesis or surgical pericardiotomy, the results had been disappointing. In the report of Ziskind et al., balloon pericardiotomy was either primary therapy, provided at the time of pericardiocentesis, or secondary, when copious drainage persisted after pericardiocentesis.

5.1   Technique

After standard catheterisation of the pericardium from the subxiphoid region and removal of most of the effusion, the pericardial cavity was opacified with 20 ml of 50 percent radiographic contrast material. A balloon 20 cm wide, 3 cm long, containing 35 percent strength of contrast was advanced until it straddled the edge of the pericardium. The balloon was inflated and withdrawn, after which successful pericardiotomy was confirmed by free flow of contrast from the pericardium to the pleura (or sometimes the peritoneum) during pericardial injection (Figure 6).

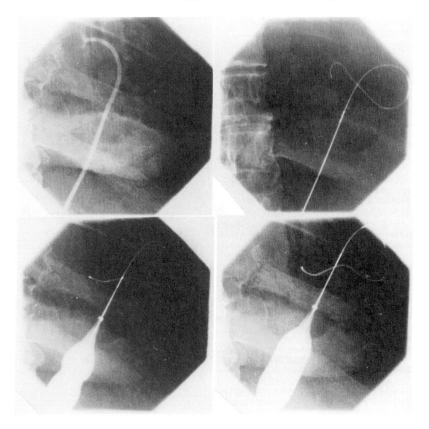

Figure 6. Balloon pericardiotomy. **Top left:** A pigtail catheter has been placed in the pericardium. **Top right:** a guide wire has been advanced beyond the tip of the catheter. **Below left:** The balloon has been partly inflated to visualise the waist to indicate the position of the parietal pericardium. **Below right:** The fully inflated balloon is shown immediately after creating the pericardiotomy. (From Palacios, Tuzcu, Ziskind, 1991, with permission)

Balloon pericardiotomy performed on 19 cadavers using the Inoue balloon created a pericardiotomy with dimensions of only 19x16 mm, with surrounding inflammation and with traumatised collagen and elastin fibers (*Chow and Chow, 1993*). A "window" of that size and in that milieu could hardly be expected to remain open for long. It is much more plausible that balloon pericardiotomy prevents recurrence of pericardial effusion by the same mechanisms as any other method of pericardiotomy, or for that matter of pericardial drainage. Injection of methylene blue into the pericardium after balloon pericardiotomy failed to stain the patient's co-existing pleural effusion (*Bertrand, Legrand, Kulbertus 1996*).

The above procedure was successful in 46 of 50 patients. Pleural effusion, caused by or added to by transfer of fluid from the pericardium to the pleura, occurred in eight patients, in six of whom it was drained by a chest tube. Two small peumothoraces occurred. A number of variations from the original technique have been described, including use of the Inoue balloon (*Chow, Chow, Yip 1996*) or double balloons (*Iaffaldano, Jones, Lewis 1995*). Although fluoroscopic guidance is usually employed, the procedure can be done with echocardiographic control (*Vora, Lokhandwala, Kale, 1992*).

Balloon pericardiotomy is a viable option for treating pericardial effusion, especially in cases of neoplastic effusion in which the least invasive methods are often appropriate. It has, however, also been used, but less commonly, in cases of nonmalignant pericardial effusion (*Thanopoulos, Georgakopoulos, Tsaousis* 1997), and for relief of cardiac tamponade (*Di Segni, Lavee, Kaplinsky 1995*).

This technique, has not, however, been embraced as enthusiastically by the cardiology community as may have been anticipated, but is done, and likely will continue to be done, in centres with an interest in it which have developed an experience and skill in its performance. Contrast agents injected into the pericardium can be quite painful, even when dilute, and pericardiostomy itself is also painful. Skilful surgeons can perform subxiphoid pericardiostomy in the same or less time than a good interventional cardiologist takes to make the pericardiostomy with a balloon. Thus, as with other options for draining the pericardium, much depends on local expertise, preferences and customs.

5.2   The PerDUCER

The perDUCER is an instrument that was devised to invade the pericardium percutaneously in cases in which pericardial effusion is not present (*Maisch, Ristic, Rupp 2001*). The device includes a channel through which the pericardium can be visualised before the puncture is made, an important asset when the pericardial space contains only a physiological amount of fluid. While it has been used in patients with pericardial effusion, this application was for the purpose of training the operators to access a dry pericardial space and is not at present an approved device for clinical use.

6.   COMPLICATIONS

6.1   Technical

Most of the complications that are related to either error in performing pericardiocentesis or are a known risk of the procedure have been mentioned in the discussion of technique. These include puncture or laceration of the heart or a coronary vessel, pneumothorax, and failure to enter the pericardium. Laceration is more likely than puncture to lead to significant bleeding and the need for prompt intervention. Puncture of a ventricle often is not followed by haemorrhage needing treatment. In addition, bleeding from inadvertent puncture of the right ventricle may be followed by formation of an intrapericardial thrombus (*Preis, Taylor, Martin 1982; Schuster and Nanda 1982*). Pneumothorax often is small and self-limiting. A large pneumothorax is treated in the standard manner with a chest tube. Arrhythmia, when it occurs, is almost never serious, although ventricular fibrillation has been reported. Even the stomach and colon have been punctured.

6.2   Pathophysiological

Disturbance of cardiac function, consequent on evacuating a pericardial effusion, is a rare but well-documented complication of pericardiocentesis and pericardiotomy (*Hamaya, Dohi, Ueda, 1993*). I have not encountered this complication either during clinical pericardiocentesis or when performing studies on experimental models of tamponade, but it is well for physicians performing pericardiocentesis to be aware that acute left ventricular failure may supervene, especially in cases where tamponade is superimposed on pre-existing myocarditis or cardiomyopathy (*Uemura, Kagoshima, Hashimoto 1995*). A suggested mechanism is that the failing left ventricle, already facing increased afterload, cannot respond physiologically to the increase in venous return that follows decompression of the right ventricle. It has been suggested that in patients with myocardial dysfunction, fluid should be removed slowly. More important, the right heart catheter and arterial cannula should be left in place and the patient should be closely monitored in the coronary care unit, where inotropic support can be given, and other measures for the management of acute left ventricular failure are readily available. Counterpulsation should be considered if the patient does not respond to these measures. However, even severe left ventricular dysfunction after pericardiocentesis may be transient (*Wolfe and Edelman 1993*). The case of a patient with myocarditis but absent ventricular dilation suggests that, in acute heart failure, the pericardium, in addition to adversely raising ventricular diastolic pressure, may support the heart by preventing excessive increase in volume (*Timmis, Daly, Monaghan 1983*). It is possible that some cases of acute left ventricular failure may, in the future, be treated by the provision of a cardiac support device (see Chapter 2).

An instructive case was that of a patient who underwent pericardiocentesis for severe cardiac tamponade, in whom tamponade recurred over the ensuing 12 hours and was treated by subxiphoid pericardiotomy, after which pulmonary oedema occurred for the second time. The tamponade was due to malignancy and the patient was considered to have hypertensive cardiomyopathy (*Vandyke, Cure, Chakko 1983*). A year later, a report of pulmonary oedema following subxiphoid pericardiotomy was published (*Shenoy, Dhar, Gittin 1984*).

Pericardiocentesis may also be followed by acute right ventricular failure (*Eyskens, Lawrenson, Moerman 1998*). The primary condition in the patient they reported was mediastinal lymphoma. The patient died almost immediately after pericardiocentesis had improved his condition. Autopsy showed that the tumour invaded the pericardium and epicardium and extended round the superior vena cava aortic arch and main pulmonary artery with compression of the proximal right coronary artery. The authors hypothesised that removal of the fluid had allowed the tumour to compress the coronary artery causing acute right ventricular failure. Acute idiopathic right ventricular dilation has also been reported as an unexpected complication of pericardiocentesis (*Armstrong, Feigenbaum, Dillon 1984*). Another and commoner situation in which tamponade may be protective is rupture of a dissecting haematoma of the ascending aorta. Pericardiocentesis must be avoided if at all possible, but, when clinical judgement dictates that it is essential, as soon as clinical improvement results, aspiration should be halted and resumed, again cautiously, if deterioration recurs before the patient can undergo sternotomy.

References

Allen KB, Faber LP, Warren WH, Shaar CJ. Pericardial effusion: subxiphoid pericardiostomy versus percutaneous catheter drainage. Ann Thorac Surg. 1999; 67:437-440

Armstrong WF, Feigenbaum H, Dillon JC. Acute right ventricular dilation and echocardiographic volume overload following pericardiocentesis for relief of cardiac tamponade. Am Heart J 1984; 107:1266-1 270.

Bertrand O, Legrand V, Kulbertus H. Percutaneous balloon pericardiotomy: a case report and analysis of mechanism of action. Cathet Cardiovasc Diagn 1996; 38:180-182

Burgess LJ, Reuter H, Taljaard JJ, Doubell AF. Role of biochemical tests in the diagnosis of large pericardial effusions. Chest 2002; 121:495-499.

Cheng TO.Ventricle or pericardial space? Ann Intern Med 1973; 78:461.

Chow LT, Chow WH. Mechanism of pericardial window creation by balloon pericardiotomy. Am J Cardiol 1993; 72:1321-1322.

Chow WH, Chow TC, Yip AS, Cheung KL. Inoue balloon pericardiotomy for patients with recurrent pericardial effusion. Angiology. 1996; 47:57-60.

Di Segni E, Lavee J, Kaplinsky E, Vered Z. Percutaneous balloon pericardiostomy for treatment of cardiac tamponade. Eur Heart J 1995; 16:184-187

Duvernoy O, Borowiec J, Helmius G, Erikson U. Complications of percutaneous pericardiocentesis under fluoroscopic guidance. Acta Radiol 1992; 33:309-313.

Eyskens B, Lawrenson J, Moerman P, Brock P, Doumoulin M, et al. Brief report. Sudden death following removal of pericardial fluid in a child presenting with mediastinal lymphoma. Med Pediatr Oncol 1998; 31:547-548.

Grewal H, Ivatury RR, Divakar M, Simon RJ, Rohman M. Evaluation of subxiphoid pericardial window used in the detection of occult cardiac injury. Injury. 1995; 26:305-310.

Hamaya Y, Dohi S, Ueda N, Akamatsu S. Severe circulatory collapse immediately after pericardiocentesis in a patient with chronic cardiac tamponade. Anesth Analg 1993; 77:1278-1281.

Iaffaldano RA, Jones P, Lewis BE, Eleftheriades EG, Johnson SA, et al. Percutaneous balloon pericardiotomy: a double-balloon technique. Cathet Cardiovasc Diagn 1995; 36:79-81.

Kilpatrick ZM, Chapman CB. On pericardiocentesis. Am J Cardiol. 1965;16:722-728.

Kondos GT, Rich S, Levitsky S. Flexible fiberoptic pericardioscopy. Chest 1986; 90:787-788.

Liu HP, Chang CH, Lin PJ, Hsieh HC, Chang JP, et al. Thoracoscopic management of effusive pericardial disease: indications and technique. Ann Thorac Surg 1994; 58:1695-1697.

Maggiolini S, Bozzano A, Russo P, Vitale G, Osculati G, et al. Echocardiography-guided pericardiocentesis with probe-mounted needle: report of 53 cases. J Am Soc Echocardiogr 2001; 14:821-824.

Maisch B, Bethge C, Drude L, Hufnagel G, Herzum M, et al. Pericardioscopy and epicardial biopsy--new diagnostic tools in pericardial and perimyocardial disease. Eur Heart J 1994; 15(Supplement C): 68-73.

Maisch B, Ristic AD. The classification of pericardial disease in the age of modern medicine. Curr Cardiol Rep 2002; 4:13-21.

Maisch B, Ristic AD, Rupp H, Spodick DH. Pericardial access using the perDUCER and flexible percutaneous pericardioscopy. Am J Cardiol 2001; 88:1323-1326.

Mann GB, Nguyen H, Corbet J. Laparoscopic creation of pericardial window. Aust N Z J Surg 1994; 64:853-855.

Mann W, Millen JE, Glauser FL. Bloody pericardial fluid. The value of blood gas measurements. JAMA 1978; 239:2151-2152.

Marfan AB. Ponction du pericarde par l'epigastre. Ann de med et chir inf 1911; 15:529-533.

Nugue O, Millaire A, Porte H, de Groote P, Guimier P, et al. Pericardioscopy in the etiologic diagnosis of pericardial effusion in 141 consecutive patients. Circulation 1996; 94:1635-41

Palacios IF, Tuzcu EM, Ziskind AA, Younger J, Block PC. Percutaneous balloon pericardial window for patients with malignant pericardial effusion and tamponade. Cathet Cardiovasc Diagn 1991; 22:244-249.

Pandian NG, Brockway B, Simonetti J, Rosenfield K, Bojar R, et al. Pericardiocentesis under two-dimensional echocardiographic guidance in loculated pericardial effusion. Ann Thorac Surg 1988; 45:99-100.

Permanyer-Miralda G, Sagrista-Sauleda J, Soler-Soler J. Primary acute pericardial disease: a prospective series of 231 consecutive patients. Am J Cardiol 1985; 56:623-630.

Preis LK, Taylor GJ, Martin RP. Traumatic pericardiocentesis: two-dimensional echocardiographic visualization of an unfortunate event. Arch Intern Med 1982; 142:2327-2329

Schuster AH, Nanda NC. Pericardiocentesis induced intrapericardial thrombus: detection by two-dimensional echocardiography. Am Heart J 1982; 104:308-311.

Seferovic PM, Ristic AD, Maksimovic R, Ostojic M, Simeunovic D, et al. Flexible percutaneous pericardioscopy: inherent drawbacks and recent advances. Herz. 2000; 25:741-747.

Shenoy MM, Dhar S, Gittin R, Sinha AK, Sabado M. Pulmonary edema following pericardiotomy for cardiac tamponade. Chest. 1984; 86: 647-648.

Soler-Soler J, Permanyer-Miralda G, Sagrista-Sauleda J. A systematic diagnostic approach to primary acute pericardial disease. The Barcelona experience. Cardiol Clin 1990; 8:609-620

Spodick DH. The Pericardium. A comprehensive textbook. New York, Marcel Dekker, Inc, 1997

Stone JR, Martin RH. Bloody pericardial fluid or intracardiac blood? A method for quick and accurate differentiation. Ann Intern Med 1972; 77:592-594

Stoner DL, Feldtman RW, Osborne D, Julian RG, Yoo JH. An alternative approach to hospital electrical safety. J Clin Eng 1978; 3:179-182

Sugimoto JT, Little AG, Ferguson MK, Borow KM, Vallera D, et al. Pericardial window: mechanisms of efficacy. Ann Thorac Surg 1990; 50:442-445

Thanopoulos BD, Georgakopoulos D, Tsaousis GS, Triposkiadis F, Paphitis CA. Percutaneous balloon pericardiotomy for the treatment of large, nonmalignant pericardial effusions in children: immediate and medium-term results. Cathet Cardiovasc Diagn. 1997; 40:97-100

Timmis AD, Daly K, Monaghan M, Jewitt DE. Pericardiocentesis in myocarditis: the protective role of the pericardium in severe heart failure. Br Med J (Clin Res Ed) 1983; 287:1348.

Tsang TS, Freeman WK, Barnes ME, Reeder GS, Packer DL, et al. Rescue echocardiographically guided pericardiocentesis for cardiac perforation complicating catheter-based procedures. The Mayo Clinic experience. J Am Coll Cardiol 1998; 32:1345-1350.

Tsang TS, Freeman WK, Sinak LJ, Seward JB. Echocardiographically guided pericardiocentesis: evolution and state-of-the-art technique. Mayo Clin Proc. 1998; 73:647-652.

Tsang TS, Oh JK, Seward JB. Diagnosis and management of cardiac tamponade in the era of echocardiography. Clin Cardiol. 1999; 22:446-452.

Tsang TS, Seward JB. Pericardiocentesis under echocardiographic guidance. Eur J Echocardiogr 2001; 2:68

Uemura S, Kagoshima T, Hashimoto T, Sakaguchi Y, Doi N, et al. Acute left ventricular failure with pulmonary edema following pericardiocentesis for cardiac tamponade--a case report. Jpn Circ J 1995; 59:55-59.

Vandyke WH Jr, Cure J, Chakko CS, Gheorghiade M. Pulmonary edema after pericardiocentesis for cardiac tamponade. N Engl J Med 1983; 309:595-596.

Vora AM, Lokhandwala YY, Kale PA. Echocardiography guided creation of balloon pericardial window. Cathet Cardiovasc Diagn 1992; 25:164-165.

West S. Purulent pericarditis treated by paracentesis and free incision, with recovery. Br Med J 1883; 1:814.

Wolfe MW, Edelman ER. Transient systolic dysfunction after relief of cardiac tamponade. Ann Intern Med 1993; 119:42-44.

Ziskind AA, Pearce AC, Lemmon CC, Burstein S, Gimple LW, et al. Percutaneous balloon pericardiotomy for the treatment of cardiac tamponade and large pericardial effusions: description of technique and report of the first 50 cases. J Am Coll Cardiol 1993; 21:1-5.

Chapter 6

CONSTRICTIVE PERICARDITIS
Hemodynamic comparisons with tamponade and restrictive cardiomyopathy

1.   HISTORICAL BACKGROUND

Dr. Hope observed that he had never examined a case after death, a case of complete adhesion of the pericardium without finding enlargement of the heart, generally hypertrophy with dilation...With deference to this high authority, I must venture to suggest that the above remarks can be applied only to one class of cases of this description - to those in which, superadded to the adhesion of the pericardial surfaces, there is also disease of the valvular passages of the heart...a sufficient number of contrary cases have occurred under my own notice, to prove that, where the valves are healthy, complete and close adhesion of the pericardial surfaces, so far from producing hypertrophy and dilatation, has a tendency to be followed by general diminution in the size of the heart and its vessels, and contraction of its cavities (Norman Chevers 1842).

Like Lower 173 years before, Chevers fully appreciated that constrictive pericarditis is a disease of diastole. His description in Guy's Hospital reports of the clinical course and autopsy findings in six cases is one of the classics of medical literature (Chevers 1842).

2. DEFINITION

Constrictive pericarditis is a condition in which a pathological lesion has obliterated the pericardial cavity, eliminating pericardial fluid. The fused parietal layers are usually greatly thickened, and invariably pericardial compliance is impaired and finally lost altogether. Less commonly, the parietal pericardium is spared; constriction is exerted by the visceral pericardium alone, in which case increased thickness of the pericardium is absent. Common causes are neoplasm, scarring that follows inflammation, and collagen vascular diseases. Which of the major causes is the most prevalent is strongly influenced by demography and selection bias. Radiation damage is a leading cause in centres treating large numbers of patients for Hodgkin's lymphoma, and this was particularly so before the introduction of modern shielding and refinements of the radiation delivery system. Series published by cancer centres naturally are dominated by neoplastic pericardial disease, whereas tuberculous pericarditis is the leading cause in India. These biases should be kept in mind when reviewing published series. The most probable aetiology of pericarditis seen by practitioners obviously depends on the speciality they practice.

3. PATHOLOGY

A recent review reported the gross and microscopic pathology of 361 specimens obtained during pericardiectomy between 1993 and 1999. The operation was performed for constrictive pericarditis in 143 of the cases in which fibrosis was found in 96 percent, but calcification in only 35 percent. Pericardial thickness ranged from 1 mm to 1.7 cm with regional thickness up to 1.9 cm. Chronic lymphocytic inflammation was seen in 73 percent. Importantly, in 4 percent, pericardial thickness was normal and fibrosis, inflammation, and calcification were absent (*Oh, Shimizu, Edwards 2001*). This last finding explains some of the difficulties encountered in making the diagnosis clinically. The prevalence of calcification has decreased in recent decades but still retains significance for diagnosis and in pericardiectomy (*Ling, Oh, Breen 2000*).

4. AETIOLOGY, AN EVOLVING SPECTRUM

Pericarditis of almost any cause may lead to constrictive pericarditis. In earlier series, the leading cause was tuberculosis (*Andrews, Pickering,*

Sellors 1948). Some forty years later, the aetiology of constrictive pericarditis in 95 consecutive patients treated by pericardiectomy at Stanford was idiopathic in 40, a complication of mediastinal radiation in 29, and of cardiac surgery in 10. The series did not include a single case of tuberculous constrictive pericarditis (*Cameron, Oesterle, Baldwin 1987*). A similar distribution of aetiology was observed in a cohort of 90 patients who had undergone pericardiectomy for constrictive pericarditis in Boston (*Spodick 1987*). These reports prompted a comparison of 135 patients who were operated on for constrictive pericarditis during the last decade of the 20th Century with 231 patients whose pericardiectomy was done in the era 1936 through 1982. The final diagnosis was idiopathic in only 33 percent of the later series as against 73 percent in the earlier series, a result different from the series reported by Cameron et al. The patients were older in the later series. The commonest cause was cardiac surgery (18%), followed by "pericarditis" (16%) and mediastinal radiation (13%). The aetiology was tuberculosis in only one patient. The changes in aetiology were associated with decreased survival and more disappointing outcome in spite of decreased operative mortality (*Ling, Oh, Schaff 1999*).

4.1   Neoplasia

Other important causes include neoplasm, the chief offenders, but by no means the only ones, being breast and lung cancer. Hodgkins disease and other lymphomas are less common causes, but still fairly frequent. Primary pericardial neoplasms such as mesothelioma are much less common, but also usually manifest as constriction (Figure 1). It is not always easy, or even possible to be certain when constriction is caused by a neoplasm, or its treatment with radiation or, less commonly, sclerotherapy.

4.2   Trauma

Prior trauma has emerged as an important cause. The trauma may have been blunt, commonly a steering wheel injury (Figure 2), or penetrating, for example, stab wounds, bullets, impalement or even self-inflicted wounds (*Keogh, Oakley, Taylor 1988*). Trauma may result in an organized haematoma causing localized constriction (*Brown and Ivey 1996*) and sometimes may simulate a tumour. Significant pericardial injury can occur but is uncommon after vigorous closed chest cardiac massage. When it has occurred, it has taken the form of bloody pericardial effusion; a rare sequel to this effusion is constrictive pericarditis (*Khan, Noah, Al-Saddique 1988*).

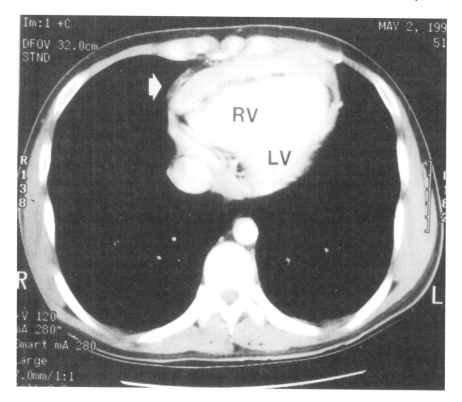

Figure 1: Computer assisted tomogram of constrictive pericardial disease due to
mesothelioma. Until tissue had been obtained during pericardiectomy, the patient was thought
to have tuberculous pericarditis. The pericardium was greatly thickened.

4.3   Complication of cardiac surgery or interventional procedure

Cardiac surgery has emerged as an important cause of constrictive
pericarditis (*Kutcher, King, Alimurung 1982*). Although this complication is
reported in only 0.1 to 0.3 cardiac operations, the large number of cardiac
operations performed annually translates into a large annual incidence of
constrictive pericarditis. It is important, therefore, to suspect postoperative
constrictive pericarditis in cases with unexplained hemodynamic
deterioration soon or, less commonly, long after a cardiac operation.
Extensive adhesions, a well-known bane of surgeons performing a
subsequent cardiac operation, are far more common than constriction.
Constrictive pericarditis has been reported in association with patch
electrodes for automatic defibrillation (*Almassi, Chapman, Troup 1987*). If
the oesophagus is perforated in the course of sclerotherapy for varicose

veins, acute pericarditis results and may be followed by constrictive pericarditis (*Brown and Luchi 1987*).

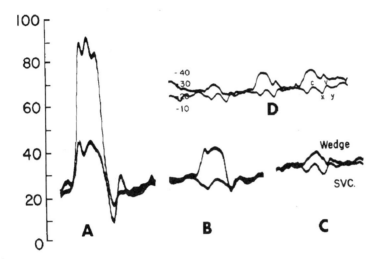

Figure 2: Cardiac catheterisation pressure recordings from a stock car driver who had sustained a major injury two years previously **A:** left and right ventricles **B:** right atrium and right ventricle showing prominent x and y descents. **C:** pulmonary wedge (upper trace) and superior vena cava. **D:** pulmonary artery and right atrium. The findings are characteristic of constriction. (From Shabetai and Grossman 1980, with permission*)*

Cardiac tamponade is much more common than constriction as a complication of cardiac surgery. It should be recalled, however, that when a significant pericardial effusion, especially haemorrhagic, develops after cardiac surgery, the course may go on to constrictive pericarditis.

4.4   Infection

Infection is now a less common cause of constrictive pericarditis, but the occasional case associated with empyema is still encountered. Staphylococcus or pneumococcus would then be likely culprits, but constrictive pericarditis may follow infection with any living organism. Tuberculosis must still be kept in mind, especially in underprivileged persons and recent immigrants from countries where the prevalence of tuberculosis is high. Histoplasmosis, especially in the Ohio valley region, and coccidiomycosis in the Western United States are fungal infections that mimic tuberculous constrictive pericarditis. *Candida albicans* may be the responsible fungus in patients who have been treated with large doses of potent antibiotics and when the immune system has been compromised by immunosuppressive therapy or AIDS. Acute viral infection seldom leads to constrictive pericarditis and usually is transient. Although rare, even *Nocardia asteroids* may invade the pericardium and cause constrictive pericarditis (*Kessler, Follis, Daube 1991*), as shown in Figure 3.

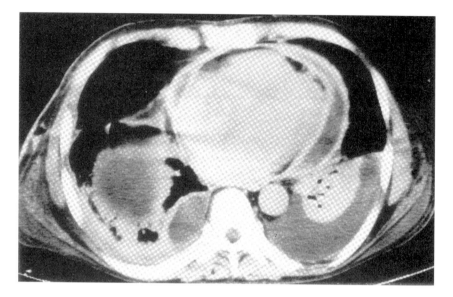

Figure 3: Contrast enhanced computed tomogram showing thick pericardium and pericardial effusion in a case of nocardial infection. (From Kessler, Follis, Daube 1991, with permission*)*

4.5   Collagen vascular disease

Almost all of the collagen vascular diseases may be complicated by constrictive pericarditis (*Cooper, Cleland, Bentall, 1978*) but chief among them are rheumatoid arthritis, lupus erythematosus, progressive systemic sclerosis and the CREST syndrome (*Panchal, Adams, Hsieh, 1996*). Rheumatoid arthritis is perhaps the commonest of these troublesome conditions to develop constrictive pericarditis (*McRorie, Wright, Errington, 1997*). Constrictive pericarditis has also been documented in dermatomyositis (*Tamir, Pic, Theodor 1988*). The series reported by Cooper et al. included lupus erythematosus.

4.6   Cardiac transplantation

Evidence for restriction or constriction is quite common after cardiac transplantation. The usual pathology is myocardial, but the lesion may be both pericardial and myocardial, or occasionally only or mainly pericardial

(*Hinkamp, Sullivan, Montoya 1994*). These authors described four patients treated by pericardiectomy, three without the benefit of improvement.

4.7   Other less common causes

A number of other associations of constrictive pericarditis and other diseases are known, but frequently the mechanism is not known. I will discuss cardiac amyloidosis in detail further on in this chapter in the discussion of restrictive cardiomyopathy; here, suffice it to mention that calcific constrictive pericarditis has been described in amiloidosis. The calcification was found within the amyloid deposits present in the thickened pericardium (*Hou 1983*). Asbestosis in which calcified pleural plaques are a long recognized feature may also be a cause of constrictive pericarditis (*Davies, Andrews, Jones 1991*). A patient with a long history of recurrent pericardial effusion due to cholesterol pericarditis eventually developed calcific constrictive pericarditis (*Stanley, Subramanian, Lie, 1980*). Constrictive pericarditis is an uncommon late manifestation of the hypereosinophilic syndrome (*Lui and Makoui 1988*). Whipple's disease is another multi-system disease that may eventuate with constrictive pericarditis (*Crake, Sandle, Crisp 1983*). Clinicians are all too familiar with cardiac tamponade in uremic pericarditis and, more relevant to the current era, in patients receiving haemodialysis. With improved survival, constrictive pericarditis has emerged as a late complication in these patients (*Ptacin 1983*). The increased thickness and calcification of the pericardium may be pronounced in the syndrome of retroperitoneal and mediastinal fibrosis (*Hanley, Shub, Lie 1984*), as illustrated by Figure 4.

Right ventricular infarction may simulate the hemodynamics of constrictive pericarditis when acute right ventricular dilation forces the heart against the pericardium which, except in some post-surgical cases, is normal (*Lorell, Leinbach, Pohost 1979*). Dressler's syndrome rarely leads to constrictive pericarditis. Constrictive pericarditis may also be found in association with secundum type atrial septal defect. The reason for this association is unknown (*Albers, Hugenholtz, Nadas, 1969*). Mulibrey nanism belongs in the category of unusual causes of constrictive pericarditis. Nanism is dwarfism, and mulibrey is an acronym for muscle-liver-brain-eye, the principal organs affected by this autosomal recessive disorder found mainly in Finland. Almost all the cases reported had pericardial constriction. Other features include yellow dots on the optic fundi, fibrous dysplasia of long bones, and abnormal shape of the skull and sella turica.

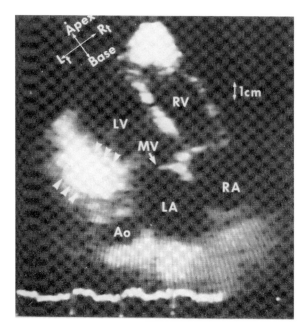

Figure 4: A 2 cm bright echodensity on the posterolateral wall of the left ventricle in a case of retroperitoneal and mediastinal fibrosis with pericardial constriction. (*From Hanley, Shub, Lie 1984, with permission*)

5.   PATHOPHYSIOLOGY

The pathophysiology of constrictive pericarditis readily explains the findings on clinical examination, echo-Doppler cardiography, and cardiac catheterisation. The pathophysiology of cardiac tamponade has important components in common with constriction, but equally important are the ways in which the two differ. Similarly, the pathophysiology of constrictive pericarditis and restrictive cardiomyopathy share many important features, but the features that differ between the two are the underlying basis of tests performed to distinguish one from the other. One cannot overemphasise the importance of a clear understanding of the pathophysiology of these three disorders of the heart and circulation. Another feature of constrictive pericarditis is that, because the pericardial space ceases to exist, pericardial pressure is unequivocally a contact pressure but, under the circumstances, it cannot be measured. Furthermore, once the pericardial space is obliterated, respiratory variation in thoracic pressure is no longer transmitted to the cardiac chambers and great vessels.

5.1   Ventricular systolic function

The combination of elevated ventricular diastolic pressure and reduced stroke volume are the major hemodynamic abnormalities in both heart failure and constrictive pericarditis, but the mechanism is quite different. In heart failure, myocardial contractility is impaired, whereas, in constrictive pericarditis, myocardial contractility is preserved and the ejection fraction is normal. Poor pump function is the direct consequence of absence of the Frank-Starling mechanism in ventricles that do not increase in volume after early rapid filling ceases. The fixed preload provides an opportunity to evaluate the force-frequency relation in a clinical environment of unchanging preload. Figure 5 shows a normal response of peak dP/dt and V_{max} when the pre-preceding interval is short (*Gaasch, Peterson, Shabetai 1974*).

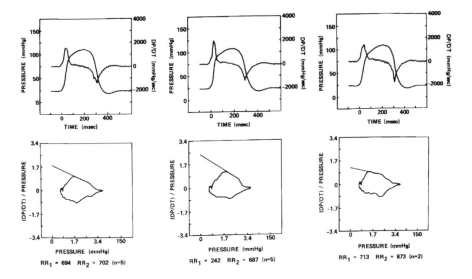

Figure 5: Plot of left ventricular pressure and dP/dt (**top**) and (dP/dt)/kP vs. total pressure (**below**). RR_1= pre-preceding R-R interval; R-R_2 preceding R-R interval. The shorter R-R_1 is associated with an increase in peak d/P/dt and Vmax. (*Gaasch, Peterson, Shabetai 1974, with permission*)

5.2   Increased ventricular interdependence

In constrictive pericarditis, the total volume of the heart is constant, being set by the non-compliant pericardium; if one chamber gets bigger, another must get smaller, that is, ventricular interdependence is far stronger than normal. In this respect, tamponade and constriction are alike. The pulmonary veins, being intrathoracic structures, are subject to respiratory variation in pressure. With inspiration, pulmonary venous pressure drops, but left ventricular diastolic pressure does not. The inevitable consequence is that the pressure gradient responsible for left ventricular diastolic pressure is reduced and ventricular diastolic volume is necessarily diminished. The terminal portions of the venae cavae and the right atrium are intrapericardial structures, and thus, like the left ventricle, do not "see" the inspiratory drop in intrathoracic pressure. Systemic venous return does not, therefore, increase, as it would have in normal subjects and patients with cardiac tamponade. Because ventricular interaction is so strong, the smaller left ventricle allows the right heart chambers to increase their volume via leftward shift of their septa.

5.2.1   Ventricular filling

An important feature of increased ventricular interdependence is markedly increased respiratory variation in ventricular filling. In clinical echo-Doppler cardiography, increased respiratory variation is measured as respiratory change in peak early rapid filling rate. Transmitral peak velocity diminishes significantly more than in normal subjects, while transtricuspid peak velocity increases to an abnormally great extent. The increased respiratory variation, opposite in direction on the two sides of the heart, is reliable evidence of abnormal ventricular interdependence. Stroke volume can be derived by multiplying the velocity-time integral of the whole velocity signal (E and A waves) by the area of the valve. This calculation of respiratory variation in stroke volume of similar magnitude to that of peak velocity confirms animal work in which stroke volume was measured directly with flow meters (*Shabetai, Fowler, Fenton,*1965). In cardiac tamponade, ventricular interaction is also very strong; therefore, the same exaggerated respiratory variation of ventricular inflow is found.

5.2.2   Ventricular diastolic pressure and volume profiles

Constrictive pericarditis constricts the heart only during the late phases of diastole. At end-systole the cardiac volume is minimal; therefore, the pericardium, although scarred and rigid, does not compress the heart. Early rapid filling is even more rapid than normal because elastic recoil of the ventricle is increased. The hemodynamic evidence for this pathophysiology is the early diastolic dip of ventricular pressure and the steep initial portion of the slope of ventricular filling. Rapid ventricular filling continues until further expansion of ventricular volume is abruptly halted by the noncompliant pericardium. From this time to the end of diastole, little or no filling of the ventricle can take place, as cardiac volume is then limited by the unyielding pericardium (Figure 6). The figure illustrates that, in a normal ventricular volume-time curve, early rapid filling, diastasis, and filling by atrial contraction can be easily distinguished. In the curve from a patient with constrictive pericarditis, early filling is more rapid than normal and diastasis lasts from the end of early rapid filling to end-diastole. The consequence of inability of the ventricular myocardium to stretch as diastole continues is that the Frank-Starling mechanism cannot operate. This means that the ventricular dysfunction is not due to impaired contractility, but to absence of the Frank-Starling response. In the more severe cases, the small end diastolic volume is another contributing factor (*Gaasch, Peterson, Shabetai 1974*). The early diastolic dip of ventricular diastolic pressure, followed by a longer plateau, together constitute the well known dip and plateau or square root sign of constrictive pericarditis and restrictive cardiomyopathy (Figure 6).

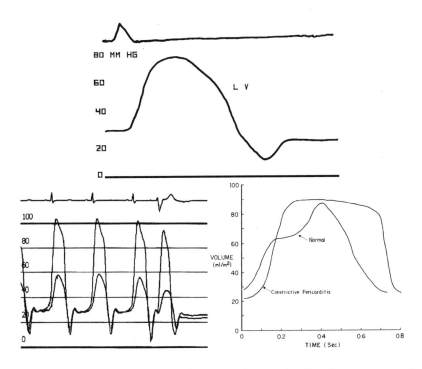

Figure 6: **Top:** The dip-and-plateau configuration of ventricular diastolic pressure recorded by micromanometry of the left ventricle in a case of severe constrictive pericarditis. **Bottom left:** Ventricular diastolic pressure recorded through a fluid filled system and an external transducer. **Bottom right:** left ventricular volume-time curves from a normal beat in a patient with normal ventricular function and a post-extrasystolic beat in a patient with constrictive pericarditis.

In severe cases this limitation is absolute; therefore a plateau is inscribed on the ventricular filling curve and on the contour of ventricular diastolic pressure. In less severe cases, while ventricular filling in late diastole is severely limited, it is not entirely absent. In such cases, a large "a" wave may be inscribed on the pressure recording, suggesting a possible small increase in ventricular end-diastolic volume.

The morphology of the right ventricular diastolic pressure curve in constrictive pericarditis was described a little over half a century ago (*Hansen, Eskildsen, Götzsche 1951*). The early diastolic dip they described was a sharply down-going wave, the nadir of which often being below the zero pressure line. The plateau following the upstroke of the dip was a relatively long flat line. The fancied resemblance of the dip and plateau to the mathematical symbol √ gave rise to another commonly used connotation, the square root sign. These authors speculated that this contour of ventricular diastolic pressure reflected the pattern of filling, but of course, at that time, methods for measuring ventricular volume had not been developed.

Generations of physicians have been brought up to recognise the square root sign as pathognomonic of constrictive pericarditis or restrictive cardiomyopathy. A word of caution is, however, in order. Under-damped tracings, obtained using a conventional fluid-filled system and an external pressure transducer during cardiac catheterisation of patients who have neither disorder, may be contaminated with an artefact that simulates the dip and plateau (Figure 7). Under-damped tracings simulating constriction or restriction of the ventricles can safely be ignored as long as the pressure is normal in mid- and late-diastole.

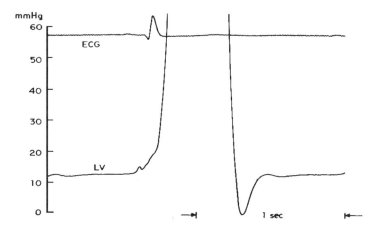

Figure 7: Left ventricular pressure tracings obtained during cardiac catheterisation of a patient with normal ventricular function and without pericardial disease. Oscillations due to under-damping are responsible for the notches on the upstroke and in early diastole.

5.3   Coronary circulation

The pattern of coronary flow is affected by constrictive pericarditis. Compared with normal, acceleration and deceleration are both considerably faster. Furthermore, coronary flow reserve is diminished. The proposed mechanisms responsible for decreased reserve are increased pressure at zero flow secondary to the high ventricular diastolic pressure, and increased resistance offered by the epicardial arteries and the small coronary vessels (*Akasaka, Yoshida, Yamamuro 1997*). Ischemia at rest or inducible by stress, however, is not a feature of constrictive pericarditis.

6.   CARDIAC CATHETERISATION

Cardiac catheterisation is often performed, especially in patients being considered for pericardiectomy. Non-invasive cardiologists, however, point out that clinical means and appropriate non-invasive imaging can make the diagnosis and an assessment of severity, reliably. The need for coronary arteriography is a common reason to include cardiac catheterisation in the evaluation. Some cardiologists favour including cardiac catheterisation when doubt exists concerning whether a patient has constrictive pericarditis, restrictive cardiomyopathy, or both. Most often, however, this distinction can be made with confidence by clinical history, standard non-invasive cardiac testing, computerised tomography or magnetic resonance imaging, and echo-Doppler cardiography. In the most obstinate cases, endomyocardial biopsy is the court of last resort. It is difficult to imagine many cardiologists performing biopsy or arteriography resisting the temptation to measure invasive hemodynamics while they are at it. Left ventriculography or angiocardiography, frequently performed in bygone times, is no longer deemed necessary, and exposes the patient to unwarranted risk. Suspicion of co-existing heart disease can be allayed or confirmed by echo-Doppler cardiography, but cardiac catheterisation may be required to help to sort out their relative contributions to the deranged hemodynamics.

6.1   Technique

Meticulous attention to technique is critical. Many laboratories are so oriented to interventional procedures and imaging that neither the technicians nor the physicians have a strong interest in, or even detailed knowledge of hemodynamics. Every attempt to correct these deficiencies where they exist should be made before performing cardiac catheterisation for constrictive pericarditis. Failing that, the patient should be referred to another laboratory.

No attempt should be made to restore the patient to "dry weight." Some oedema and elevation of venous pressure in severe cases is acceptable, indeed preferable. If excessive amounts of powerful diuretics were used in preparation for the procedure and caused hyponatremic alkalosis or hypokalemia, catheterisation should be postponed. The principal hemodynamic abnormalities are easily predicted from the foregoing discussion of the pathophysiology.

Constrictive pericarditis most often is global; therefore, diastolic pressure is equal in both ventricles, the right atrium and the pulmonary wedge position or left atrium. In addition, the pulmonary arterial diastolic pressure is the same as this common pressure, as in cardiac tamponade. It is commonly stated in the literature that these pressures should agree within 5 mmHg. It is therefore important to be certain that the pressure recording systems are equisensitive and that all pressure transducers are at exactly the same hydrostatic height. Respiratory changes in peak left and right ventricular, and in aortic and pulmonary arterial pressures are almost 180 degrees out of phase (*Hurrell, Nishimura, Higano 1996*) even when these changes are of insufficient magnitude to meet criteria for pulsus paradoxus. Many cardiologists and fellows concentrate on demonstrating equal diastolic pressures on the two sides of the heart. They therefore tend to neglect to record simultaneous left and right ventricular pressures at low, as well as at high gain, an error comparable to looking at a pathology slide under oil immersion before looking at it at low power. The effects of respiration on hemodynamics are extremely helpful when evaluating pericardial compressive diseases. Pressure recordings of patients being investigated for pericardial disease must therefore be accompanied by a reliable record of the phase of respiration. Ideally, a rapidly responding respirometer (*Adolph and Frommer 1966*) is used for this purpose, but failing that, wedge pressure should be recorded simultaneously with the pressure of interest, because it tracks the respiratory cycle quite faithfully.

6.2   Characteristic pressure recordings

The inability of the scarred pericardium to transmit respiratory changes in thoracic pressure to the cardiac chambers is the basis for many of the characteristic findings typical of constriction. Right atrial pressure does not decline during inspiration; therefore, mean right atrial pressure does not display the respiratory variation found in normal subjects and preserved in cardiac tamponade in which respiratory variation in thoracic pressure is transmitted to the heart; the *y* descent, however, is deeper and steeper with inspiration. The mechanism underlying the alteration of the *y* descent has not, to my knowledge, been explained. Failure of the central venous pressure to fall during inspiration is the *forme fruste* of Kussmaul's sign. In addition to describing the paradoxical pulse for the first time, and whose name is associated with air hunger, Adolph Kussmaul showed that central venous pressure may increase during inspiration (*Kussmaul 1878*).

6.2.1 Right atrial pressure

The *a, c,* and *v* waves of the right atrial pressure are less prominent than the *x* and *y* descents, which therefore assumes a W-like configuration. Either of the nadirs may predominate but often the *y* in early diastole, corresponding with the early diastolic dip of right ventricular diastolic pressure, is deeper than the *x,* which is inscribed during ventricular ejection (Figure 8).

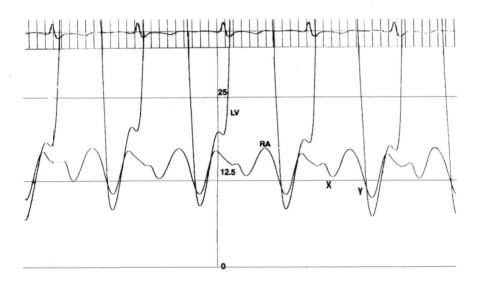

Figure 8: Pressure recorded simultaneously in the left ventricle and right atrium showing the x descent during ventricular ejection and the y corresponding with the early diastolic dip of ventricular pressure.

As in the case of tamponade, ventricular diastolic and atrial pressures are equal in the two sides of the heart. In cardiac tamponade, this equalization is tight throughout the respiratory cycle, but in constrictive pericarditis, the pulmonary wedge pressure falls in inspiration, whereas the right atrial pressure does not. Tracking of the two pressures therefore is not as tight, usually being confined to the period of inspiration (Figure 9). Acceptable simultaneous records from the right atrium and pulmonary wedge position, or other combinations of right heart pressure can be obtained via the proximal and distal ports of a Swan Ganz catheter.

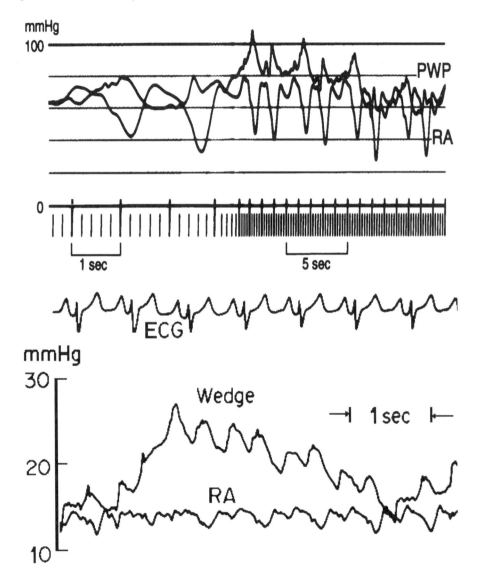

Figure 9: Two examples to show the effect of respiration on how right atrial and pulmonary wedge pressures track. **Top:** The patient did not have dyspnoea at rest. **Bottom:** The patient's breathing was laboured.

6.2.2   Ventricular diastolic pressure

A faithful recording of the dip and plateau can be obtained with the use of a transducer mounted on the catheter to eliminate the problems with damping inherent in conventional fluid-filled recording systems (Figure 6). Using this technique, the early diastolic dip does not reach subatmospheric levels and the pattern is unmistakable. In clinical practice, this ideal usually is not practical. The resulting tracings can certainly be diagnostic, even when not aesthetically pleasing. With careful attention to details, better quality tracings can be obtained (Figure 10). Catheters with a large internal diameter are suitable for angiography, but their use is not conducive to high quality pressure recording. The operator should be willing to exchange catheters as the need arises and not to measure pressure with an angiographic catheter. A number 6 or 7 multipurpose catheter yields pressure records of acceptable quality, and is more readily available today than the Cournand catheter which used to be the ideal catheter through which to obtain good pressure records. It goes without saying that failure to flush all bubbles from the system compromises the quality of pressure recordings. Tubing connecting the catheter to the transducers should be as short as possible; the internal diameter should be small and the walls rigid.

Spurious "dip and plateau" patterns are frequently caused by catheter fling (Figure 7), especially in patients with tachycardia or whip, and in patients with a hyperdynamic circulation and tachycardia. These artefacts can mar the data, whatever recording system is used. When a fluid-filled system is used, the appearance of the tracings may improve when a small amount of radio-opaque contrast is added to the catheter, or the stopcock is turned slightly to reduce the orifice size. The problem with such techniques is that real data may be lost in the process, even though the operator ensures that the records do not look over-damped. If the recording system stores data, a powerful means to eliminate "white," or random noise is signal averaging. The signal is often remarkably clean after averaging as few as three beats. Of course, an artefact that occurs regularly would not be eliminated.

6.2.2.1   Elastic constrictive pericarditis

In some cases of constrictive pericarditis without extensive calcification, the pericardium retains limited elasticity. When this is present, the ventricular volume and peak systolic pressure increase in response to atrial systole (Figure 11), indicating less impairment of preload reserve, whereas, with typical severe restriction, no filling occurs in the latter two thirds of diastole. Thus when some elasticity is preserved, ventricular performance can increase via the Starling mechanism. In non-elastic constrictive pericarditis, unavailability of the Starling response is the major reason that pump function is impaired (*Gaasch, Peterson, Shabetai, 1974*).

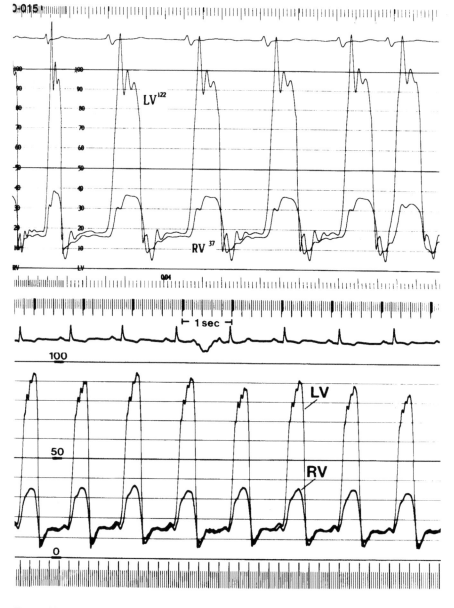

Figure 10: **TOP:** Left and right ventricular pressures in a patient with constrictive pericarditis recorded using a fluid-filled system. The tracings are diagnostic but include artefacts.
BOTTOM: An example of improved quality ventricular pressure records; attention had been paid to the technical details discussed above.

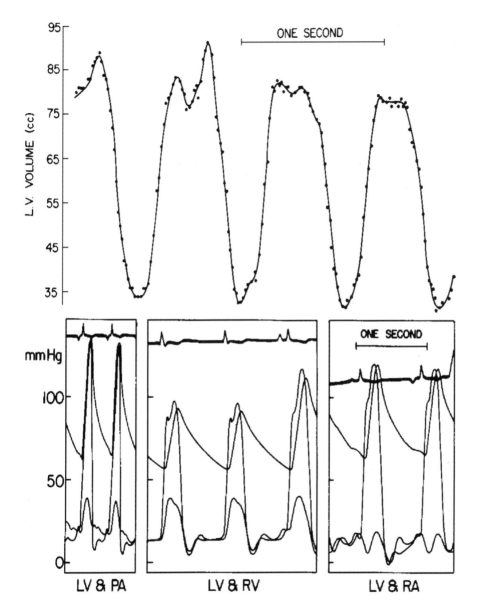

Figure 11: **TOP:** Left ventricular time plots during sinus rhythm (first two beats) and spontaneous junctional rhythm, in the absence of atrial contraction. **BOTTOM:** Simultaneously recorded high fidelity pressures in both ventricles, and the left ventricle and pulmonary artery and right atrium. The contribution of atrial systole to end-diastolic and developed systolic pressure in this non-compliant heart is illustrated by the transition from junctional bradycardia to sinus rhythm (**middle panel). (**From Gaasch, Peterson, Shabetai, 1974, with permission)

Inspiration diminishes the pressure difference between the pulmonary wedge pressure and left ventricular diastolic pressure more than in other patients (*Hurrell, Nishimura, Higano 1996*). The pathophysiological significance of this observation is that, in constrictive pericarditis, it is the reason for diminished left ventricular volume with inspiration whereas, in tamponade, it is one of two mechanisms. This is because, in tamponade, an important mechanism is increased right ventricular filling during inspiration causing the septum to bulge into the left ventricle. In patients with restrictive cardiomyopathy, left ventricular diastolic and pulmonary venous pressures fall to the same extent with inspiration; therefore, the decrease in ventricular volume does not exceed normal.

6.2.3   Coronary arteriography

The angiographic appearance of the coronary arteries is characterised by decreased accordion-like motion through the cardiac cycle (*Alexander, Kelley, Cohen, 1979*) and the vessels are at a distance from the cardiac borders in all projections (*Ramsey, Sbar, Elliott 1970*). The abnormalities of the coronary flow profile and coronary reserve have been mentioned under pathophysiology. Coronary arteriography is not justified, however, when the sole purpose is to strengthen the diagnosis of constrictive pericarditis.

7.   IMAGING.

Imaging has long played an important role in the diagnosis of constrictive pericarditis, and its importance continues to evolve (*Nishimura 2001*). Transthoracic echocardiography is not always helpful in showing the pathologic changes, but echo-Doppler has proven to be a highly valuable diagnostic tool by virtue of its ability to lay out the pathophysiology. Computerised tomography (*Sechtem, Tscholakoff, Higgins 1986*) is the most frequently employed imaging modality for measuring pericardial thickness although magnetic resonance imaging *(White 1995)* is just as accurate but is used less often, because it is more cumbersome and is less well tolerated by some patients; its advantage is that contrast enhancement is unnecessary. More recently, trans-oesophageal echocardiography has been found to be as accurate as computerised tomography (*Ling, Oh, Tei 1997*).

7.1   Echocardiography

Both M mode and real time echocardiography have been helpful for the diagnosis and understanding of constrictive pericarditis. Both techniques show the characteristic abnormal motion of the interventricular septum. With inspiration, the septum bulges toward the left ventricle with consequent increase in the size of the right ventricle and diminution of the left ventricle. This shift in septal position during the respiratory cycle reflects enhanced ventricular interdependence, and is dramatic when seen in real time, earning for itself the epithet "septal bounce."

Systolic septal motion was normal in only half of a series of 40 patients (*Engel, Fowler, Tei 1985*). In this classic study, the investigators described the mechanisms underlying abnormal notching of the septum. When the results in these patients were compared with those in 40 subjects who were free from heart disease, abnormal septal notching was not recorded in any. Of the 29 patients in sinus rhythm, a posteriorly directed notch coincident with atrial systole was present in 10. A posterior notch occurred in the mid portion of early diastole in 18 of the 40 patients, and an anterior notch in 13. Thus, an abnormal notch in early diastole was seen in most of the patients. Lack of anterior motion of the posterior wall in mid- and late- diastole, after an abrupt anterior motion in early diastole, was a frequent finding. In the most severe cases, the pulmonary valve opens prematurely during inspiration, that is, with atrial systole, because the right ventricular end-diastolic pressure may briefly exceed pulmonary arterial pressure, inspiration being associated with a decrease in pulmonary arterial, but not right ventricular diastolic pressure in constrictive pericarditis (*Vandenbossche, Jacobs, Decroly 1985*).

7.1.1   Mechanism of abnormal septal notching

Engel et al. proposed that the notches are caused by transient reversal of the trans-septal pressure gradient in early diastole and pre-systole related to the rapid ventricular filling characteristic of constrictive pericarditis and asynchronous opening of the tricuspid and mitral valves (Figure 12). In a subsequent study in which some of the same investigators participated (*Tei, Child, Tanaka, 1983),* the pressure was measured on both sides of the ventricular septum to establish the relation of notching to transient reversal of the pressure gradient.

Motion of the posterior wall of the left ventricle is also abnormal and again the abnormality reflects the pathophysiology. The brisk anterior motion due to the abnormally rapid rate of early diastolic filling, and the absence of any increase in ventricular volume for the remainder of diastole, reflect the restrictive filling pattern.

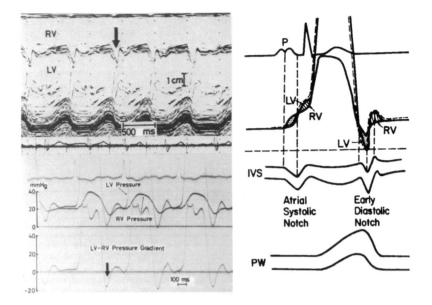

Figure 12: **Left:**. M mode echocardiogram, ventricular pressure, and difference in pressure between the ventricles. in a patient with constrictive pericarditis and atrial fibrillation. The early diastolic notch **(thick arrow)** is seen in the upper panel and the pressure reversal **(thinner arrow)** in the lower panel. The notch and pressure reversal disappeared after pericardiectomy, but the absence of motion of the posterior wall in mid- and late-diastole persisted. **Right:** Schematic diagram to illustrate the hemodynamics of atrial notching. Each atrium contracts asynchronously against a high ventricular diastolic pressure. (*Modified from Tei, Child, Tanaka 1983, with permission*)

7.1.2   Anatomical findings

The ventricles and great arteries are of normal size and the valves are normal, unless the patient also has cardiac disease. The atria are mildly enlarged, but less than in restrictive cardiomyopathy. The inferior vena cava is dilated and fails to diminish in diameter with inspiration when constriction is moderate or severe. As in cardiac tamponade and heart failure, this sign indicates very high systemic venous pressure (*Himelman, Kircher, Rockey 1988*). When pericardial thickness is greatly increased or calcification is abundant, these abnormalities may readily be identified (Figure 13) but in a series of 85 patients who had pericardiectomy or were examined at autopsy within six months, the pericardial abnormality was recognized in only 35 percent. On the other hand, over-interpreting "increased pericardial brightness" is a common error. Therefore, unless the findings are obvious, caution is necessary before making or rejecting the diagnosis of constrictive pericarditis on these grounds (*Hinds, Reisner, Amico 1992*). In an experimental study, pericardial thickness was estimated by two-dimensional echocardiography and correlated poorly when compared with measurements of the gross pathological specimens or the surgeon's operative report. Transesophageal echocardiography increased sensitivity to 95 percent and specificity to 86 percent (*Ling, Oh, Tei 1997*).

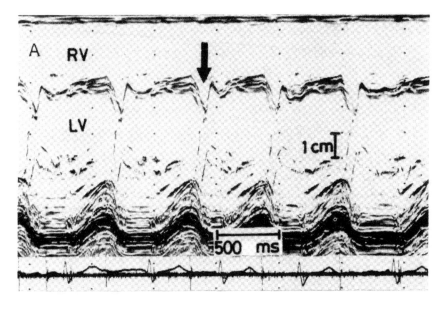

Figure 13: M-mode echocardiogram of constrictive pericarditis. The thick echo-dense pericardium moves with the heart, an indication of its adherence to the myocardium. Arrow = septal notch. (From Shabetai R, 1994*)*

7.1.3   Doppler findings

A number of Doppler abnormalities are found in constrictive pericarditis. The combination of a rigid pericardium that shields the cardiac chambers from respiratory fluctuation of thoracic pressure and strengthens ventricular interdependence with sparing of the ventricular and atrial septa is the basis for the abnormalities of trans-valvular velocities and the role that altered curvature of the septum plays in constrictive pericarditis. In patients without cardiac tamponade, constrictive pericarditis or obstructive lung disease, breathing quietly, peak early diastolic transmitral velocity varies less than 5 percent (*Spodick 1983; Oh, Hatle, Seward, 1994)*. In patients with constrictive pericarditis, respiratory variation in peak early filling velocity is 25 to 45 percent (*Oh, Hatle, Seward 1994*), as illustrated in Figure 14, taken from Sun, Abdalla, Yang 2001. When chronic lung disease is responsible for increased respiratory variation of ventricular inflow, similar variation is also present in flow through the superior vena cava *(Boonyaratavej, Oh, Tajik, 1998).*

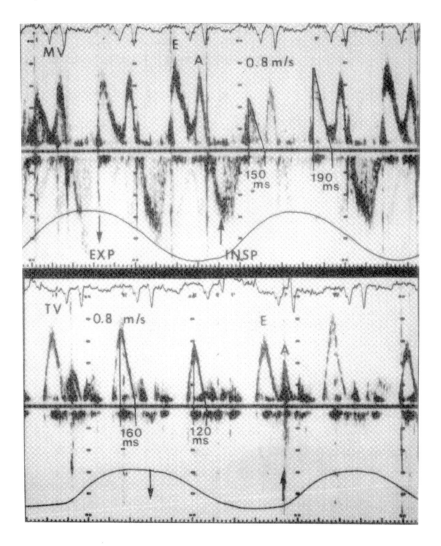

Figure 14: Dopppler records of mitral and tricuspid inflow to show increased respiratory variation opposite in direction on the two sides of the heart. Respiratory variation of peak E wave velocity was 17%. MV = mitral and TV = tricuspid inflow velocity. (From Sun, Abdalla, Yang 2001, with permission)

Although increased respiratory variation is a highly valuable sign of constrictive pericarditis, it is not present in perhaps 10 percent of patients, in some of whom respiratory variation is inhibited by high left atrial pressure and opening of the mitral valve on a steep portion of the diastolic pressure volume curve (*Oh, Tajik, Appleton 1997*). When sound reasons to suspect constrictive pericarditis exist, Doppler examination should be repeated after lowering preload to reduce left atrial pressure. Most often, head-up tilting achieves this, but diuresis is an alternative method. The study by Oh et al. demonstrated that, after reducing preload, abnormal respiratory variation can be restored in many of the cases. Good technique calls for inclusion of a respirometer tracing, as the maximal change in transvalvular velocity is seen with the first beat in inspiration.

Respiratory variation of pulmonary venous flow likewise increases and the variation is greater than that of transmitral velocity (*Tabata, Kabbani, Murray 2001*) and Figure 15. Atrial fibrillation impedes beat-to-beat analysis of hemodynamic parameters but, by averaging six beats in the patients who had atrial fibrillation, the authors were able to show that respiratory variation in pulmonary venous flow retains its diagnostic value. Other abnormalities of pulmonary venous flow include significantly increased velocities in both systole and diastole. Respiratory variation of pulmonary venous blood flow and velocity reverts to normal soon after pericardiectomy (*Sun, Abdalla, Yang 2001*).

Respiratory changes in the spectral signal of tricuspid regurgitation may help to make the diagnosis. Investigators have used trans-oesophageal studies during cardiac catheterisation for this purpose (*Klodas, Nishimura, Appleton 1996*). That technique would be optimal for clinical care, but other considerations often determine that trans-thoracic examination must suffice. We have seen that, during inspiration, left ventricular filling is impaired and that the chamber volume therefore diminishes. Ventricular interaction causes the ventricular septum to bulge leftward, and since total pericardial volume cannot change, volume is shifted from the left to the right ventricle. Right ventricular pressure increases as a result, and therefore the velocity and duration of tricuspid regurgitation and hence the time-velocity index increase. This phenomenon is not present in heart failure, but may be present in severe obstructive lung disease. The latter is readily recognized on other grounds.

Increased respiratory variation of left ventricular and pulmonary vein flow is highly specific for compressive disorders of the heart, once severe lung disease has been ruled out (Figure 15). This abnormal variation is the most critical of the various Doppler abnormalities for diagnostic purposes. Ventricular interdependence is not increased in restrictive cardiomyopathy, making increased respiratory variation particularly useful in the differential diagnosis (*vide infra*). Dominant flow during diastole, like severe reduction of the mitral E/A ratio and decreased deceleration time, however, are non-specific signs of diastolic dysfunction.

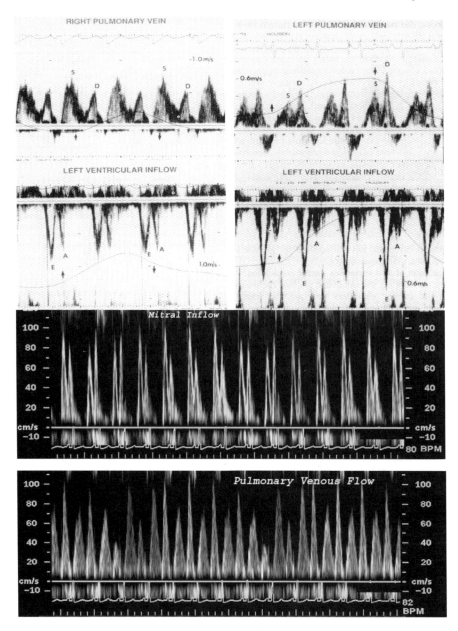

Figure 15: **TOP; Left:** Normal subject, pulmonary venous and left ventricular inflow. Minimal respiratory variation in either record. **Right:** Constrictive pericarditis. Note: increased respiratory variation in pulmonary vein flow is more pronounced than in left ventricular inflow (**up arrows:** inspiration); (**down arrows:** expiration). (From Klein, Cohen, Pietrolungo 1993, with permission). A striking example of greater respiratory variation of pulmonary vein flow than mitral inflow is shown in the lower two panels (Courtesy of Dan Blanchard, MD University of California, San Diego)

7.2   Computer assisted tomography

For the purpose of imaging the pericardium, computer-assisted tomography is the method of choice in most institutions, and has much to commend it. The normal pericardium is not always visible on standard tomograms (Figure 16); the dorsal aspect is visualised less frequently. The pericardium is seen clearly on electron beam tomography although, again, the dorsal region may be missed. The density is similar to that of the myocardium, but the epicardial fat delimits the pericardium, which is 1 to 2 mm thick, except in the region of the pericardio-diaphragmatic ligament, where it may be 3 to 4 mm thick.

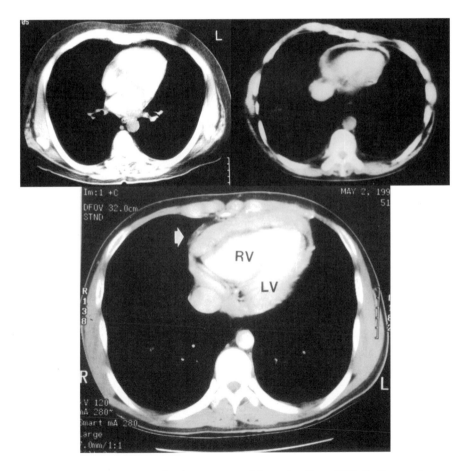

Figure 16: Computer-assisted tomograms of the pericardium. **TOP; Left:** normal pericardium; **Right:** typical constrictive pericarditis; **BOTTOM:** unusually thick pericardium of a patient with mesothelioma presenting as severe constrictive pericarditis.

The pericardium of constrictive pericarditis is clearly demonstrated by standard tomography without contrast enhancement (Figure 16) and is typically at least 3 mm thick, and separated from the heart by a fat pad of variable thickness. It is important to recall, however, that a normal appearing pericardium, or failure to visualise the pericardium does not exclude the diagnosis of constrictive pericarditis. Constriction is a physiological concept, as well as an anatomic one.

A promising method for diagnosing both the anatomy and pathophysiology is cine-computed tomography. In a recent study using this technique, five patients with proven constrictive pericarditis, seven with cardiomyopathy and normal pericardium, and seven normal volunteers underwent this procedure. The pericardial thickness of patients with constriction averaged 10 mm +/-2, and 1 mm in all the other subjects. The study clearly documented the typical filling pattern of constrictive pericarditis, with much more complete filling in the first third of diastole than in the other two groups. (*Oren, Grover-McKay, Stanford 1993*).

7.3   Magnetic resonance imaging

Magnetic resonance imaging is also an established tool for evaluating the pericardium. The normal pericardium is seen on T1 weighted images. It is black because, like the blood pool, its signal intensity is low, but is easy to see, because it is sandwiched between the high intensity signals of epicardial and pericardial fat (Figure 17). Thus the pericardium is at opposite ends of the grey scale when magnetic resonance imaging is compared with computer-assisted tomography. Portions of the pericardium may not be identifiable in areas where fat may be absent or scanty, for example, over the right atrium and the postero-lateral wall of the left ventricle. Likewise, it is not seen where the pericardium and lung are contiguous. Comparing computer-assisted tomography with magnetic resonance imaging, calcium is identified only on the former, but the latter allows for imaging in multiple planes. It should be recalled that calcification does not necessarily mean constriction is present, emphasising yet again that any test must be interpreted in the proper context.

8.   CLINICAL FEATURES

The clinical features are those of right heart failure although myocardial systolic function is normal in the vast majority and diastolic dysfunction is not intrinsic to the myocardium, but imposed by the greatly increased external restraint. As in heart failure generally, the symptoms and signs are due to retention of fluid and, as in right heart failure, systemic congestion is predominant. This similarity in clinical findings does not mean that the pathophysiology is the same. The heart is overloaded in heart failure, but unloaded by constrictive pericarditis, and although diuretics have a role in treatment, in other respects treatment is different.

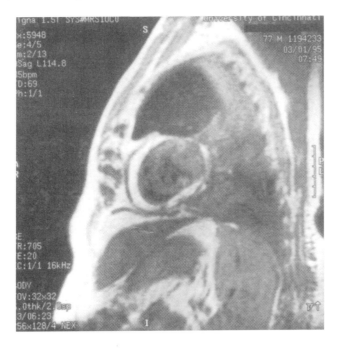

Figure 17: Spin-echo image. Increased, but variable thickness of the pericardium. (From Hoit 1997, with permission)

8.1   Symptoms.

Mild cases are asymptomatic and usually discovered in the course of the evaluation for other problems or during a routine physical examination. The chief complaint most often relates to fluid retention and may range from swelling of the lower extremities to increased abdominal girth with associated discomfort. Exercise capacity is limited by both dyspnoea and fatigue. Muscle weakness, due to cachexia, is a complaint in advanced cases. Late in the course, patients may also complain of dyspepsia caused by liver dysfunction and congestion of the gastrointestinal tract. When atrial fibrillation supervenes, again late in the course, the patients may note palpitation and decreased exercise tolerance. Chest pain is unusual in chronic constrictive pericarditis, but may be a feature of subacute constriction.

8.2   Clinical examination

8.2.1   General appearance and vital signs

The findings on examination can be predicted from the pathophysiology. If the case is not longstanding, the patient does not appear acutely or chronically ill, but in longstanding severe cases, cachexia may be profound and the abdomen may be greatly swollen. The patient may appear slightly icteric because of severe chronic hepatic congestion and, for the same reason, may have spider angiomata about the upper chest and neck. These features, together with swollen lower extremities, present a picture reminiscent of severe malnutrition of beriberi (Figure 18). This clinical picture is becoming less common with improved methods for early diagnosis and safety of pericardiectomy. The wasted neck and high venous pressure often make jugular pulsations obvious even before the formal examination commences.

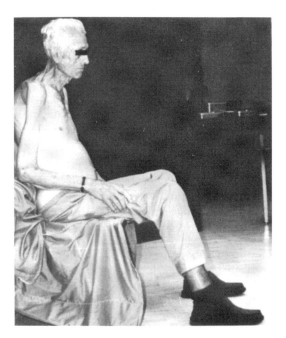

Figure18: Clinical photograph of a patient with "end-stage" constrictive pericarditis. The patient underwent pericardiectomy, but long after hope had passed for substantial benefit. He died a few weeks later.

The jugular pulse shows all the characteristics seen on right atrial catheterisation. Central venous pressure is elevated, the degree depending on the severity of the disease but also, to a lesser extent, on the state of hydration. In the most severe cases, venous pressure exceeds 20 cm. In that circumstance, venous pressure should be estimated while the patient is sitting straight up; otherwise, the pulsations are damped and may become invisible. In less severe cases, elevation of the thorax should be decreased. Trial and error determines the optimal posture of the patient for assessing venous pressure.

The most striking of the pulsations is the *y* descent, easily recognised as such by its occurrence after the carotid pulse, which should be palpated or observed on the contra-lateral side of the neck. A *v* wave is also likely to be present, but is less steep, and reaches its apex more slowly. These features are detectable even when the patient has atrial fibrillation, but tachycardia may make detection difficult or impossible. The systemic arterial pulse is often of low volume and, in advanced cases, is irregular because of atrial fibrillation. The pulse pressure may be low, reflecting reduced stroke volume. All these signs are attenuated in less severe cases; often, the only abnormalities are mild peripheral oedema and a jugular pressure of approximately 10 cm.

The abnormalities of the venous pulse, although highly characteristic, are not specific for constrictive pericarditis. Similar findings may be found in tricuspid regurgitation, especially when the enlarged right atrium is compliant, and in right heart failure or severe volume overload. Kussmaul's venous sign, usually as the *forme fruste,* is also present in these conditions.

8.2.2   Thoracic examination

In severe chronic cases, the ribs are clearly evident. In some patients, systolic retraction replaces the usual apex beat. The most striking abnormality is the protodiastolic sound known as the pericardial knock. Readers may be interested to know that the knock was first described by Dominic Corrigan (1802-1880), better known for his description of the pulse in aortic regurgitation. In 1842 he wrote, "In this case there had been bruit to frappement (frapper = to knock (French)) when the patient lay on his back; when he sat up, it was diminished and sometimes altogether disappeared."

8.2.2.1   Mechanism of the pericardial knock
This sound occurs later than the opening snap of mitral stenosis, but earlier than the typical third heart sound of heart failure, in which early diastolic filling is not quite as rapid. It coincides with the abrupt halting of

filling and therefore with the nadir or upstroke of the early diastolic dip of ventricular pressure (*Mounsey 1955*).

The murmur of tricuspid regurgitation may be present but, more commonly, tricuspid regurgitation is silent, but detected by Doppler. In severe cases, dullness and decreased intensity of the breath sounds may be found, denoting pleural effusion that may be bilateral. In less severe cases, the lungs are normal on clinical examination. While the patient is sitting up, the examiner should check for sacral oedema.

8.2.3   Abdominal examination

The findings are highly dependent on the stage to which the disease has progressed. In early cases, the examination is normal. Further in the course, the liver is enlarged and, when the venous pressure elevation is severe, it may pulsate in synchrony with the jugular pulse (Figure 19). This finding may be obvious; otherwise, it can be detected by bimanual palpation, with one hand over the right costal margin and the other behind it. The patient should be asked to hold in a deep breath, but without straining down. In the most advanced cases, the liver may be shrunken by cardiac cirrhosis. Signs of ascites may be present, but, in the era of abdominal scanning, proficiency in eliciting signs of peritoneal fluid by clinical examination, never very sensitive, is diminishing.

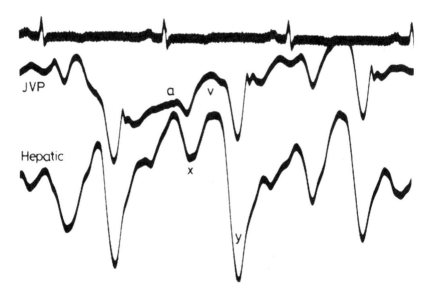

Figure 19: The electrocardiogram and transcutaneous tracings of the jugular **(top)** and hepatic pulsations in a patient with constrictive pericarditis. (From Magna, Vythilingum, Mitha 1984, with permission))

8.3   Laboratory findings

8.3.1   Electrocardiogram

The typical findings are flat or inverted T waves, with or without ST segment depression, and low voltage (Figure 20). In the more severe cases, p mitrale is evident denoting atrial conduction defect, secondary to left atrial enlargement. In more advanced cases, the atrial pathology leads to atrial fibrillation, often treated with digoxin, in which case ST and T changes may be due, in whole or in part, to digitalis effect. Depolarisation abnormalities are distinctly uncommon, but rarely, in chronic cases with heavy calcification, the coronary arteries may be involved in the fibrosis or calcification, causing bundle branch block (*Levine 1973*).

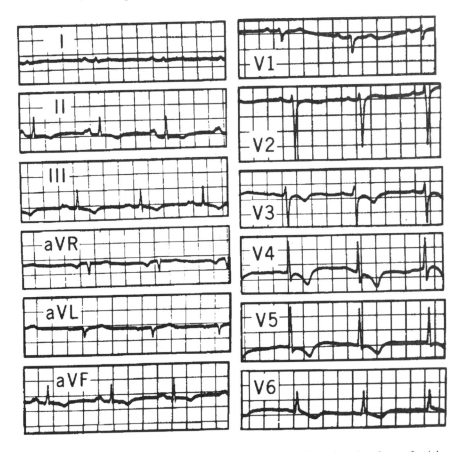

*Figure 20: T*ypical electrocardiogram of constrictive pericarditis before the advent of atrial fibrillation

8.3.2   Chest Radiogram

The cardio-thoracic ratio is not necessarily normal. The thickened pericardium may contribute to the cardiac silhouette, and atrial enlargement can be a cause of cardiomegaly. In other cases, cardiac enlargement is explained by pre-existing heart disease. The right heart border may be slightly more prominent than normal, and the left main bronchus may be somewhat elevated, due respectively to right and left atrial enlargement, but massive atrial enlargement is not a feature of constrictive pericarditis. Calcification of the pericardium, best seen by cardiac fluoroscopy, may also be visible on the plain films, especially in the lateral projection (Figure 21). If it is not clear that calcification is in fact in the pericardium, cardiac fluoroscopy will help to identify whether calcification is in the pericardium, the myocardium, coronary arteries, a mural thrombus, or is valvular. Pleural effusion is common in the more severe cases.

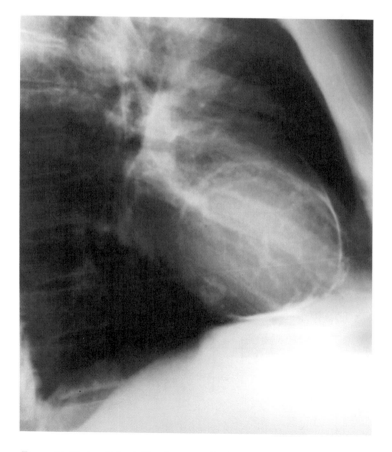

Figure 21: Pericardial calcification seen clearly on a lateral chest radiogram.

9. SYNDROMES OF CONSTRICTIVE PERICARDITIS

Most of what has been written so far in this chapter refers to chronic constrictive pericarditis, in which the manifestations vary considerably in relation to severity and chronicity. In the following paragraphs, I discuss so-called occult constrictive pericarditis, effusive constrictive pericarditis and transient constrictive pericarditis. It is important also to recall that the hemodynamics simulating constrictive pericarditis may be present in acute volume overload, for instance, acute rupture of the mitral valve apparatus, acute tricuspid regurgitation secondary to traumatic rupture or avulsion during endomyocardial biopsy, or right ventricular infarction and carcinoid of the tricuspid valve (*Johnston, Johnston, O'Rourke, 1999*). The explanation for this simulation is that acute cardiac dilation forces the heart against the less compliant pericardium, thereby increasing contact pressure.

9.1 Occult constrictive pericarditis

This was described first in a report of 19 patients with non-specific chest pain, dyspnoea and fatigue (*Bush, Stang, Wooley 1977*). Twelve of the 19 gave a history of acute pericarditis (recurrent in 5). In 2, the pericardium was calcified, and in 16 the electrocardiogram showed repolarisation changes. A plausible aetiology for pericardial disease was noted in 10. The authors hypothesised that mild constrictive pericarditis could be present despite the absence of clinical signs or laboratory evidence (available in that era). They used fluid challenge in 6 patients, 12 subjects with other heart disease, and 12 normal subjects, to determine whether it would bring out the typical hemodynamic findings of constrictive pericarditis in the patients but not in the controls.

All subjects received a large rapid saline infusion. The response in the patients with occult constriction was elevation and equalization of the ventricular diastolic pressures and the development of atrial and ventricular diastolic waveforms consistent with constrictive pericarditis (Figure 22). Ventricular filling pressures and diastolic pressure waveforms were unaltered in the normal subjects. The patients with myocardial disease showed unequal elevation of their ventricular filling pressures. Eleven of those diagnosed as occult constrictive pericarditis were submitted to pericardiectomy, which improved them dramatically. All of these had pathological or histological evidence of chronic pericarditis.

Based on these findings, the authors advised pericardiectomy for disabling symptoms. However, I have reservations about this study, even though it was well conducted, using micromanometer-tipped catheters to obtain high fidelity tracings in a laboratory with a record of excellence in hemodynamic studies.

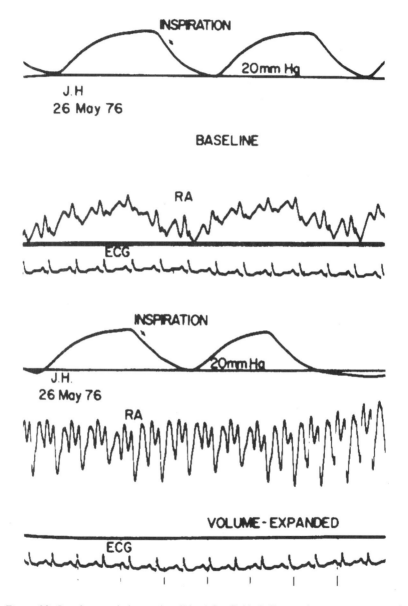

Figure 22: Occult constrictive pericarditis. After fluid challenge, the venous pressure is higher, x and y descents become prominent, and respiratory variation is lost. (Redrawn from Bush, Stang, Wooley 1977 for Shabetai R, Hemodynamics in constrictive and effusive pericarditis versus restrictive cardiomyopathy. UpToDate 10.2 2002.)

The authors did not (probably because they could not) explain how such mild constriction could cause disabling symptoms, or why the patients had chest pain, normally absent in constrictive pericarditis. Furthermore, dramatic relief following pericardiectomy is not supported by increased cardiac output or significantly lower venous pressure. These results have not been consistently reproducible (*Ilia, Weizman, Gueron 1991*). Another concern is that their results in normal subjects are not consonant with those obtained by volume loading in animals (*Holt, Rhode, Kines 1960*). My view is that this test is seldom required and that the results should seldom be the rationale for advising pericardiectomy.

9.2   Effusive constrictive pericarditis

The pericardial cavity is obliterated in constrictive pericarditis; pericardial fluid is totally absent. In some cases, however, pericardial fluid is present between the parietal and visceral layers of the pericardium, either or both of which may be scarred. When this fluid is under increased pressure, the compression of the heart is due in part to constrictive pericarditis and in part to tamponade. This syndrome was named, described, and explained by Hancock, a long-time student of the pericardium and its diseases (*Hancock, 1971 and 1980*). In the first of these papers, he was discussing the findings in 24 patients who had undergone pericardiectomy for constrictive pericarditis, 9 of whom also had pericardial effusion.

In theory, at least, any constrictive pericarditis may have an effusive-constrictive phase, but more common aetiologies include idiopathic pericarditis (especially those with a small, if innocuous, effusion), radiotherapy, tuberculosis, rheumatoid arthritis and neoplasia.

Often the jugular pulse is more like that of constriction, showing somewhat prominent *x* and *y* descents, rather than abolition or attenuation of the *y*. In Hancock's experience and also in mine, the diagnosis often becomes apparent during pericardiocentesis for apparently straightforward cardiac tamponade. Despite having lowered pericardial pressure to normal, right atrial pressure remains elevated with features characteristic of constriction (Figure 23). Even in uncomplicated tamponade, right atrial pressure may be elevated to 5 or 6 mmHg after successful pericardiocentesis, but the waveform and respiratory variation are normal. A persistently elevated right atrial pressure may, however, also be evidence of myocardial or valvular disease, for example, right heart failure or tricuspid valve disease. Likewise, failure of the wedge pressure to normalise in these circumstances indicates either heart disease or effusive constrictive pericarditis. Wedge and right atrial pressures, equally elevated, strongly supports the diagnosis of effusive constrictive pericarditis, whereas, when wedge pressure is more elevated than the right atrial pressure, the patient is most likely to have cardiomyopathy.

9.2.1   Treatment

It is critically important to understand that constriction in these cases is not caused by the scarred parietal pericardium, but by the visceral pericardium. Consequently, the essential component of surgical treatment is visceral pericardiectomy.

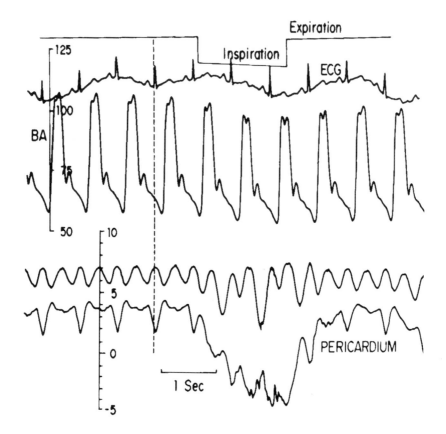

Figure 23: Effusive constrictive pericarditis. A substantial volume of fluid aspirated resulted in a profound fall of pericardial pressure, but the waveform of the slightly elevated right atrial pressure without respiratory variation of mean pressure is consistent with an element of effusive constrictive pericarditis.

A case of severe effusive constrictive pericarditis is demonstrated by the following brief case description. The patient was a young man with rheumatoid arthritis who presented with a large pericardial effusion and severe tamponade. Pericardiocentesis relieved the symptoms, abolished the physical signs and returned the hemodynamics to normal. He then went abroad for a protracted period, only to be brought home nearly in extremis from what we assumed was tamponade and *e coli* infection. The hemodynamic data before and after pericardiocentesis are presented in Table 1. The pericardial fluid grew abundant *e coli*.

Table 1. Effusive-constrictive pericarditis: Hemodynamic data.

Source	Hemodynamic variables before pericardiocentesis	Hemodynamic variables after pericardiocentesis
Pericardium	18	**minus 2**
Right atrium	18	18
Right ventricle	36/18	35/17
Pulmonary artery	36/19	36/18
Pulmonary arterial wedge	20	20
Aorta	130/82	125/78
Cardiac index l/m_2	2.7	2.6

The hemodynamics were not changed because constriction was significantly more severe than tamponade, which was therefore masked.

9.3   Transient constrictive pericarditis

Some patients with acute effusive pericarditis go through a transient phase of constriction before normal hemodynamics are restored (*Sagrista-Sauleda, Permanyer-Miralda, Candell-Riera 1987*). Constriction in this series was not severe, but subsequently I have seen quite impressive transient constriction in the course of subacute effusive pericarditis. In their series of 16 patients, Sagrista-Sauleda et al. reported that not all the features of constriction were present in every case, but they observed pericardial knock, near-equalisation of left and right ventricular pressures, characteristic central venous pressure contours, and serial echocardiographic changes within the cohort (Figure 24).

The possibility that constriction may be a transient phenomenon should be kept in mind, especially in subacute effusive pericarditis. Treatment with an anti-inflammatory agent reduces the extent of exudate and, by this means, reduces the element of constriction. Transient constrictive pericarditis usually resolves in a matter of weeks, but may require several months. The whole clinical course determines how long it is appropriate to withhold pericardiectomy. The operation should be performed before the advent of calcification of the pericardium when venous pressure elevation of 15 or more mmHg persists.

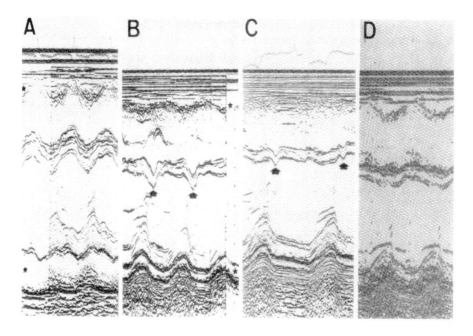

Figure 24: Transient constrictive pericarditis. Serial M-mode echocardiograms. **A:** early, acute effusive pericarditis, pericardial effusion. **B:** 30 days, persisting small effusion, early diastolic notching (arrows) and parallel pericardial echoes. **C:** 44 days, constrictive pattern, no effusion remains. **D:** 33 months, the echocardiogram is normal. (* marks pericardial effusion). (From Sagrista-Sauleda, Permanyer-Miralda, Candell-Riera, 1987, with permission)

9.4   Localised constriction

Constrictive pericarditis is normally a generalised pathological process with the scar surrounding all the heart, which accounts for the classic hemodynamics. As is the case with tamponade, but much less frequently, the process may be localised; the findings are then highly atypical. In South Africa, pericardial disease is quite common, and a series of 200 cases was reported (*Schrire, Gotsman, Beck 1968*). These authors encountered two patients with a murmur typical of tricuspid stenosis with a pan-diastolic pressure gradient across the tricuspid valve. Right ventricular obstruction in a patient treated at the Mayo clinic was caused by calcific constrictive pericarditis, predominantly over the right side of the heart (*Nishimura, Kazmier, Smith, 1985*). Severe compression of the right ventricular outflow tract was demonstrated by right ventriculography. Surgical debridement reduced the systolic pressure difference across the pulmonary valve from 40 to 6 mmHg. Figure 25 illustrates a case of our own. The patient developed constrictive pericarditis two months after rupture of the oesophagus into the pericardium. The venous pressure was elevated and he had a pulmonary ejection systolic murmur. The operative findings confirmed constrictive pericarditis with a band of scar tissue compressing the right ventricular outflow tract. Resection abolished the systolic pressure gradient and normalised the contour of pulmonary arterial pressure pulse.

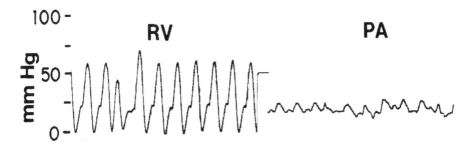

Figure 25: Pressure recorded as the catheter was pulled across the pulmonary valve of the patient with extrinsic pulmonary stenosis due to a band of constriction around the outflow tract of the right ventricle.

10.   COMPARISON OF CONSTRICTIVE PERICARDITIS WITH CARDIAC TAMPONADE

Both are compressive diseases of the heart, and therefore primarily affect diastolic function and, in both, total pericardial space is invariable and chamber interdependence is greatly intensified. In the vast majority, the whole heart is evenly compressed. This shared pathophysiology is the basis for features that the two disorders have in common.

In cardiac tamponade, respiratory fluctuations in intrathoracic pressure are in part transmitted through the pericardium and the contained fluid into the cardiac chambers, permitting systemic venous return to increase in the normal manner during inspiration. The pericardial scar of constrictive pericarditis, on the other hand, blocks transmission of changes in thoracic pressure from being transmitted to the heart, thus preventing increased systemic venous return during inspiration. In cardiac tamponade, the heart is compressed for the entire cardiac cycle, whereas in constrictive pericarditis compression exists only from the end of early rapid filling until end-diastole (Figure 26). Isolation of the heart from pressure changes in the thorax and freedom from constriction in early diastole are the bases for features of

constrictive pericarditis and cardiac tamponade that differ in the two
diseases.

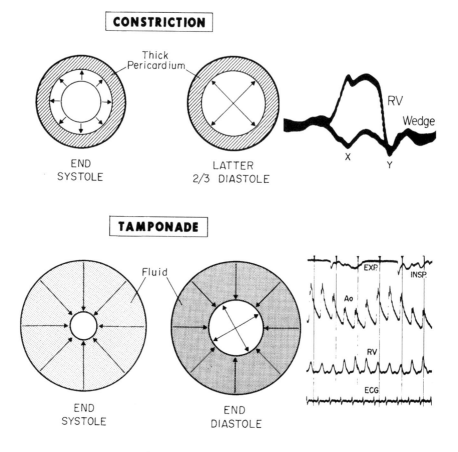

Figure 26: Schematic to differences between constrictive pericarditis and cardiac tamponade.
In constrictive pericarditis the heart is free until the end of rapid filling, after which filling
ceases, creating the dip-and-plateau pattern of ventricular diastolic pressure and the y wave of
atrial pressure. In tamponade the fluid compresses the heart throughout the cardiac cycle.
Venous return occurs only during ventricular systole.

A diagram to compare the respiratory effects on cardiac pressures and
ventricular volumes (Figure 27) shows that in normal subjects, tamponade
and restrictive cardiomyopathy, inspiration lowers pericardial and left
ventricular diastolic pressure by a few mmHg, but in constriction, the
pericardial space is obliterated, pulmonary venous pressure drops normally,
but left ventricular diastolic pressure is not lowered.

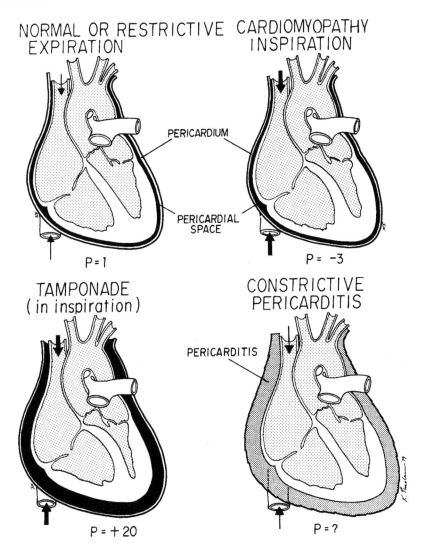

*Figure 27: Comparison of the effects of respiration on the hemodynamics of cardiac tamponade, constrictive pericarditis and restrictive cardiomyopathy. **The top panels** represent normal physiology or restrictive cardiomyopathy in which inspiration lowers intrathoracic pressure, causing pericardial pressure to fall, for example, from 1 to -3 mmHg, systemic venous return to increase (arrows). The compressive disorders are shown and contrasted in **lower panels.** **Left:** Tamponade. With inspiration, systemic venous return increases (heavier black arrows) and pericardial pressure falls from 20 to 18 mmHg and right heart volume increases due to septal bulging. **Right:** Constrictive pericarditis. Systemic venous return does not increase (arrows). The pericardial space is obliterated and therefore intrathoracic pressure changes are not transmitted to the cardiac chambers, impairing left heart filling. The smaller left ventricle causes the septum to shift to the left, increasing the size of the right heart.*

10.1   Clinical

Patients with tamponade are more likely to complain of dyspnoea and chest discomfort, whereas the major complaint of patients with constrictive pericarditis is often ankle and abdominal swelling, although they also have dyspnoea and fatigue. Tachypnoea and orthopnoea are more common in tamponade.

In both conditions the jugular pressure is elevated, but in tamponade declines with inspiration and the y descent is absent. With constriction the jugular pressure does not fall with inspiration, and may even increase when the patient is asked to breathe deeply. Both x and y are prominent. A friction rub is uncommon in tamponade and rare in constriction. Systolic retraction is a finding in some cases of constriction, not in tamponade. A pericardial knock means constriction, even in the presence of pericardial effusion. Pleural effusion is common in severe untreated constriction, but is not a feature of tamponade. Atrial fibrillation is common in late stage constriction, but usually absent in tamponade. Pulsus paradoxus is more common and more pronounced in tamponade. Evidence of fluid retention, ranging from peripheral oedema to anasarca, is characteristic of constrictive pericarditis, but is less common and less severe in tamponade.

10.2   Laboratory findings

Imaging has been discussed extensively in preceding sections. Of course, impressive cardiomegaly would favour tamponade. In both conditions, respiratory variation in ventricular inflow are increased, but in tamponade ventricular filling continues throughout diastole, whereas in constrictive pericarditis it is limited to the first third of diastole. In tamponade, systemic venous return is limited to the ejection period of systole when cardiac volume is minimal and therefore pericardial pressure is a little less. In constriction, flow peaks are present in systole and early diastole. Thus, the dip-and-plateau configuration of ventricular diastolic pressure is an important diagnostic finding in constriction, but is not seen in tamponade.

11.   DIAGNOSIS AND DIFFERENTIAL DIAGNOSIS

In severe and advanced cases, the cause of anasarca must be elucidated. The error of diagnosing hepatic cirrhosis is still prevalent in spite of many warnings in the literature (*Van der Merwe, Dens, Daenen, 2000*). Patients in the advanced stages of the disease certainly look like patients with cirrhosis of the liver and have many of the same complaints. To compound the problem, liver function tests are abnormal, serum albumen is low in patients who have the complication of protein losing enteropathy (*Kumpe, Jaffe, Waldmann 1975*) and liver biopsy may show "cardiac cirrhosis." This error can be avoided by careful attention to the height and pressure contour of the jugular pressure. If doubt remains, an abdominal scan or an echocardiogram will resolve it, because in constriction severe enough to cause massive oedema, the inferior vena cava is greatly dilated. Other possible sources of confusion include the nephrotic syndrome, lymphoedema and idiopathic oedema (*Kuchel and Ethier 1998*). Significant pulmonary venous hypertension is not a feature of any of these conditions.

11.1 Distinguising constrictive pericarditis from restrictive cardiomyopathy

Restrictive cardiomyopathy is a subset of the large set of diastolic dysfunction due to heart diseases of many aetiologies. Most cases of diastolic dysfunction of cardiac aetiology would be recognised as such by a competent clinician, and so-called restrictive ventricular filling pattern is by no means synonymous with restrictive cardiomyopathy. The group designated as restrictive cardiomyopathy earned its name because the cases so closely simulate constrictive pericarditis. In these cases, the heart is not enlarged or hypertrophied, diastolic dysfunction is often extreme, the physical examination is identical to that in constrictive pericarditis, and the two conditions have many hemodynamic abnormalities in common (*Ammash, Seward, Bailey 2000*).

A lot of recent writing focuses on laboratory studies applicable to cases where the distinction is difficult. In many instances, however, the differentiation is not difficult; it therefore behooves the clinician to approach the question along traditional lines and order special studies, when needed, in the context of information gleaned from the initial evaluation. In many instances the special tests are only confirmatory, but in others they are critical for arriving at the correct diagnosis. Although the problem of this differential diagnosis does not arise frequently in the clinical practice of cardiology, the correct answer is, for obvious reasons, critically important. Here I must mention that the most difficult therapeutic as well as diagnostic decisions revolve around cases who have both constrictive pericarditis and myocardial damage.

11.1.1   History

The history can be very helpful. Evidence of a past history of pericarditis or pericardial effusion points strongly to constrictive pericarditis. Any systemic disease that often involves the pericardium or prior chest injury (see aetiology) is a good clue to constrictive pericarditis. Ionising radiation often injures the pericardium but is a leading cause of mixed pericardial and myocardial injury. Neoplastic disease with clinically manifest cardiovascular manifestations is much more likely to cause constrictive pericarditis than myocardial dysfunction. Anything suggesting amyloidosis (*Meaney, Shabetai, Bhargava 1976*), glycogen storage disorder (*Kushwaha, Fallon, Fuster 1997*), haemochromatosis (*Wasserman, Richardson, Baird 1962*), or the presence of a cardiac allograft (*Hinkamp, Sullivan, Montoya 1994*) makes the diagnosis of constrictive pericarditis extremely improbable. Both constrictive pericarditis and restrictive cardiomyopathy may be "idiopathic." The hypereosinophilic syndromes may also cause restrictive cardiomyopathy (*Ommen, Seward, Tajik 2000*).

11.1.2   Clinical examination

By definition this is unlikely to be helpful, but pulsus paradoxus would make constrictive pericarditis the more likely diagnosis. There are abnormalities that strongly suggest cardiomyopathy, but other abnormalities may be found in either condition. Thus bundle branch block, especially left, atrio-ventricular conduction delay, or pathological Q waves would indicate the likelihood of myocardial over pericardial disease. On the other hand, inversion or flattening of the T waves and deviation of the ST segment from the baseline are not specific and may be the only abnormalities in restrictive cardiomyopathy. Evidence of left atrial enlargement or atrial fibrillation may be found in either condition. Low voltage also may be seen in both conditions. The paradoxical presence of low voltage but greatly increased thickness of the left ventricular myocardium is an important clue to the diagnosis of cardiac amyloidosis (*Carroll, Gaasch, McAdam 1982*).

11.1.3   Chest radiography

Like the electrocardiogram, this may or may not be helpful, but it can be virtually diagnostic. A dense ring of pericardial calcification will convince the clinician that the patient has constrictive pericarditis, not restrictive cardiomyopathy. Absence of calcification of the pericardium is of no help either way. After these enquiries the diagnosis may have become apparent, but in a number of cases the results are ambiguous.

11.1.4   Other imaging modalities

The next logical step is to image the pericardium, for which purpose computer-assisted tomography is usually the simplest and most convenient, but equally satisfactory measurements can be obtained by magnetic resonance or trans-oesophageal echocardiography. An abnormally thick or calcified pericardium is incontrovertible evidence of constrictive pericarditis but, as with the electrocardiogram and the chest radiogram, failure to find the pathognomonic change does not exclude the possibility of constrictive pericarditis. Indeed, pericardial thickness is normal in some 20 percent of cases.

Both the images and the Doppler may furnish crucial information, much of it based on the aforementioned presence of enhanced ventricular interdependence in constrictive pericarditis, but not in restrictive cardiomyopathy in which interdependence, if anything, is less than normal because the septa are involved in the cardiomyopathy and therefore are less capable of responding to even the normally occurring increased or decreased load on one or other side.

Impressive biatrial enlargement speaks strongly for restrictive cardiomyopathy. Other features favouring this diagnosis are left ventricular hypertrophy or pseudohypertrophy, and glittering or other abnormal appearance of the myocardium, as in cardiac amyloidosis. Early diastolic notching of the ventricular septum should be absent in restrictive cardiomyopathy. Of greater significance in restrictive cardiomyopathy, respiration does not cause reciprocal changes in left and right ventricular dimension, and the septal bounce is absent, but is a key finding in constrictive pericarditis in which ventricular interdependence is an important feature of the pathophysiology. Rapid increase in left ventricular dimension followed by little or no further increase in mid- and late-diastole is found in both conditions, since in both, compliance in early diastole is normal, but in later diastole is greatly decreased.

The presence or absence of enhanced ventricular interdependence dictates that exaggerated and reciprocal respiratory variation in the velocity of ventricular inflow should be anticipated in constrictive pericarditis, but not in restrictive cardiomyopathy (Figure 28). While this is generally true, the respiratory variation may be normal in 10 to 20 percent of the cases of constrictive pericarditis. This number can be improved upon by lowering preload by means of head-up tilting, and seeking this finding in the pulmonary veins, where it is more sensitive. If a patient with restrictive cardiomyopathy has laboured breathing for another reason such as asthma or chronic obstructive lung disease, respiratory variation in ventricular inflow is increased.

Both constrictive pericarditis and restrictive cardiomyopathy are characterised by the "restrictive pattern," which really indicates high ventricular diastolic pressure. Peak velocity of the early diastolic E wave usually exceeds 100 mm/sec, and the peak velocity of the diminutive A wave is characteristically less than 400 mm/sec. The E wave deceleration time is very short in both diseases, more so in restrictive cardiomyopathy. It is impossible to tell the two patterns apart by this means alone.

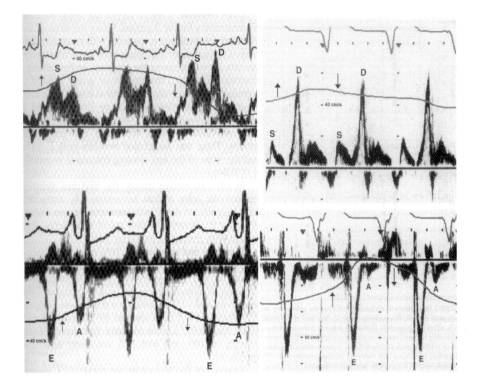

Figure 28: **Left:** Constrictive pericarditis. TEE of the left pulmonary venous flow (top) and mitral inflow (bottom). The respiratory variation of systolic (S) flow is 27% and diastolic (D) flow is 43%. Respiratory variation of mitral peak early (E) filling velocity (bottom) is less, but clearly excessive, at 15%. **Right:** Restrictive cardiomyopathy. Respiratory variation of pulmonary venous flow (top) and mitral inflow (bottom) is within normal limits. Up arrows = inspiration, down arrows = expiration. (From Rajagopalan, Garcia, Rodriguez 2001, with permission)

Attention must also be paid to flow in the systemic veins. Spectral flow in the superior vena cava is seen from the jugular notch and in a hepatic vein in the subcostal imaging plane. As is the case with the pulmonary veins, flow and velocity should be dominantly systolic in normal subjects. In patients with diastolic dysfunction, including both constrictive pericarditis and restrictive cardiomyopathy, flow and velocity are dominant in diastole. In both conditions flow reversals are appreciably greater than the normal maximum of 20 percent. In constriction, however, the reversals are mostly during expiration, but in restrictive cardiomyopathy reversals are mostly in inspiration.

The traditional Doppler indices used to distinguish impaired early diastolic relaxation from restriction of ventricular filling by reduced ventricular compliance, while they constituted a notable advance and proved clinically useful, have important limitations that have been recognised for several years. Transmitral blood flow is influenced by atrial as well as ventricular compliance, mitral inertance, and left atrial pressure.

The Doppler ventricular filling pattern is a function of both early relaxation and ventricular compliance. During progressive left ventricular dysfunction, the diastolic pressure and therefore left atrial pressure increase, with the result that the velocity of early rapid filling denoted by the amplitude of the E wave increases until it exceeds the amplitude of the A wave. This phenomenon, termed *pseudonormalisation (Appleton, Hatle, Popp 1988)*, is often an intermediate stage of progression from delayed relaxation to frank restriction (*Whalley, Doughty, Gamble, 2002*). When good quality Doppler records of pulmonary flow are available, increased atrial reversal velocity may help tell normal from pseudonormal, but is unreliable in children and young adults in whom early diastolic filling is so rapid that the pattern simulates restriction (the reason for the physiological third heart sound). Colour M mode and tissue Doppler (*Palka, Lange, Donnelly 2000*) measure the velocity of blood flow from the left ventricular inflow area toward the apex, and the velocity of myocardial motion respectively. These parameters are relatively insensitive to load and therefore are helpful in distinguishing between pseudonormal and truly normal, and between constrictive pericarditis and restrictive cardiomyopathy (*Garcia, Thomas, Klein 1998*).

In constrictive pericarditis, diastolic compliance is reduced by the pericardial lesion, but myocardial velocity is supernormal; therefore, propagation of blood from the mitral orifice toward the left ventricular apex is not slow, but is more rapid than normal. The Doppler signal of transmitral blood flow has a tall, narrow E wave depicting rapid inflow to the left ventricle, and the colour M mode depicts rapid intraventricular transit of blood. The two signals are thus congruent. In restrictive cardiomyopathy, on the other hand, while blood enters the left ventricle with great rapidity, it traverses slowly towards the apex. This slow transit is demonstrated by colour M mode. In restrictive cardiomyopathy, the transmitral Doppler E wave looks like that of constrictive pericarditis, but the colour M mode is entirely different; the transmitral signal and the colour M mode signals are discordant (Figure 29).

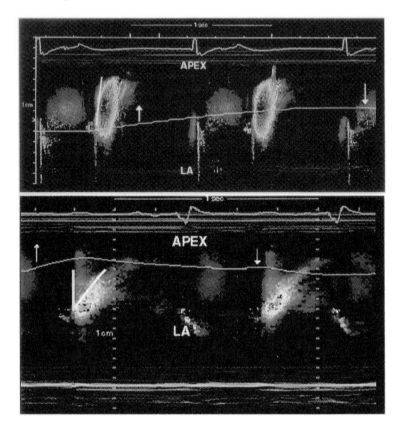

Figure 29: Black and white representation of colour M-mode echocardiography of diastolic flow from the left atrium (LA) toward the left ventricular apex. **TOP:** *constrictive pericarditis;* **BOTTOM:** *restrictive cardiomyopathy. Up arrows on respirometer tracing = inspiration, down arrows = expiration. The flow propagation slope of the first aliasing contour (white line) is steep in constrictive pericarditis, but the slope is considerably slower in restrictive cardiomyopathy. (From Rajagopalan, Garcia, Rodriguez 2001, with permission)*

Tissue Doppler measures the velocity of myocardial contraction and relaxation, not blood flow velocity. Myocardial velocity associated with early rapid relaxation is recorded as a tissue E wave (E_m or E'). Myocardial movement caused by atrial contraction is recorded as a wave synchronous with the transmitral A wave (A_m or A'). In constrictive pericarditis E and E_m are both prominent and considerably larger than A and A_m. In restrictive cardiomyopathy, the scarred and relatively non-compliant myocardium cannot move rapidly or far; therefore E_m is diminutive; that is, E and E_M are not congruent (Figure 30). It has been shown for patients with heart failure, but not pericardial disease, that a ratio E/E_m above 15 identifies a high left ventricular diastolic pressure. In constrictive pericarditis, E_m is deep, and the high myocardial velocity that it depicts is helpful in recognizing that a patient is more likely to have constriction than restriction. The deep E_m in constrictive pericarditis is due to exaggerated longitudinal movement of the mitral annular region. The more severe the constriction, and thus the left ventricular diastolic pressure, the deeper the E_m. The consequence is that in constrictive pericarditis, the ratio E/E_m correlates *inversely* with left ventricular diastolic pressure, so-called annulus paradoxus (*Ha, Oh, Ling 2001*). The principal echo-Doppler images used to separate cardiac tamponade from constrictive cardiomyopathy have been reviewed in a recent publication (*Asher and Klein 2002*).

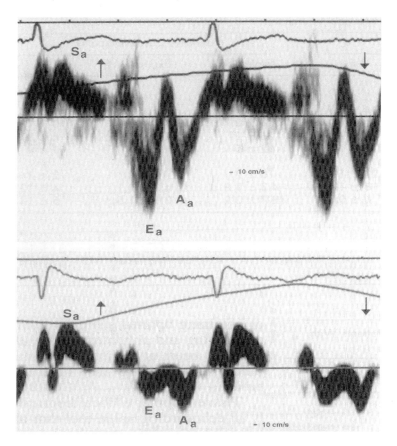

Figure 30: Tissue Doppler in constrictive pericarditis (top) and restrictive cardiomyopathy (below), with respirometer tracing (inspiration, up arrow). Peak systolic velocities are 10 cm/sec in both. The early diastolic velocity is 15 cm/sec in constrictive pericarditis but only 5 cm/sec. in restrictive cardiomyopathy. (From Rajagopalan, Garcia, Rodriguez 2001)

11.1.5   Cardiac catheterisation

When the left and right ventricular pressures differ by more than five mmHg, and scrupulous attention has been paid to technique, restrictive cardiomyopathy is the most probable diagnosis (Figure 31). It is important, however, to emphasise that the two ventricular diastolic pressures are equal in many, perhaps most, cases of restrictive cardiomyopathy. Equal diastolic pressures in the two ventricles, therefore, must never be taken as absolute evidence for constrictive pericarditis, as was shown in a landmark paper in which the invasive hemodynamic of 16 patients with severe constrictive pericarditis were compared with 17 patients with severe restrictive cardiomyopathy and the results of endomyocardial biopsy were reported (*Schoenfeld, Supple, Dec 1987*). In this study, the hemodynamics were identical in both groups. The cardiac index averaged 2.5 ml/m^2, right atrial pressure was 15 mmHg, the ejection fraction was 59, and pulmonary arterial systolic pressure did not exceed 50 mmHg, regardless of the diagnosis. Likewise, equilibration of the ventricular diastolic pressures was found in both groups. Biopsy disclosed the cause of cardiomyopathy in 15 of the 38 patients: 11, amyloidosis and 4, myocarditis. The dip-and-plateau configuration of ventricular diastolic pressure, as shown in Figure 31, depicts the pull-back tracing from a woman with cardiac amyloidosis.

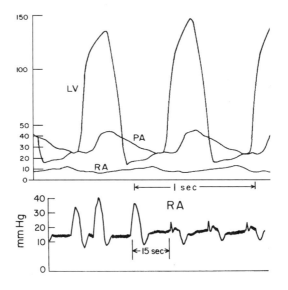

Figure 31: **Top:** Left ventricular, right atrial and pulmonary pressures in a case of restrictive cardiomyopathy. Right atrial pressure is elevated, but is substantially lower than left ventricular diastolic pressure. **Bottom:** Ventricular diastolic pressure contour identical to constrictive pericarditis.

I recommend endomyocardial biopsy in any case in which the correct differential diagnosis has not been made after completion of all the available diagnostic tests, but not when the diagnosis has been clearly established.

11.1.5.1 Provocative tests

Mention of rapid infusion of a large volume of fluid to bring out the hemodynamics of constrictive pericarditis has already been made (see occult constrictive pericarditis). It would seem logical to predict that in patients with restrictive cardiomyopathy, the infusion would unbalance the equal ventricular diastolic pressures in the ventricles. Infusion, as well as the post-extrasystolic response and pacing have been tested in small numbers of patients with variable results; consequently, we lack information on their value.

12. TREATMENT

Not every patient with constrictive pericarditis needs a pericardiectomy. When the right heart filling pressure is less than 10 mmHg, the patient can safely be watched and treatment can be delayed until there is a further increase in central venous pressure, dyspnoea, fatigue, or evidence of fluid retention. I usually do not recommend pericardiectomy for patients who have no, or minimal symptoms who do not require diuretic, or strict limitation of fluid intake. Patients with proven constrictive pericarditis but less than the expected elevation of central venous pressure, but have oedema, fatigue or dyspnoea should have good exercise tolerance, demonstrated by objective exercise testing before withholding pericardiectomy.

In elderly patients with far advanced disease the operative risk is significantly higher and the outcome of pericardiectomy much less satisfactory. It is then advisable to encourage participation in the decision by the patient, the family, and personal physician. All should understand that neither the quality of life nor the survival would necessarily be better than with medical treatment. Medical management thus is appropriate when the disease is too mild to merit operative treatment, or too far advanced to anticipate a high probability of success. These classes of patients will be described separately, as their medical management is obviously quite different.

12.1   Mild or early constrictive pericarditis

Patients who are symptom free and whose exercise tolerance is not significantly impaired do not need drug treatment. A moderately reduced sodium intake should be the first step for patients with oedema. When the response to modifying the diet is not satisfactory, diuretic therapy constitutes the best management for patients with symptoms and signs, and for those with somewhat higher venous pressure who are unwilling to accept, or wish to postpone operative treatment. The dose should be enough to remove most oedema. The need for escalating doses, or adding potent agents like metolazone signals the need to reconsider pericardiectomy. Vasodilators, beta adrenergic antagonists and inotropic agents have no place in the treatment regimen, except that digoxin can be used as help to manage atrial fibrillation.

12.2   Late stage disease

Patients in the advanced stage of the disease who refuse or are not accepted for operation present a more difficult problem. Often the pericardium is heavily calcified and the cardiac rhythm is atrial fibrillation. Much larger doses of diuretic and combinations of diuretics with differing sites of action in the nephron are needed, a difficulty compounded by poor absorption due to gastrointestinal congestion. Spironolactone in diuretic doses can be a useful adjunct. An excellent means of treating severe refractory anasarca is ultrafiltration (*Ronco, Bellomo, Ricci 2001*). This option deserves serious consideration.

Atrial fibrillation should be treated with drugs to regulate the heart rate and with anticoagulants. Cardioversion is unlikely to be successful and these patients would not be candidates for ablation therapy or atrio-ventricular node modification.

12.3   Pericardiectomy

12.3.1   Historical background

A detailed history of pericardiectomy can be found in a text on the history of thoracic surgery (*Meade 1961*). The idea was first considered, as early as 1649, by Riolanus, famous for his disagreements with William Harvey. In France, Weill predicted: "It will one day come within the province of surgery to deliver the heart from the shell that strangles it." In the early part of the last century, the ever flamboyant Viennese thoracic surgeon Sauerbruch resected a portion of the pericardium for a patient bedridden with dyspnoea and generalised oedema. The real impact, however, in the U.S. followed Churchill's description of his first pericardiectomy (*Churchill, 1929*), which was the first such operation to be performed there. The Hunterian lecture delivered by Holmes Sellors in 1944 to the Royal College of Surgeons is a classic on the aetiology and treatment of constrictive pericarditis.

12.3.2   Indications

Standard treatment is pericardiectomy, which should be as complete as possible. The operation is recommended for most patients whose central venous pressure has reached the range of 12 to 15 mmHg. Pressures appreciably higher than that call for surgery in every case, unless there is an overriding contraindication. When venous pressure is even higher, the operation becomes urgent. Another urgent indication is hepatic dysfunction, when it can be proven that the cause is passive congestion, not intrinsic liver disease.

12.3.3   Relative contraindication

The question of what to do with patients with "end-stage" constrictive pericarditis has already been raised. Constrictive pericarditis resulting from prior mantle radiation requires even finer clinical judgement. Almost all surgical series published in the literature point out that, because of associated myocardial injury, the operative risk is greater in these patients and that the result may be disappointing. The critical question then is how severe and how extensive is the myocardial scar; for upon this depends the surgical outcome. I advise endomyocardial biopsy. It is possible that quantitative assessment of the fibrosis would be helpful, as has been done to assess prognosis in the cardiomyopathies, but I am not aware of data pertaining to the suitability of patients with radiation-induced constrictive pericarditis for pericardiectomy. Increased levels of atrial naturetic peptide were found in a series of patients who had received radiation treatment for Hodgkins' lymphoma or mammary carcinoma, compared with controls (*Wondergem, Strootman, Frolich 2001*) but, surprisingly, the series included no instances of constrictive pericarditis. Magnetic resonance imaging, as used for assessing myocardial viability, may prove useful for quantifying myocardial post-radiation damage (*van der Wall, Vliegen, de Roos 1996*).

12.3.4   Operative details and results

Preoperatively, it is important not to administer excessive doses of diuretic, because reducing the central venous pressure below 10 or so cm in severe cases is detrimental. The lungs usually are not severely congested and a degree of peripheral oedema, or small serous effusion, is well tolerated. When the operation is performed for late stage disease, manifest by anasarca, cachexia, or liver dysfunction with low serum albumin, intravenous hyperalimentation is sometimes recommended to optimise the patient's condition before operation, but achieving the desired nutritional and fluid balance is difficult.

Most surgeons use median sternotomy, although some prefer anterior thoracotomy. Cardiopulmonary bypass must always be ready, but may not need to be used in cases with little or no calcification and in whom fibrosis is not dense. Cardiopulmonary bypass is used in other cases, probably a large majority, and is essential when visceral pericardiectomy has to be done. In this connection, I deplore the term epicardium when the visceral pericardium is meant, because it encourages the idea that the inner layer of the pericardium is not amenable to resection. In a significant proportion of cases, it is the visceral pericardium that constricts and must be resected, despite the fact that the dissection plane between the visceral pericardium and the epicardium requires expert dissection. Stripping as completely as possible the visceral pericardium is much preferred over the "waffle procedure" in which tension of the visceral pericardium is decreased by multiple incisions (*Kao and Chang 2001)*. The best results are obtained from radical pericardiectomy in which the pericardium is resected anteriorly between the phrenic nerves from the level of the great vessels to the diaphragm, along the left lateral border posterior to the phrenic nerve, inferiorly along the diaphragmatic surface and posteriorly up to the atrio-ventricular ring. The presence of an open coronary graft, especially an internal mammary artery, adds to the operative risk. Bilateral anterior thoracotomy with splitting of the sternum is then a safer operative approach (*Okamoto, Morita, Fujimoto 1998)*. Bypass grafting can be done at the same time as pericardiectomy (*Sugimoto, Ogawa, Asada 1996*).

The last two decades have witnessed a progressive decline in the operative risk, the mortality in good hands now being approximately 5 percent (*DeValeria, Baumgartner, Casale 1991)*. The outcome of pericardiectomy in 58 surgically confirmed cases showed, as had many previous studies, that the maximal benefit may not be seen for several months (*Senni, Redfield, Ling 1999)*. At three months, echo-Doppler investigation of these patients showed either constrictive or restrictive physiology in 45 and 19 percent respectively. At 21 months, the percentages were 34 and 9, an improvement, but still a matter for concern. As in other series, many of the patients with evidence of restriction had been operated on for radiation-induced constrictive pericarditis. Again, concordant with other studies, advanced age, severe disease, and chronicity correlated with less satisfactory outcomes.

12.3.5 Complications

In a minority of patients, significant left ventricular systolic dysfunction may follow pericardiectomy and may persist for several months. The causes of this syndrome are not known but, like the slow improvement in diastolic function, may be related to the sudden removal of a strong external constraining force on the atrophic myocardium *(Dines, Edwards, Burchell 1958)*. It responds to standard treatment for heart failure and, in my experience, always eventually resolves. Mitral and tricuspid regurgitation may worsen after pericardiectomy *(Johnson, Bauman, Josephson, 1993)*.

References

Adolph RJ, Frommer JC. A transducer for recording the instantaneous respiratory waveforms in animals and man. J Appl Physiol 1966; 21:737-740.

Akasaka T, Yoshida K, Yamamuro A, Hozumi T, Takagi T, et al. Phasic coronary flow characteristics in patients with constrictive pericarditis: comparison with restrictive cardiomyopathy. Circulation 1997; 96:1874-1881

Albers WH, Hugenholtz PG, Nadas AS. Constrictive pericarditis and atrial septal defect, secundum type. With special reference to left ventricular volumes and related hemodynamic findings. Am J Cardiol 1969; 23:850-857

Alexander J, Kelley MJ, Cohen LS, Langou RA. The angiographic appearance of the coronary arteries in constrictive pericarditis. Radiology 1979; 131:609-617

Almassi GH, Chapman PD, Troup PJ, Wetherbee JN, Olinger GN. Constrictive pericarditis associated with patch electrodes of the automatic implantable cardioverter-defibrillator. Chest 1987; 8:369-371

Ammash NM, Seward JB, Bailey KR, Edwards WD, Tajik AJ. Clinical profile and outcome of idiopathic restrictive cardiomyopathy. Circulation. 2000; 101:2490-2496

Andrews GWS, Pickering GW Sellors TH. The aetiology of constrictive pericarditis with special reference to tuberculous pericarditis, together with a note on polyserositis. Q J Med 1948; 17:291-321

Appleton CP, Hatle LK, Popp RL. Relation of transmitral flow velocity patterns to left ventricular diastolic function: new insights from a combined hemodynamic and Doppler echocardiographic study. J Am Coll Cardiol 1988; 12:426-440.

Asher CR, Klein AL. Diastolic heart failure: restrictive cardiomyopathy, constrictive pericarditis, and cardiac tamponade: clinical and echocardiographic evaluation. Cardiol Rev 2002; 10:218-229.

Boonyaratavej S, Oh JK, Tajik AJ, Appleton CP, Seward JB. Comparison of mitral inflow and superior vena cava Doppler velocities in chronic obstructive pulmonary disease and constrictive pericarditis. J Am Coll Cardiol 1998; 32:2043-2048.

Brown DL, Ivey TD. Giant organized pericardial hematoma producing constrictive pericarditis: a case report and review of the literature. J Trauma 1996; 41:558-560.

Brown DL, Luchi RJ. Cardiac tamponade and constrictive pericarditis complicating endoscopic sclerotherapy. Arch Intern Med 1987; 147:2169-2170

Bush CA, Stang JM, Wooley CF, Kilman JW. Occult constrictive pericardial disease. Diagnosis by rapid volume expansion and correction by pericardiectomy. Circulation. 1977; 56:924-930.

Cameron J, Oesterle SN, Baldwin JC, Hancock EW. The etiologic spectrum of constrictive pericarditis. Am Heart J 1987; 113:354-360.

Carroll JD, Gaasch WH, McAdam KPWJ: Amyloid cardiomyopathy: characterization by a distinctive volume/mass relation. Am J Cardiol 1982; 49:9-13.

Chevers N. Observations on the diseases of the orifice and valves of the aorta. Guys Hosp Rep 1842; 7:387-439)

Churchill ED: Decortication of the heart for adhesive pericarditis. Arch Surg 1929; 19:1457-1469.

Cooper DK, Cleland WP, Bentall HH. Collagen diseases as a cause of constrictive pericarditis. Thorax. 1978; 33:368-371.

Crake T, Sandle GI, Crisp AJ, Record CO. Constrictive pericarditis and intestinal haemorrhage due to Whipple's disease. Postgrad Med J 1983; 59:194-195

Davies D, Andrews MI, Jones JS. Asbestos induced pericardial effusion and constrictive pericarditis. Thorax. 1991; 46:429-432.

DeValeria PA, Baumgartner WA, Casale AS, Greene PS, Cameron DE, et al. Current indications, risks, and outcome after pericardiectomy. Ann Thorac Surg 1991; 52:219-224.

Dines DE, Edwards JE, Burchell HB. Myocardial atrophy in constrictive pericarditis. Proceedings of the Staff Meetings of the Mayo Clinic. 1958; 33:93-99

Engel PJ, Fowler NO, Tei CW, Shah PM, Driedger HJ, et al. M-mode echocardiography in constrictive pericarditis. J Am Coll Cardiol 1985; 6:471-474.

Gaasch WH, Peterson KL, Shabetai R. Left ventricular function in chronic constrictive pericarditis. Am J Cardiol 1974; 34:107-110

Garcia MJ, Thomas JD, Klein AL. New Doppler echocardiographic applications for the study of diastolic function. J Am Coll Cardiol 1998; 32:865-875

Ha JW, Oh JK, Ling LH, Nishimura RA, Seward JB, et al. Annulus paradoxus: transmitral flow velocity to mitral annular velocity ratio is inversely proportional to pulmonary capillary wedge pressure in patients with constrictive pericarditis. Circulation 2001; 104:976-978.

Hancock EW. Effusive constrictive pericarditis. In Pericardial Diseases, PS Reddy, DF Leon JA Shaver (eds). pp 357-369. Raven Press, 1980, New York.

Hancock EW. Subacute effusive-constrictive pericarditis. Circulation 1971; 43:183-192.

Hanley PC, Shub C, Lie JT. Constrictive pericarditis associated with combined idiopathic retroperitoneal and mediastinal fibrosis. Mayo Clin Proc 1984; 59:300-304

Hansen AT, Eskildsen P, Götzsche H. Pressure curves from the right auricle and the right ventricle in chronic constrictive pericarditis. Circulation 1951; 3:881-888

Himelman RB, Kircher B, Rockey DC, Schiller NB. Inferior vena cava plethora with blunted respiratory response: a sensitive echocardiographic sign of cardiac tamponade. J Am Coll Cardiol 1988; 12:1470-1477

Hinds SW, Reisner SA, Amico AF, Meltzer RS. Diagnosis of pericardial abnormalities by 2D-echo: a pathology-echocardiography correlation in 85 patients. Am Heart J 1992; 123:143-150.

Hinkamp TJ, Sullivan HJ, Montoya A, Park S, Bartlett L, et al. Chronic cardiac rejection masking as constrictive pericarditis. Ann Thorac Surg 1994; 57:1579-1583

Hoit BD. Pericardial heart disease. Curr Probl Cardiol 1997; 22:353-400.

Holt JP, Rhode EA, Kines H. Pericardial and ventricular pressure. Circ Res 1960; 8:1171-1181.

Hou HD. A case of heart amyloidosis accompanied by chronic pericarditis and calcification within the amyloid. Chin Med J (Engl) 1983; 96:549-550

Hurrell DG, Nishimura RA, Higano ST, Appleton CP, Danielson GK, et al. Value of dynamic respiratory changes in left and right ventricular pressures for the diagnosis of constrictive pericarditis. Circulation 1996; 93:2007-2013.

Ilia R, Weizman S, Gueron M. Effects of rapid volume expansion on the right filling pressures after prosthetic valve surgery. Cathet Cardiovasc Diagn 1991; 23:169-171.

Johnson TL, Bauman WB, Josephson RA. Worsening tricuspid regurgitation following pericardiectomy for constrictive pericarditis. Chest 1993; 104:79-81.

Johnston SD, Johnston PW, O'Rourke D. Carcinoid constrictive pericarditis. Heart 1999; 82:641-643.

Kao CL, Chang JP. Modified method for epicardial constriction: the electric-Waffle procedure. J Cardiovasc Surg (Torino) 2001; 42:643-646.

Keogh BE, Oakley CM, Taylor KM. Chronic constrictive pericarditis caused by self-mutilation with sewing needles. A case report and review of published reports. Br Heart J 1988; 59:77-80

Kessler R, Follis F, Daube D, Wernly J. Constrictive pericarditis from Nocardia asteroides infection. Ann Thorac Surg 1991; 52:861-862

Khan MA, Noah MS, Al-Saddique A, Sharaf el-Deane MS. Constrictive pericarditis as a complication of closed chest injury. Injury 1988; 19:39-40

Klein AL, Cohen GI, Pietrolungo JF, White RD, Bailey A, et al. Differentiation of constrictive pericarditis from restrictive cardiomyopathy by Doppler transesophageal echocardiographic measurements of respiratory variations in pulmonary venous flow. J Am Coll Cardiol 1993; 22:1935-1943.

Klodas E, Nishimura RA, Appleton CP, Redfield MM, Oh JK. Doppler evaluation of patients with constrictive pericarditis: use of tricuspid regurgitation velocity curves to determine enhanced ventricular interaction. J Am Coll Cardiol 1996; 28:652-657.

Kuchel O, Ethier J. Extreme diuretic dependence in idiopathic edema: mechanisms, prevention and therapy. Am J Nephrol 1998; 18:456-459

Kumpe DA, Jaffe RB, Waldmann TA, Weinstein MA. Constrictive pericarditis and protein losing enteropathy. An imitator of intestinal lymphangiectasis. Am J Roentgenol Radium Ther Nucl Med 1975; 124:365-373

Kushwaha SS, Fallon JT, Fuster V. Restrictive cardiomyopathy. *New Engl Med J* 1997; 336:267-276

Kussmaul A: Ueber schwielige Mediastino-Pericarditis und den paradoxen Puls. Berliner *Klinische Wochenschrift* 1878; 10:461-464

Kutcher MA, King SB 3rd, Alimurung BN, Craver JM, Logue RB. Constrictive pericarditis as a complication of cardiac surgery: recognition of an entity. Am J Cardiol 1982; 50:742-748

Levine HD. Myocardial fibrosis in constrictive pericarditis: electrocardiographic and pathologic observations. Circulation 1973; 48:1268-1281.

Ling LH, Oh JK, Breen JF, Schaff HV, Danielson GK, et al. Calcific constrictive pericarditis: is it still with us? *Ann Intern Med* 2000; 132:444-450.

Ling LH, Oh JK, Schaff HV, Danielson GK, Mahoney DW, et al. Constrictive pericarditis in the modern era: evolving clinical spectrum and impact on outcome after pericardiectomy. Circulation 1999; 100:1380-1386.

Ling LH, Oh JK, Tei C, Click RL, Breen JF, et al. Pericardial thickness measured with transesophageal echocardiography: feasibility and potential clinical usefulness. J Am Coll Cardiol 1997; 29:1317-1323

Lorell B, Leinbach RC, Pohost GM, Gold HK, Dinsmore RE, Hutter AM Jr, Pastore JO, Desanctis RW. Right ventricular infarction. Clinical diagnosis and differentiation from cardiac tamponade and pericardial constriction. Am J Cardiol 1979; 43:465-471.

Lui CY, Makoui C. Severe constrictive pericarditis as an unsuspected cause of death in a patient with idiopathic hypereosinophilic syndrome and restrictive cardiomyopathy. Clin Cardiol 1988; 11:502-504.

Magna P, Vythilingum S, Mitha AS. Pulsatile hepatomegaly in constrictive pericarditis. Br Heart J 1984; 52:465-467.

McRorie ER, Wright RA, Errington ML, Luqmani RA. Rheumatoid constrictive pericarditis. Br J Rheumatol 1997; 36:100-103.

Meade RH. Surgery of the pericardium, in A History of Thoracic Surgery. Springfield Illinois, Charles C Thomas, 1961.

Meaney E, Shabetai R, Bhargava V, Shearer M, Weidner C, et al. Cardiac amyloidosis, constrictive pericarditis and restrictive cardiomyopathy. *Am J Cardiol* 1976; 38:547-556.

Mounsey P. The early diastolic sound of constrictive pericarditis. Br Heart J 1955; 17:143-152

Nishimura RA. Constrictive pericarditis in the modern era: a diagnostic dilemma. Heart 2001; 86:619-623.

Nishimura RA, Kazmier FJ, Smith HC, Danielson GK. Right ventricular outflow obstruction caused by constrictive pericardial disease. Am J Cardiol 1985; 55:1447-1448

Oh JK, Hatle LK, Seward JB, Danielson GK, Schaff HV, et al. Diagnostic role of Doppler echocardiography in constrictive pericarditis. J Am Coll Cardiol 1994; 23:154-162

Oh JK, Tajik AJ, Appleton CP, Hatle LK, Nishimura RA, et al. Preload reduction to unmask the characteristic Doppler features of constrictive pericarditis. A new observation. Circulation 1997; 95:796-799.

Oh KY, Shimizu M, Edwards WD, Tazelaar HD, Danielson GK. Surgical pathology of the parietal pericardium: a study of 344 cases(1993-1999). Cardiovasc Pathol 2001; 10:157-168.

Okamoto H, Morita S, Fujimoto K, Niimi T, Yasuura K. The "T-shaped" thoracotomy for pericardiectomy after midline crossed IMA grafting. J Thorac Cardiovasc Surg 1998; 46:97-98.

Ommen SR, Seward JB, Tajik AJ. Clinical and echocardiographic features of hypereosinophilic syndromes. Am J Cardiol. 2000; 86:110-113

Oren RM, Grover-McKay M, Stanford W, Weiss RM. Accurate preoperative diagnosis of pericardial constriction using cine computed tomography. J Am Coll Cardiol 1993; 22:832-838

Palka P, Lange A, Donnelly JE, Nihoyannopoulos P. Differentiation between restrictive cardiomyopathy and constrictive pericarditis by early diastolic doppler myocardial velocity gradient at the posterior wall. Circulation 2000; 102:655-662.

Panchal P, Adams E, Hsieh A. Calcific constructive pericarditis: a rare complication of CREST syndrome. Arthritis Rheum 1996; 39:347-350

Ptacin MJ. Uremic constrictive pericarditis: case report. Mil Med 1983; 148:603-605.

Rajagopalan N, Garcia MJ, Rodriguez L, Murray RD, Apperson-Hansen C, et al. Comparison of new Doppler echocardiographic methods to differentiate constrictive pericardial heart disease and restrictive cardiomyopathy. Am J Cardiol 2001; 87:86-94.

Ramsey HW, Sbar S, Elliott LP, Eliot RS. The differential diagnosis of restrictive myocardiopathy and chronic constrictive pericarditis without calcification. Value of coronary arteriography. Am J Cardiol 1970; 25:635-638

Ronco C, Bellomo R, Ricci Z. Hemodynamic response to fluid withdrawal in overhydrated patients treated with intermittent ultrafiltration and slow continuous ultrafiltration: role of blood volume monitoring. Cardiology 2001; 96:196-201.

Sagrista-Sauleda J, Permanyer-Miralda G, Candell-Riera J, Angel J, Soler-Soler J. Transient cardiac constriction: An unrecognized pattern of evolution in effusive acute idiopathic pericarditis. Am J Cardiol 1987; 59:961-966.

Schoenfeld MH, Supple EW, Dec GW Jr, Fallon JT, Palacios IF. Restrictive cardiomyopathy versus constrictive pericarditis: role of endomyocardial biopsy in avoiding unnecessary thoracotomy. Circulation 1987; 75:1012-1017.

Schrire V, Gotsman MS, Beck W. Unusual diastolic murmurs in constrictive pericarditis and constrictive endocarditis. Am Heart J 1968; 76:4-12.

Sechtem U, Tscholakoff D, Higgins CB. MRI of the abnormal pericardium. AJR Am J Roentgenol 1986;147:245-252.

Senni M, Redfield MM, Ling LH, Danielson GK, Tajik AJ, et al. Left ventricular systolic and diastolic function after pericardiectomy in patients with constrictive pericarditis: Doppler echocardiographic findings and correlation with clinical status. J Am Coll Cardiol 1999; 33:1182-1188.

Shabetai R. Diseases of the pericardium, In: Hurst's, The Heart. RW Alexander, R Schlant, V Fuster, eds., 9th edition, New York, McGraw Hill, 1994. pp 2169-2203.

Shabetai R, Fowler NO, Fenton JC, Masangkay M. Pulsus paradoxus. J Clin Invest 1965; 44:1882-1898.

Shabetai R, Grossman W. Profiles in constrictive pericarditis, restrictive cardiomyopathy and cardiac tamponade, in Cardiac Catheterization and Angiography, 2nd edition. Wm Grossman (ed.). Philadelphia, Lee & Febiger, 1980

Spodick DH. Etiologic spectrum of constrictive pericarditis. Am Heart J 1987; 114:1529-1530

Spodick DH. The normal and diseased pericardium: current concepts of pericardial physiology, diagnosis and treatment. J Am Coll Cardiol 1983; 1:240-251

Stanley RJ, Subramanian R, Lie JT. Cholesterol pericarditis terminating as constrictive calcific pericarditis. Follow-up study of patient with 40 year history of disease. Am J Cardiol 1980; 46:511-514

Sugimoto T, Ogawa K, Asada T, Mukohara N, Higami T, et al. Pericardiectomy and coronary artery bypass grafting for constrictive pericarditis after heart surgery. Jpn Circ J 1996; 60:177-180

Sun JP, Abdalla IA, Yang XS, Rajagopalan N, Stewart WJ, et al. Respiratory variation of mitral and pulmonary venous Doppler flow velocities in constrictive pericarditis before and after pericardiectomy. J Am Soc Echocardiogr 2001; 14:1119-1126.

Tabata T, Kabbani SS, Murray RD, Thomas JD, Abdalla I, et al. Difference in the respiratory variation between pulmonary venous and mitral inflow Doppler velocities in patients with constrictive pericarditis with and without atrial fibrillation. J Am Coll Cardiol 2001; 37:1936-1942.

Tamir R, Pick AJ, Theodor E. Constrictive pericarditis complicating dermatomyositis. Ann Rheum Dis 1988; 47:961-963.

Tei C, Child JS, Tanaka H, Shah PM. Atrial systolic notch on the interventricular septal echogram: an echocardiographic sign of constrictive pericarditis. J Am Coll Cardiol 1983; 1:907-912

van der Wall EE, Vliegen HW, de Roos A, Bruschke AV. Magnetic resonance techniques for assessment of myocardial viability. J Cardiovasc Pharmacol 1996; 28(Suppl 1):S37-44.

Vandenbossche JL, Jacobs P, Decroly P, Primo G, Englert M. Significance of inspiratory premature opening of pulmonic valve in constrictive pericarditis. Am Heart J 1985;110:896-898

Van der Merwe S, Dens J, Daenen W, Desmet V, Fevery J. Pericardial disease is often not recognised as a cause of chronic severe ascites. J Hepatol 2000; 32:164-169.

Wasserman AJ, Richardson DW, Baird CL, Wyso EM. Cardiac hemochromatosis simulating constrictive pericarditis. Am J Med 1962; 32:316-323

Whalley GA, Doughty RN, Gamble GD, Wright SP, Walsh HJ, et al. Pseudonormal mitral filling pattern predicts hospital re-admission in patients with congestive heart failure.J Am Coll Cardiol 2002; 39:1787-1795.

White CS. MR evaluation of the pericardium. Top Magn Reson Imaging 1995; 7:258-266

Wondergem J, Strootman EG, Frolich M, Leer JW, Noordijk EM. Circulating atrial natriuretic peptide plasma levels as a marker for cardiac damage after radiotherapy. Radiother Oncol 2001; 58:295-301.

Chapter 7

PULSUS PARADOXUS
Respiratory effects on hemodynamics

1. HISTORICAL BACKGROUND

Knowledge of respiratory variation of the amplitude of the pulse in pericardial disease dates back a long way. Some early observers of this phenomenon had remarkably "modern" ideas concerning the underlying mechanisms. In 1619, when describing the case of a young woman with constrictive pericarditis, Lower (See Chapter 6) stated, "...the pulse was weak and *intermittent,"* and that "...the pericardium had become thick, opaque and almost callous." He concluded that the movement of the diaphragm during breathing was the reason why the pulse disappeared during inspiration. This conclusion brought him close to the mechanism of pulsus paradoxus proposed by *Auenbrugger (1958), Dock (1961)* and *Wood 1961),* but subsequently disproved (*Shabetai, Fowler, Fenton 1965).*

The term, pulsus paradoxus, was introduced into clinical medicine by Adolf Kussmaul (*Kussmaul 1873),* a reproduction of whose original smoked drum tracing appears in Figure 1. Vierodt had reported a weaker pulse during inspiration in a case of purulent pericarditis in 1854 in his book *Die Lehre Vom Arterien.* In Kussmaul's patients, however, pulsus paradoxus was total, which is to say that the pulse disappeared entirely at the height of inspiration. The heartbeat remained regular; therefore the paradox to which Kussmaul was referring was a regular heartbeat with an irregular pulse. This was an unfortunate use of the term paradoxical, because in clinical medicine, it usually refers to a response opposite from normal, as for example in paradoxical splitting of the second heart sound. Systemic arterial pressure normally declines during inspiration, but pulsus paradoxus is an exaggerated drop in the pressure when the patient inspires, not, as the term implies, a decrease when an increase would be normal.

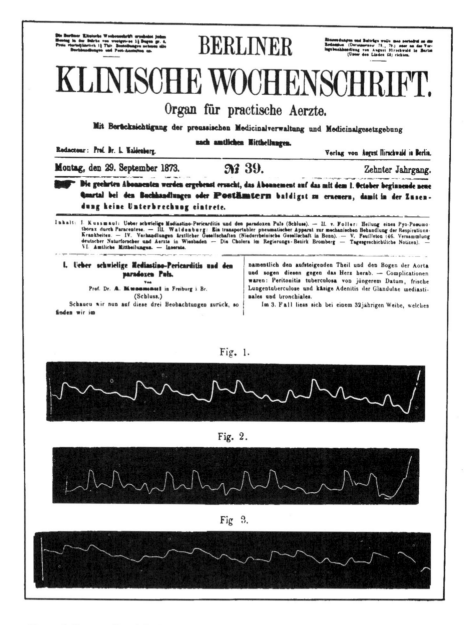

Figure 1. Kussmaul's original tracings on a smoked drum illustrating three cases of pulsus paradoxus

2. DEFINITION

A commonly employed definition is a drop in systolic blood pressure exceeding 10 mmHg (*Fowler 1976*). This value is somewhat arbitrary, depending as it does on the pattern and depth of respiration, but is useful. A definition that takes into consideration the blood pressure (*Reddy 1978)* is given by

((Expiratory systolic pressure) - (inspiratory systolic pressure)) x 100/ (expiratory systolic pressure).

This more rigorous definition is, however, not often used, because the more established one has the sanction of long custom, the advantage of simplicity and it has proved practical.

3. MEASUREMENT

The ideal is to measure pulsus paradoxus with an intra-arterial needle or cannula, find the highest and lowest systolic and diastolic pressures over several respiratory cycles, and average the results. More often, sphygmomanometry suffices for clinical purposes. The measurement must be made with the patient breathing as normally as possible. It is an error to have the patient increase the depth of respiration, as this manoeuvre exaggerates the degree of respiratory variation of the blood pressure.

Severe pulsus paradoxus can be recognized by palpation of the radial or another pulse by diminution or disappearance during inspiration, but when considering the diagnosis or following the course of cardiac tamponade, an objective measure is needed.

The method for measuring pulsus paradoxus by sphygmomanometry is to inflate the cuff to a pressure that eliminates the brachial pulse and all blood pressure sounds. The cuff is next *slowly* deflated until the first Korotkoff sound becomes audible. Deflation should then proceed slowly and evenly while respiratory movements are observed or palpated. At first the Korotkoff sound is heard only during expiration, but as deflation continues it becomes audible throughout the respiratory cycle. Pulsus paradoxus is present when the difference in systolic pressure between these two points exceeds 10 mmHg, and may range from slightly above 10 to more than 40 mmHg.

4.   PATHOPHYSIOLOGY

Pulsus paradoxus attracted the attention of many clinicians and physiologists for much of the last century. In a classic paper, Katz and Gauchat *(1924)* postulated that, in the normal condition, inspiration would have little effect on the net (transmural) filling pressure of the right heart, but that during cardiac tamponade, net filling pressure would decrease because of failure to transmit the full effect of the inspiratory pressure drop of the thorax to the pericardium.

The authors used a canine model of acute tamponade to test this hypothesis. The animals were breathing spontaneously after recovering from thoracotomy when catheters were placed in the pleural and pericardial spaces to measure the pressures using optical devices or reading the level of menisci in glass tubes. In the control state, pleural and pericardial pressures fell to the same extent with inspiration, but after raising pericardial pressure by injecting fluid into the space, intrapericardial pressure fell substantially less than intrapleural pressure (Figure 2).

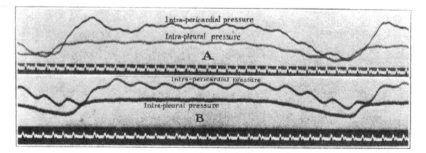

Fig. 12 (Exper. 315-10, 15).—Simultaneous optical records of intrapleural and pericardial pressures. *A*, control, no saline in pericardium; *B*, 70 c.c. of saline in pericardium. Time in tenths of a second.

	Intrapleural Pressure (in Mm. of Saline)			Intrapericardial Pressure (in Mm. of Saline)		
	Inspiration, Mm.	Expiration, Mm.	Variation, Mm.	Inspiration, Mm.	Expiration, Mm.	Variation, Mm.
A...................	—60	—24	36	—60	—25	35
B...................	—56	—16	40	+36	+56	20

Figure 2. Control, respiratory variation of intrapleural pressure was 3.6 cm H_2O and in pericardial pressure 3.5 cm H_2O. In tamponade, respiratory variation in intrapleural pressure was 4 cm H_2O, but in pericardial pressure it was only 2 cm H_2O. (From Katz and Gauchat, 1924, with permission)

To test the significance of this observation, they measured pressure in an extrapericardial region of the superior vena cava, comparing it with right atrial pressure. They found that the two pressures fell to an equal extent in the control condition, but in tamponade, right atrial pressure fell less, thus the pressure head (gradient) responsible for right heart filling was less during inspiration than during expiration (Figure 3).

Katz and Gauchat considered that with the instrumentation available to them, it would be too difficult to perform the equivalent studies on the left side of the heart to demonstrate that inspiration also creates an unfavourable pressure gradient from the pulmonary veins to the left atrium when tamponade is present. They postulated, however, that this was the probable mechanism of pulsus paradoxus.

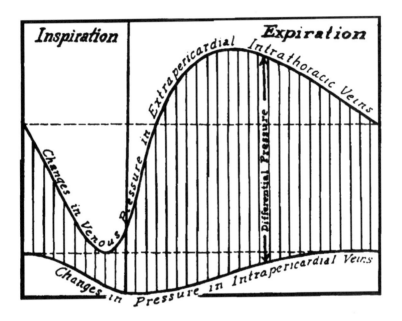

Figure 3. Another illustration from Katz and Gauchat that they used to illustrate their hypothesis regarding the effect of respiration on the filling pressure of the right heart during cardiac tamponade.

It should be noted that the hypothesis proposed by Katz and Gauchat did not allow for the possibility and, in fact, excluded the possibility that systemic venous return increases during inspiration in spite of the elevated pericardial pressure that defines cardiac tamponade. Furthermore, in spite of one's admiration for their classic study, one must concede that their system for measuring pressure differences was probably not accurate enough, considering that the differences were in the range of only one or two cm of water. Subsequent studies have shown that the mechanism proposed by Katz and Gauchat was a contributory one and not the chief cause of pulsus paradoxus.

4.1   Competition for space in the pericardium

That inspiration is associated with an increase in systemic venous return was appreciated by investigators who were among the first to explain pulsus paradoxus on the basis of competition between the two sides of the heart for room in the pericardial space that is invariable throughout the cardiac cycle in tamponade; in other words, ventricular interdependence (*Dornhorst, Howard, Leathart, 1952*). They therefore rejected the hypothesis that when a patient with cardiac tamponade inspires, the effective filling pressure of the right heart falls. They accepted the view that left ventricular filling is impaired by cardiac tamponade, but their explanation for this phenomenon differed from that of Katz and Gauchat. Instead, they proposed that the increase of systemic venous return distended the right heart, thereby increasing pericardial pressure, and it was this increase in pericardial pressure that reduced left ventricular filling. In their own words, "Increased filling of one ventricle will increase intrapericardial pressure and hence tend to hinder filling of the other. With inspiration, the intrapericardial pressure starts to fall, but does not fall as far as the intrathoracic pressure, because of increased right ventricular filling. Decreased left ventricular filling thus occurs." They confirmed their clinical observations and their resulting theory using a mechanical model (Figure 4). Thin rubber represented the ventricles and relatively elastic plastic sheeting represented the pericardium. These elements were contained in a box, and pressure in the box could be lowered to simulate inspiration. By this means, they confirmed the hypothesis that when the right ventricle is enlarged, intrapericardial pressure is increased, which adversely affects filling of the left ventricle.

4.2   The pulmonary vein to left heart pressure gradient

An invasive study of a patient with malignant effusive constrictive pericarditis was carried out to determine whether inspiration lessens the pressure gradient responsible for left ventricular filling in patients with cardiac tamponade (*Sharp, Bunnell, Holland 1960*). The authors measured the relation between pulmonary wedge pressure and pericardial pressure as a surrogate for left atrial pressure during several levels of cardiac tamponade, induced by injecting fluid into an indwelling pericardial catheter that had been placed in order to obviate frequent needle pericardiocenteses. They confirmed that inspiration decreased the pressure gradient progressively as the severity of tamponade was increased.

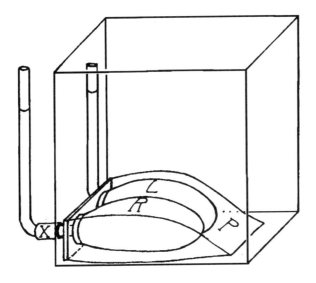

Figure 4. Model constructed by Dornhorst et al. When pressure in the "pericardium" P was slack, lowering pressure in the box caused increased filling of R, but no change in L. When the "pericardium" was made taut by filling it with fluid, lowering the box pressure caused an emptying of L. This effect was abolished when the entry to R was clamped at X.

The data are difficult to interpret because the patient's pericardium was heavily invaded by tumour. We now know that constriction effectively prevents transmission of intrathoracic pressure changes to the pericardium and heart. It is therefore not possible to determine to what extent tamponade contributed to this finding in this particular patient.

An ingenious study used imaging of pulmonary venous flow long before the development of Doppler cardiography (*Golinko, Kaplan, Rudolph 1963*). The aim of this study again was to investigate the possibility that in cardiac tamponade, a disturbance of the pressure gradient between the pulmonary venous pressure and left atrial pressure during inspiration was the cause of pulsus paradoxus in cardiac tamponade. They used spontaneously breathing dogs in which catheters had been placed in the left atrium, a pulmonary vein, and the pericardium. Intrathoracic pressure was estimated via an oesophageal balloon, or was measured via an intrapleural catheter.

In this study, tamponade greatly reduced respiratory fluctuations of pericardial pressure that became similar to left atrial pressure. Pulmonary venous pressure was slightly higher than left atrial pressure throughout the respiratory cycle, but slightly more during expiration. With tamponade, left atrial and pericardial pressures usually fluctuated less than pulmonary venous pressure with respiration. During inspiration, pulmonary venous pressure was equal to or, in some cases, lower than left atrial pressure.

The contrast employed was oil. In the controls, oil injected into the inferior vena cava moved towards the right atrium during all phases of respiration, but with maximal velocity during inspiration. Before inducing cardiac tamponade, following injection into the left pulmonary vein, the droplets moved in the antegrade direction in all phases of respiration, but with maximum velocity during expiration. During tamponade sufficient to cause pulsus paradoxus, however, movement of the droplets was reduced throughout the respiratory cycle and was virtually halted, or even reversed during inspiration. In one instance, the investigators injected a substantial volume of the oil into the left atrium, allowing them to observe its motion for several respiratory cycles. The globule remained entirely within the left atrium during expiration, but during inspiration, the globule moved retrograde towards the pulmonary veins. The authors concluded that tamponade prevents effective transmission of intrathoracic pressure variations to the pericardium and therefore, during inspiration, the pressure gradient from pulmonary veins to left atrium is diminished. They further concluded that this is the mechanism of pulsus paradoxus in cardiac tamponade.

The angiographic portion of their study is frequently cited in papers on the mechanism of pulsus paradoxus in tamponade. Their explanation did not include ventricular interdependence and seems not to have taken into consideration the role of increased systemic venous return. They concluded, as had Katz and Gauchat in 1924, that the decrease in the pressure gradient from the pulmonary veins to the left heart was simply that tamponade blocks transmission of respiratory variation of thoracic pressure to the pericardium and left heart. They did not discuss the alternative possibility that the reason that the pulmonary vein to left heart pressure gradient falls during inspiration is that the simultaneous increase in right heart volume raises pericardial pressure, thereby impeding left heart filling via chamber interdependence. This latter explanation is the major cause of the pulsus paradoxus of tamponade. A decline in the pressure head for left heart filling does, however, contribute.

4.3   Role of the diaphragm

Wenckebach, better known to most readers for his studies on atrioventricular conduction, wrote concerning pulsus paradoxus in cardiac tamponade, "The more the diaphragm and the chest wall try to move apart from each other, the more the heart is caught in the squeezer" (*Wenckebach 1910*). This explanation was endorsed by the late Paul Wood, who made seminal contributions to the clinical interpretation of hemodynamics:

"During inspiration, descent of the diaphragm stretches the already taut pericardium and increases the pressure within it; cardiac filling is then impaired and stroke volume and pulse pressure fall" (*Wood 1961*). Typically, Wood cited no evidence or publication to support a conclusion that to him seemed obvious.

This theory was subsequently tested experimentally (*Dock 1961*). For Dock's experiment, the pericardium of fresh human cadavers was cannulated and connected to a 1-litre fluid-filled bottle and manometer. By raising the bottle, the pericardium was filled with a known volume and the resulting pressure was measured. At any given point, the bottle could be clamped off, and a change in pressure, caused by lifting the sternum or pulling down on the central tendon of the diaphragm, could be measured. With the pericardium empty, and all pericardial pressures at less than 10 cm H_2O, there was little effect from either lifting the sternum forward, or pulling the diaphragm down. When pericardial pressure was increased to 10 cm H_2O, lifting the sternum still had no appreciable effect on pericardial pressure, but pulling the diaphragm down increased pericardial pressure by a further 4 cm H_2O. Pericardial pressure was then raised to 20 cm H_2O by adding more fluid from the bottle. Pulling down 3 or 4 cm on the diaphragm without moving the sternum increased pericardial pressure another 12 to 22 cm H_2O. Thus, simulating inspiration by pulling the diaphragm down, when the pericardium was slack, had no effect on pericardial pressure; however, when the pericardium had been rendered taut by fluid injection in amounts sufficient to raise pericardial pressures to levels comparable to those seen in severe tamponade, tugging down the diaphragm increased pericardial pressure considerably (Figure 5).

4.4   Stroke volume

Pulsus paradoxus in cardiac tamponade is a drop in systolic and pulse pressures during inspiration, with little or no change in diastolic pressure, a finding that suggested to many investigators that left ventricular stroke volume also declines with inspiration. This hypothesis was subsequently proven in our laboratory (*Shabetai, Fowler, Gueron 1963*) (Figure 6). By the end of the 1960s, although there were many competing theories to explain pulsus paradoxus in tamponade, there was general agreement that pulse pressure and stroke volume decline, pulmonary venous pressure falls less than left heart chamber pressures, and right heart volume increases during inspiration.

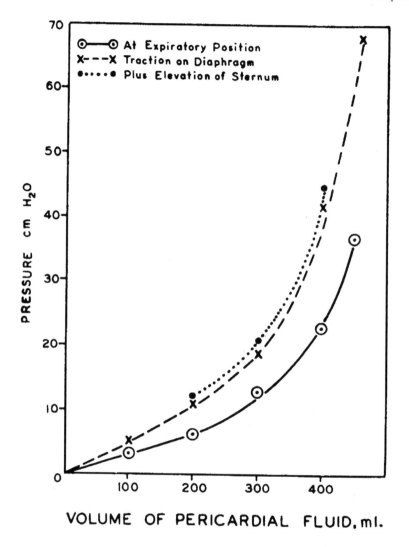

Figure 5. A figure from Dock's study carried out to prove that inspiratory descent of the diaphragm is the cause of pulsus paradoxus. He postulated that this action should increase the severity of cardiac compression during inspiration and this is the reason why pulsus paradoxus is a finding in cardiac tamponade. (From Dock, 1961, with permission)

On the other hand, the reason why pulmonary venous pressure declines more than left atrial pressure during inspiration had not been clarified, the importance of inspiratory increase in systemic venous return had not been worked out, and the contribution of inspiratory descent of the diaphragm had not been established. Fowler and Shabetai, therefore, initiated studies to address these issues.

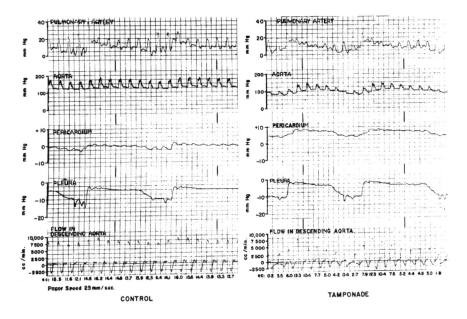

Figure 6. Aortic pressure and flow in a canine model of acute cardiac tamponade. **Left:** control, **Right:** tamponade. (From Shabetai, Fowler, Gueron 1963, with permission)

We and others have also shown increased respiratory variation in stroke volume corresponding with pulsus paradoxus in patients with cardiac tamponade or constrictive pericarditis (Figure 7).

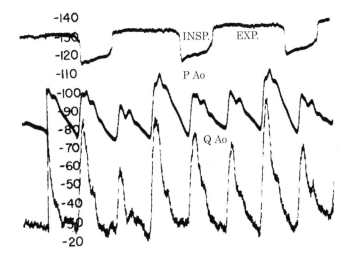

Figure 7. A case of constrictive pericarditis with pulsus paradoxus, shown in the records of aortic pressure (PAo) and stroke volume (Qao).

4.5   The effect of inspiration on systemic venous return

Inspiration in normal subjects lowers pressure in the thorax and in the intrathoracic portion of the great veins, and also in the pericardium and the cardiac chambers, increasing filling from the extrathoracic venous reservoirs. Right ventricular stroke volume increases during inspiration, but the augmented right ventricular stroke volume does not arrive at the aorta for another two or three cardiac cycles. Thus, in general, pulmonary arterial pressure and right ventricular stroke volume increase during inspiration and aortic pulse pressure and left ventricular pericardial pressure decrease with inspiration. In cardiac tamponade, inspiration has the same hemodynamic effect on right heart filling as in normal subjects. If, in cardiac tamponade, pulsus paradoxus were *only* a matter of competition for room in a fixed pericardial volume, aortic and pulmonary arterial peak systolic pressures would be exactly 180° out of phase. Other factors influence these pressures, so they are often nearly, but not precisely, 180° out of phase (Figure 8). In addition, recent literature has emphasised that, in patients with strong ventricular interdependence, the first beat that occurs after the onset of inspiration is characterised by minimal left-sided peak systolic pressure, and maximal right-sided peak systolic pressure. It should be understood, however, that the correlation of respiration and hemodynamics also depends on the rate and pattern of respiration and on the phase relation of the respiratory cycle to the cardiac cycle.

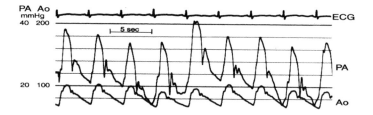

Figure 8. A case of tamponade showing nearly, but not exactly, 180° phase difference between left and right ventricular systolic pressures. The inspiratory change in stroke volume can be inferred from the decrease in aortic pulse pressure.

We studied the effects of respiration on the velocity of blood flow in the superior and inferior venae cavae, using snugly fitted electromagnetic flow probes, before and after inducing acute tamponade. Blood flow velocity in both venae cavae increased during inspiration, both in control and with tamponade. Superior vena caval flow increased 61 percent in control and 47 percent with tamponade. Inferior vena caval flow increased 53 percent in control and 62 percent with tamponade. The heart rate did not increase, because the anaesthetic was Pentothal sodium (Figure 9).

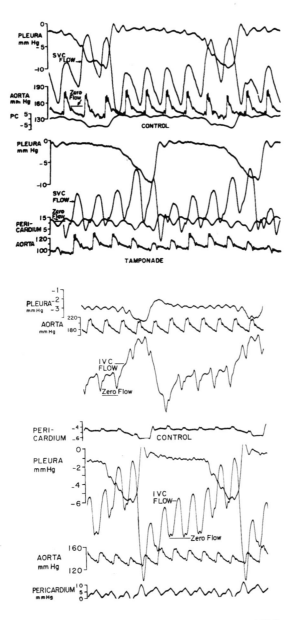

Figure 9. The effect of inspiration on systemic venous return **TOP:** superior caval flow, **Bottom:** inferior caval flow. The tracings show marked increase in flow during inspiration in both cavae in tamponade as well as in control. (From Shabetai, Fowler, Fenton 1965, with permission)

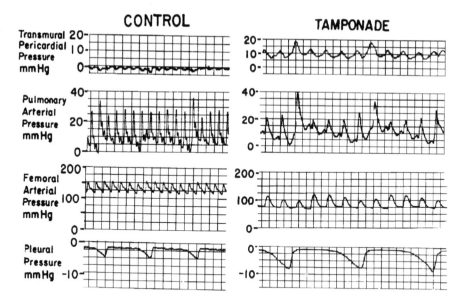

Figure 10. Transmural pericardial pressure in cardiac tamponade. In the control, there is no significant change in transmural pericardial pressure with respiration, but in tamponade, transmural pericardial pressure increases with inspiration. Note also that, in tamponade, the respiratory variation of femoral arterial and pulmonary arterial pressure is close to but not precisely 180° out of phase. (From Shabetai, Fowler, Fenton 1965, with permission)

Increase in transmural pericardial pressure is critically important to our understanding of cardiac tamponade. We and many other investigators have consistently documented this phenomenon by simultaneously recording pleural and pericardial pressures (*Shabetai, Fowler, Fenton 1965*) (Figure 10).

Having shown that cardiac tamponade does not limit respiratory variation of systemic venous return, we performed a canine experiment in which we used an extracorporeal pump to see whether pulsus paradoxus would not occur if we prevented respiratory variation of systemic venous return (Figure11). Systemic venous return was diverted from the venae cavae to an open dependent reservoir after ligating the azygos vein. The effluent from the reservoir was returned to the right to the superior vena cava by a totally occlusive sigmamotor pump via a cannula directed towards the right atrium. The only violation of the pericardial sac was the insertion of two tiny polyethylene tubes, one to allow infusion of fluid to induce tamponade and the other to record pericardial pressure. The right heart bypass tubing, the pericardial tubes and a chest tube were brought out by stab wounds in an intercostal space. The thoracotomy was closed, the skin and muscles were secured in airtight fashion around the tubes, and free air was aspirated from the pleura.

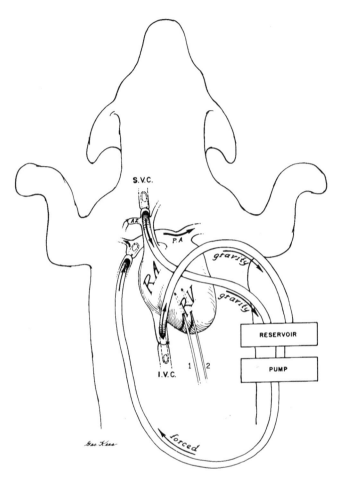

Figure 11. Closed chest preparation employed for studies with controlled constant venous return to the right atrium. 1 and 2 denote the pericardial tubes.

Several hours after the dogs had resumed spontaneous respiration, with constant venous return, and both low and high flow rates, raising pericardial pressure even to 20 mmHg did not increase respiratory variations in aortic pressure (Figure 12). This experiment finally disproved the Katz hypothesis that the cause of pulsus paradoxus in tamponade is solely an inspiratory drop in the pressure gradient from the pulmonary veins to the left ventricle, due to failure of the inspiratory decline to transmit through the pericardial effusion, and that inspiratory increase in systemic venous return has nothing to do with it, being prevented by tamponade. Indeed, the experiment shows that when the inspiratory increase in right heart volume is prevented, by making systemic venous return constant, the drop in pleural and pericardial pressures is equal, that is to say, the inspiratory increase in transmural pericardial pressure characteristic of cardiac tamponade no longer occurs.

Since the dogs were breathing spontaneously, diaphragmatic descent was present, disposing of Dock's theory of the mechanism of pulsus paradoxus. We proved conclusively that, in tamponade, pulsus paradoxus does not occur without respiratory variation in systemic venous return. The data support the view that respiratory variation is the dominant mechanism causing pulsus paradoxus in cardiac tamponade via cardiac chamber interdependence.

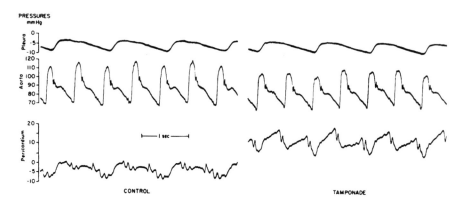

Figure 12. The effects of cardiac tamponade on aortic pressure when systemic venous return is held constant. In control, a pleural pressure decline of 4.5 mmHg during inspiration is accompanied by a fall in systolic aortic pressure of 7 mmHg. During tamponade, pericardial pressure is elevated 14 mmHg above control: during inspiration, pleural pressure falls 4.5 mmHg, and aortic systolic pressure falls 8 mmHg. Transmural pericardial pressure did not change with respiration. Blood flow was 48 ml/K/min. (From Shabetai, Fowler, Fenton, 1965, with permission)

4.6   Simulating the hemodynamic effects of respiration

Our next step was to simulate the hemodynamic effect of inspiration during a period of apnoea. We did the study in open chest dogs, employing the same modified right heart bypass we had used to study the effects of abolishing respiratory variation in systemic venous return. Pressure was measured in the pericardium, the aorta and the pulmonary artery. After a steady state lasting at least several minutes, the respirator was disconnected for a brief period, and approximately 10 ml of blood was injected into the systemic venous return line to simulate the hemodynamic effect of an inspiration. This intervention caused a prompt increase in pulmonary arterial pressure, followed two or three heartbeats later (representing the pulmonary transit time) by an increase in aortic pressure (Figure 13). At the instant when the pulmonary arterial pressure increased, there was no change in the pressure of the lax pericardium, or in the aorta.

When the experiment was repeated during cardiac tamponade, significant differences in the result were observed. The addition of volume to the venous return line caused a prompt increase in pulmonary arterial pressure, as in the control, but now there was a simultaneous drop in aortic pressure and increase of pressure in the taut pericardium. Thus, the effect of a sudden brief increase in systemic venous return during tamponade was more complex than in control, where it was a simple transit time phenomenon. Augmenting right heart volume caused the pressure in the stretched pericardium to rise and, therefore, aortic pressure fell. This drop in aortic pressure was followed after two or three heartbeats by an increase, larger than in the control, when the augmented right heart output appeared in the aorta.

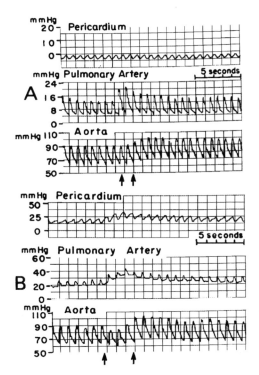

Figure 13. Hemodynamic simulation of inspiration. For description, see text. The arrows indicated the time during which supplemental volume was added to the venous return.

In another group of dogs breathing spontaneously after recovering from instrumentation, we measured pulmonary arterial flow with a snugly fitted electromagnetic probe, and pressure in the left atrium, pleura, pericardium, and aorta. In the controls, pulmonary arterial flow increased 47 percent with inspiration, and in tamponade 84 percent (Figure 14). Also, in the controls, pericardial pressure fell briefly and briskly near the onset of inspiration, and left atrial pressure varied in a more sinusoidal manner with the respiratory cycle. During tamponade, the dogs developed pulsus paradoxus and the fall in left atrial and pericardial pressures was less than in the control state.

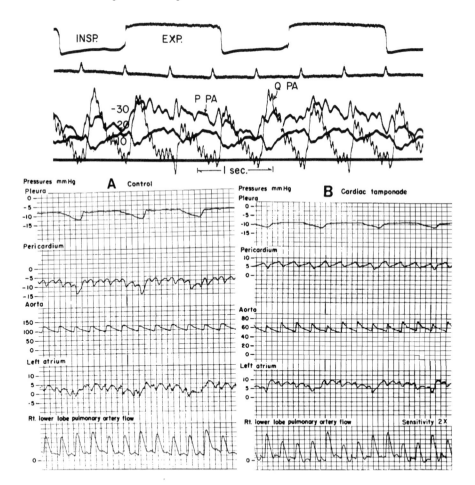

Figure 14. **TOP:** Pulmonary arterial pressure (PPA) and flow (QPA) in a patient with cardiac tamponade; pulmonary arterial flow increases with inspiration. **BOTTOM:** The effect of respiration on flow through a major pulmonary arterial branch in a dog with experimental cardiac tamponade. The inspiratory augmentation of pulmonary flow is greater than in tamponade.

4.7 The effect of leftward bulging of the ventricular septum

In both constrictive pericarditis and cardiac tamponade, the ventricular septum bulges from right to left with inspiration. This positional change, when left ventricular diastolic volume is small, unloads the septum which ceases to assist left ventricular ejection during inspiration. This loss of systolic ventricular interaction has been proposed as another mechanism contributing to pulsus paradoxus in cardiac tamponade (*Savitt, Tyson, Elbeery 1993*).

4.8 Summary and conclusions

(1) Cardiac tamponade does not abolish inspiratory augmentation of systemic venous return. (2) Respiratory variation of systemic venous return is an essential, and probably the most important mechanism causing pulsus paradoxus in cardiac tamponade. (3) The increase in right heart volume that occurs with inspiration does not affect pressure in the normal pericardium but, in the presence of tamponade, the augmented right heart volume causes the pressure in the taut, inelastic pericardium to rise with inspiration. (4) This inspiratory increase in right heart volume lowers the pulmonary vein to left heart pressure gradient that diminishes left heart filling. (5) Inspiratory traction caused by descent of the diaphragm is insufficient to increase pericardial pressure in cardiac tamponade, and thus is not a cause of pulsus paradoxus. (6) Lack of augmentation of left ventricular function by the ventricular septum during inspiration, when it bulges leftward, may also contribute to pulsus paradoxus, at least in tamponade. (7) Pooling in the pulmonary vascular bed does not contribute to pulsus paradoxus.

The last conclusion is warranted because, when systemic venous return was kept constant, the effect of inspiration on aortic pressure did not differ between control and tamponade, even when cardiac output was maintained at a deliberately low level. Furthermore, in contrast to tamponade with normal respiration, when systemic venous return is constant throughout the respiratory cycle, transmural pericardial pressure does not increase during inspiration, a finding also incompatible with the idea that pericardial traction caused by descent of the diaphragm contributes to pulsus paradoxus.

4.9 Transmission of thoracic pressure to the circulation

In addition to the mechanisms discussed thus far, respiratory variation of thoracic pressure is directly transmitted to the heart and circulation. With normal respiration, direct transmission causes fluctuation of systemic and pulmonary arterial pressure of only a few mmHg, and thus its effect on pulsus paradoxus is negligible. When, however, breathing is laboured, as it may be in lung disease or severe heart failure, wide fluctuation of thoracic pressure that can amount to 20 or 30 mmHg, contribute significantly to pulsus paradoxus. To study this aspect of respiratory variation of arterial blood pressure, we performed two experiments.

In the first of these, we modified respiration, either by increasing airways resistance in spontaneously breathing dogs with an endotracheal tube in place, by partially clamping the tube, or by vagotomy. In the dogs with airways obstruction, the respiratory swing of thoracic pressure exceeded 20 mmHg in most of the experiments. Similar changes were recorded in the pericardium, pulmonary artery and aorta (Figure 15 B). In this instance, however, diastolic pressure changed to the same extent as systolic pressure, and therefore pulse pressure was not affected, as it is in cardiac tamponade (Figure 15 C). After vagotomy, without airways obstruction, both phases of respiration were greatly prolonged, and the altered pattern was clearly seen in the pericardium, aorta and pulmonary artery (Figure 15A). The clinical significance of these observations is discussed in a later section.

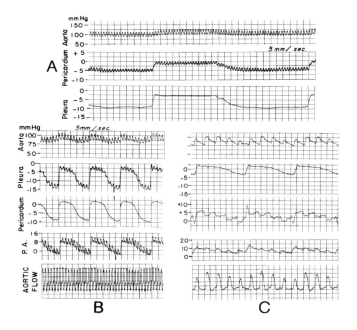

Figure 15. The effect of altered respiration on cardiovascular pressures. For description, see the text. The paper speed was 25 mm/sec for all records. **A**: vagotomy. **B**: tracheal obstruction. **C**: cardiac tamponade. Only tamponade reduced aortic stroke volume.

For the second set of experiments, we made a canine model in which the descending aorta was perfused at a constant rate by a sigmamotor pump, while the ascending aorta was perfused in the normal manner by the left ventricle, and compared respiratory variation of pressure in these isolated vascular beds, both in controls and tamponade. The experimental setup is shown below (Figure 16) but for ease of interpretation, does not indicate that the chest was closed and all tubes were brought to the exterior through tightly sealed stab wounds.

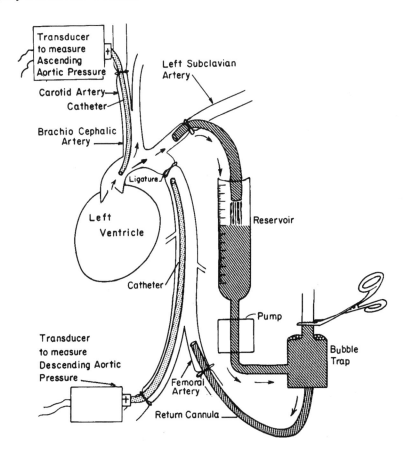

Figure 16. Model used to assess the contribution of thoracic pressure variation to lowering aortic pressure in the controls and during tamponade.

In the controls, respiratory variation of pressure in the ascending and descending aorta both equalled that in pleural pressure. With tamponade, pulsus paradoxus developed in the ascending aorta, but pressure in the descending aorta remained the same as that of pleural pressure (Figure 17).

The contribution of transmission of pressure is small in this example, but clearly would be significant in patients with respiratory distress.

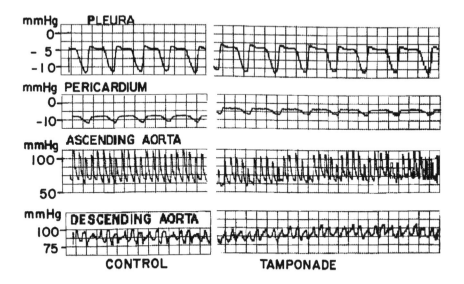

Figure 17. Contribution of transmission of thoracic pressure to aortic respiratory variation in aortic pressure calculated from the model shown in Figure 16.

4.10   Cardiac output

Cardiac output is depressed in severe cardiac tamponade *(Craig, Whalen, Behar 1968)*. An inspiratory drop in stroke volume of a given magnitude therefore represents a higher percentage drop. This proportionate change may be another factor in the genesis of pulsus paradoxus. Another consequence of tamponade is a reduction of ventricular diastolic volume. Therefore, the pressure-volume relation is steep, because the ventricles then operate on the steep portion of the ascending limb of the Starling curve. The increased effects of changing volume on systolic pressure would thus increase, contributing to pulsus paradoxus *(Friedman, Sakurai, Choe* 1980).

4.11   Inspiration and ventricular loading

4.11.1   Clinical implications of the pathophysiology.

Inspiration increases right ventricular preload and stroke volume without an instantaneous effect on left ventricular ejection. Inspiration, by lowering external pressure, also increases transmural pressure; that means that left ventricular afterload increases, and therefore ejection decreases, thereby adding to the other causes of decreased arterial systolic pressure during inspiration (*McGregor 1979*). Inspiration, because it reduces thoracic pressure, can be visualised as lowering the venous reservoir below the level of the arterial reservoirs (Figure 18), obliging the left ventricle to develop more force if it were to achieve the same systolic pressure as in expiration. If the ventricle does not develop additional force, the result is a lower aortic pressure during inspiration.

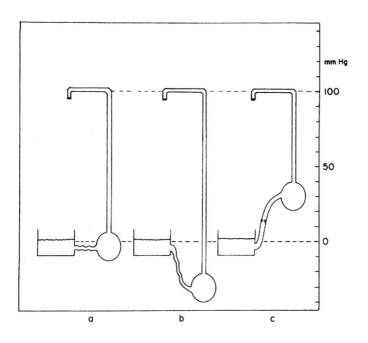

Figure 18. Representation of the effects of changing pleural pressure on right ventricular inflow and left ventricular outflow. **a:** Normal: The heart and lungs are shown as a single pump-oxygenator filled from a venous reservoir at a pressure of 2 mmHg via collapsible tubes. The pump expels blood into the systemic arteries to achieve a pressure head of 100 mmHg. **b:** Müller Manoeuvre: Reducing pleural pressure to minus 30 mm is comparable to lowering the pressure within the heart-lung pump by an equivalent amount relative to the systemic arterial reservoirs. The left ventricle must develop more force to "raise" the pressure of blood to the previous arterial pressure. Filling of the right ventricle is potentiated by the more favourable venous return gradient. **c:** Valsalva Manoeuvre: Elevating the thoracic pressure to 30 mmHg. has the opposite effect. The heart-lung pump has been "raised" relative to the systemic reservoirs. Systolic ejection is facilitated, since less energy is required to raise aortic blood to the level of the previous arterial pressure. Venous return to the right heart is impeded by the adverse gradient. (From McGregor 1979, with permission)

4.11.2   Normal subjects

In healthy adults, ventricular interdependence is weak; therefore, other mechanisms may underlie normal respiratory effects on blood pressure. A study of 30 normal children and young adults, aged between 5 and 47 years, demonstrated reciprocal variation of the right and left ventricle (Figure 19). That result could have been because changes in a single dimension do not necessarily reflect changes in volume, or be due to movement of the heart in relation to the transducer *(Brenner and Waugh, 1978)*. An alternative explanation is that the reciprocal respiratory variation of ventricular dimensions resulted from the transit time from the pulmonary veins to the systemic arteries *(Guntheroth, Morgan, Mullins 1967)*. Pulsus paradoxus has also been reported in normal subjects subjected to 60° head up tilting or rotation in the vertical axis when seated *(Urschel 1967)*.

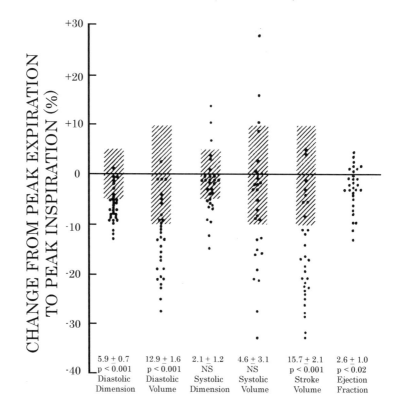

Figure19. Respiratory variation in the dimensions and calculated volumes of the left ventricle in a 17-year-old lad, derived from an M mode echocardiographic study. (From Brenner and Waugh 1978, with permission)

4.12   Absence of anticipated pulsus paradoxus

In a number of conditions, pulsus paradoxus is absent in spite of severe cardiac tamponade. Left ventricular diastolic pressure, elevated beyond pericardial pressure because of other heart disease, is one of the commoner examples, as is late stage renal disease requiring dialysis. Pulsus paradoxus develops when tamponade increases pericardial pressure and the diastolic pressure of both ventricles to the same level. The two ventricles then fill against a common stiffness, but reciprocal variation of systemic and pulmonary venous pressures alternately favour filling of one or the opposite ventricle (*Reddy, Curtiss, O'Toole, 1978*). When another disease has increased left ventricular diastolic pressure to a higher level than the current pericardial pressure, a prerequisite for the development of pulsus paradoxus is absent. In the same way, cardiac tamponade does not cause pulsus paradoxus when right heart failure or right ventricular hypertrophy with right ventricular diastolic pressure exceeds the pressure common to the left ventricle and pericardium. In animal laboratories, heart worms may be the reason for the same phenomenon.

Atrial septal defect is another condition that, when large enough, prevents pulsus paradoxus in spite of tamponade *(Winer and Kronzon 1979)*. The reason is that most of the pulmonary flow is accounted for by the left to right shunt. All of the shunt flow is intrathoracic and therefore does not vary with respiration; thus, respiratory variation of total inflow to the right heart no longer increases significantly with inspiration, removing a prerequisite for pulsus paradoxus in tamponade.

Two mechanisms underlie absence of pulsus paradoxus in patients with severe aortic regurgitation who also have cardiac tamponade. In the first place, this valvular abnormality often increases left ventricular diastolic pressure, and secondly, the regurgitant fraction does not vary with respiration; thus, much of left ventricular filling does not vary with the respiratory cycle. Absence of pulsus paradoxus in cases of dissecting haematoma of the aorta that has progressed retrograde and caused severe aortic regurgitation and acute haemopericardium is important, because the intrapericardial bleeding complicating the dissection may be missed.

5.   PULSUS PARADOXUS IN OTHER CONDITIONS

The features of pulsus paradoxus in experimentally induced airways obstruction, described in Section 4.9, may also apply clinically (Figure 20). We studied patients with chronic obstructive lung disease, measuring pressure and flow in the brachial artery that had been exposed for the purpose of performing coronary arteriography and recording the phase of respiration. We found substantial variation in the pressure, without appreciable change in the flow. Hyperventilation in patients with lung disease may exaggerate the increase in systemic venous return to the extent that reciprocal changes in left and right ventricular dimension are seen during the respiratory cycle. In such cases, right ventricular enlargement occurs during inspiration and, as in tamponade, encroaches on the left ventricle, impairing its filling and emptying, and contributing to pulsus paradoxus *(Settle, Engel, Fowler 1980)*. Pulsus paradoxus is a feature of severe bronchial asthma. It correlates with arterial pCO_2 and has prognostic value, especially in children *(Frey and Freezer 2001)*. Six asymptomatic subjects, prone to asthma, underwent pulmonary function testing, radionuclide angiography and measurement of oesophageal pressure, during normal breathing, asthma induced by inhaling cold air, and loaded respiration *(Blaustein, Risser, Weiss, 1986)*. These investigators concluded that pulsus paradoxus, during periods of increased airways resistance, results from exaggeration of the normal respiratory variation of stroke volume, mediated mostly by the influence of thoracic pressure on the preload of the two ventricles. This conclusion is supported by the demonstration of reciprocal variation of mitral and tricuspid flow in chronic lung disease *(Hoit, Sahn, Shabetai 1986)*. In a study of 12 patients with obstructive lung disease, breathing against increased expiratory and inspiratory load, increased fluctuations of intrathoracic pressure increased left ventricular afterload, causing pulsus paradoxus by the mechanism described by McGregor in 1979 *(Viola, Puy, Goldman 1990)*.

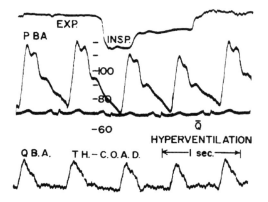

Figure20 Pulsus paradoxus recorded from the brachial artery in a patient with chronic lung disease. Note absence of respiratory variation in brachial arterial blood flow and pulse pressure. Compare with Figure 10 (tamponade).

I was once asked to evaluate cardiac tamponade in a young man with Hodgkin's disease who was admitted for newly discovered cardiomegaly on a chest x-ray, and pulsus paradoxus. On examination, I found a normal jugular pressure, and severe stridor. Examining the chest film more closely, the trachea appeared to be narrowed (Figure 21). Tracheal narrowing was confirmed by a close-up view. The patient received irradiation to shrink the offending lymph nodes. Pulsus paradoxus then disappeared, and thereafter the pericardial effusion resolved spontaneously. The case illustrates the importance of not arriving at a diagnosis only on the basis of two physical signs and a likely aetiology. Simple clinical evaluation rapidly disclosed the correct diagnosis.

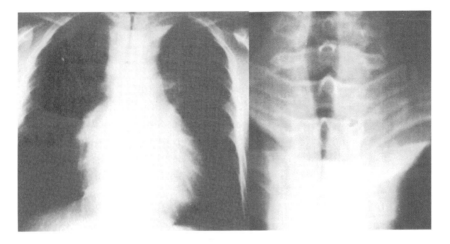

Figure 21. Radiological study of the patient described above. **Left:** anterior-posterior projection of chest x-ray showing apparent cardiomegaly due to pericardial effusion and narrowing of the distal trachea. **Right:** Trachea, close-up.

5.1 Pulmonary embolism

Pulsus paradoxus may be a feature of pulmonary embolism (*Cohen, Kupersmith, Aroesty 1973*). In this condition, there may be an expiratory increase in venous pressure (Kussmaul's venous sign) and pulsus paradoxus, as in some cases of constrictive pericarditis (Figure 22). Cohen et al. suggested that increased respiratory variation of venous return to the left heart is caused by the combination of blockage of the pulmonary arterial tree and depletion of the pulmonary veins. Thus, when inspiration increases the capacity of the pulmonary bed, right ventricular output fails to increase to fill it. The left ventricle is therefore underfilled in inspiration, resulting in pulsus paradoxus.

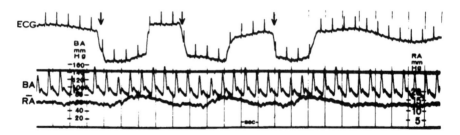

Figure 22. Large pulmonary embolism. Pulsus paradoxus is accompanied by an increase in right atrial pressure. Inspiration: downward deflection of the ECG. Systemic arterial pressure falls and right atrial pressure increases. (From Cohen, Kupersmith, Aroesty 1973, with permission)

5.2 Shock

Shock is another condition in which pulmonary blood flow is drastically reduced. In one study, pulsus paradoxus was found in 30 of 61 patients (*Cohn, Pinkerson, Tristani, 1967*). In the patients with pulsus paradoxus, blood volume and inspiratory right atrial pressure were lower, whereas systemic vascular resistance was higher than in those without this sign. Rapid administration of intravenous fluid abolished pulsus paradoxus, whereas vasoconstrictors accentuated it. To better understand these phenomena, the authors next studied the effects of respiration on flow in the aorta, pulmonary artery and great veins in closed chest, anaesthetised dogs. Upon depleting blood volume, respiratory variation of pulmonary arterial flow disappeared or greatly diminished, but pulsus paradoxus appeared. Thus, depletion of the systemic venous reservoir could no longer supply increased venous return with inspiration and therefore the left ventricle did not increase in volume in early expiration.

References

Auenbrugger L. Novum Inventum Ex Percussione. Vienna, 1761. Quoted by East T. The Story of Heart Disease. Wm Dawson & Sons, Ltd, 1958. p 28.

Blaustein AS, Risser TA, Weiss JW, Parker JA, Holman BL, et al. Mechanisms of pulsus paradoxus during resistive respiratory loading and asthma. J Am Coll Cardiol 1986; 8:529-536.

Brenner JI, Waugh RA. Effect of phasic respiration on left ventricular dimension and performance in a normal population. An echocardiographic study. Circulation 1978; 57:122-127.

Cohen SI, Kupersmith J, Aroesty J, Rowe JW. Pulsus paradoxus and Kussmaul's sign in acute pulmonary embolism. Am J Cardiol 1973; *32:271-275.*

Cohn JN, Pinkerson AL, Tristani FE. Mechanism of pulsus paradoxus in clinical shock. J Clin Invest 1967; 46:1744-1755.

Craig RJ, Whalen RE, Behar VS, McIntosh HD. Pressure and volume changes of the left ventricle in acute pericardial tamponade. *Am J Cardiol* 1968; 22:65-74.

Dock W. Inspiratory traction on the pericardium. *Arch Intern Med* 1961; 108:837-840.

Dornhorst AC, Howard P, Leathart GI. Pulsus paradoxus. *Lancet* 1952; 1:746-748.

Fowler NO. Cardiac Diagnosis and Treatment (ed 2). New York, Harper & Row, 1976. pp 865-866.

Frey B, Freezer N. Diagnostic value and pathophysiologic basis of pulsus paradoxus in infants and children with respiratory disease. Pediatr Pulmonol 2001; 31:138-143

Friedman HW, Sakurai H, Choe SS, Lajam F, Celis A. Pulsus paradoxus: a manifestation of a marked reduction of left ventricular end-diastolic volume in cardiac tamponade. J Thorac Cardiovasc Surg 1980; 79:74-82

Golinko RJ, Kaplan N, Rudolph AM. The mechanism of pulsus paradoxus during acute pericardial tamponade. J Clin Invest 1963; 42:249-257.

Guntheroth WG, Morgan BC, Mullins GL. Effect of respiration on venous return and stroke volume in cardiac tamponade. Mechanism of pulsus parodoxus. Circ Res 1967; 20:381-390

Hoit B, Sahn DJ, Shabetai R. Doppler-detected paradoxus of mitral and tricuspid valve flows in chronic lung disease. J Am Coll Cardiol 1986; 8:706-709.

Katz LN, Gauchat HW: Observations on pulsus paradoxus (with special reference to pericardial effusions). *Arch Intern Med* 1924; 33:371-393.

Kussmaul A. Mediastino-pericarditis und den paradoxen. *Klinische Wochenschrift* 1873; 10:433-464.

McGregor M. Current concepts: pulsus paradoxus. N Engl J Med 1979; 301:480-482

Reddy PS, Curtiss EI, O'Toole JD, Shaver JA. Cardiac tamponade: Hemodynamic observations in man. *Circulation* 1978; 58:265-272

Savitt MA, Tyson GS, Elbeery JR, Owen CH, Davis JW, et al. Physiology of cardiac tamponade and paradoxical pulse in conscious dogs. Am J Physiol 1993; 265(6Pt2):H1996-H2008.

Settle HP Jr, Engel PJ, Fowler NO, Allen JM, Vassallo CL, et al. Echocardiographic study of the paradoxical arterial pulse in chronic obstructive lung disease. Circulation 1980; 62:1297-1307.

Shabetai R, Fowler NO, Fenton JC, Masangkay M. Pulsus paradoxus. *J Clin Invest* 1965; 44:1882-1898.

Shabetai R, Fowler NO, Gueron M. The effects of respiration on aortic pressure and flow. Am Heart J 1963; 65:525-533.

Sharp JT, Bunnell IL, Holland JF, Griffith GT, Greene DG: Hemodynamics during induced cardiac tamponade in man. *Am J Med 1960;* 29:640-646.

Urschel CV. Pulsus paradoxus: Effect of gravity and acceleration in its production. Am J Cardiol 1967; 19:360-364.

Viola AR, Puy RJ, Goldman E. Mechanisms of pulsus paradoxus in airway obstruction. J Appl Physiol. 1990; 68:1927-1931.

Wenckebach KF. Beobachtungen bei exsudativer und adhasiver Perikarditis. Zeitschrift Klin Med 1910; 71:402-420.

Winer HE, Kronzon I. Absence of paradoxical pulse in patients with cardiac tamponade and atrial septal defects. Am J Cardiol 1979; 44:378-380.

Wood P. Chronic constrictive pericarditis. *Am J Cardiol* 1961; 7:48-61.

Chapter 8

ACUTE PERICARDITIS
Viral and idiopathic pericarditis

1. HISTORICAL BACKGROUND

"This, the most common form, occurs usually as a secondary process, and is distinguished by the small amount of fluid exudation, which does not, as in the next variety, give special characters to the disease. It is a benign form, and rarely, if ever, of itself proves fatal." (Osler 1892)

2. DEFINITION

Acute pericarditis is an acute inflammation of the pericardium. The syndrome is characterized by pain, a pericardial friction rub, displacement of the PR and ST segments on the electrocardiogram and systemic signs of acute infection or inflammation. This chapter, for the most part, is limited to pericarditis in which pericardial effusion is small or absent.

3. PATHOLOGY

The essential pathological change is acute inflammation with fibrinous deposits widely distributed over the pericardium. Macroscopically, this gives rise to a shaggy appearance of the membrane, referred to in the older literature as a "bread and butter" appearance from its superficial resemblance to the inside surface of a bread and butter sandwich after the two pieces have been pulled apart. Laennec, in his treatise on diseases of the chest in 1821, wrote, *"Sometimes the knobbed appearance of this exudation is very like what would result from the sudden separation of two pieces of slab joined by a pretty thick layer of butter; at other times, it is more like the internal surface of the second stomach of the calf, an observation made in one case by M Corvisart"* (Laennec 1821).

The pericardium may also appear reddened, and a small exudate may be present. Adhesions may be found between the outer aspect of the pericardium and the mediastinum and the chest wall, and fibrinous material may accumulate between the layers of the pericardium. In some cases, the superficial myocardium is inflamed, which, when recognised, qualifies the case as an acute myopericarditis. The histology confirms heavy fibrin deposition and, in addition, shows the standard changes of acute inflammation, leucocytic infiltration and increased vascularity.

4.   AETIOLOGY

Acute pericarditis may accompany, or be a part of a disconcerting number of disorders. In some, pericarditis is the only obvious manifestation. In these cases, the patient presents with symptoms and signs of acute pericarditis but without those of the underlying disease. The causative disease may then not be disclosed until sought by laboratory testing, or may become apparent only later in the clinical course. In other cases, the clinical picture is made up of the features of acute pericarditis combined with those of the underlying condition. Rarely, acute pericarditis is the initial manifestation of a systemic disease.

In this chapter, I will consider only the manifestations of acute pericarditis, regardless of whether it is an isolated disease, or a component of a more general disease, and defer consideration of pericarditis of specific aetiology until Chapter 9. For the most part, the present chapter will deal with acute viral or idiopathic pericarditis and pericarditis complicating an occult or silent systemic disease.

In a well-known series of 231 cases of acute pericarditis from Spain (*Permanyer-Miralda, Sagrista-Sauleda, Soler-Soler 1985*), the vast majority were classified as idiopathic in spite of a painstaking attempt to arrive at the aetiology. This experience is still the norm. The true prevalence of viral pericarditis remains unknown because of the difficulties in making the diagnosis objectively. Another prospective study of 100 patients, also from Spain, using a similar diagnostic protocol, found a specific aetiology in only 22 percent. The remaining 78 were classified as "idiopathic" (*Zayas, Anguita, Torres*, 1995).

It is necessary to exclude cardiac murmurs or mediastinal crunch owing to air in the mediastinum. The crunch (Hammond's sign), a frequent finding soon after a thoracic operation, can be confused with hydropericardium and artefacts produced by bed clothes, the patient's garment, or the skin. Cardiac murmurs should be distinguished easily by their acoustic qualities and timing. Murmurs caused by specific lesions have characteristics that allow easy recognition. It is difficult to confuse the high-pitched early diastolic murmur of aortic regurgitation, or the rumbling mid-diastolic murmur of mitral stenosis with a friction rub. On the other hand, some systolic murmurs, notably those of mitral and tricuspid regurgitation, may be misinterpreted and thought to be a pericardial friction rub. Pericardial friction rubs fail to behave in the anticipated manner to manoeuvres designed to alter cardiac murmurs. Patients with mediastinal crunch frequently also have palpable subcutaneous emphysema that generates additional crackles,.

By far the commonest viral pericardial infections are with *coxsackie* virus, especially group B, and *echovirus*, especially type 8. Other implicated viral infections include influenza, adenoviruses, infectious mononucleosis, mumps and chicken pox (*Fowler and Manitsas 1973*).

5. CLINICAL EXAMINATION

The pathognomonic sign is a pericardial friction rub. This is a scratching superficial sound that has been likened to the creaking of new leather. It may be audible anywhere over the precordium, but the most favourable sites are at the lower left sternal border, and between there and the cardiac apex. The stethoscope diaphragm, pressed firmly, should be used for auscultation. Posture may make a difference; therefore, the patient should be examined supine, in the left lateral decubitus and sitting up. The intensity varies from faint to very loud. The quality of the rub is also variable, sometimes being fine, but at other times coarse, even to the point of being palpable. Palpable rubs are particularly associated with uremic pericarditis. Pericardial rubs are notoriously evanescent; therefore, auscultation must be repeated frequently when pericarditis is suspected.

In some cases, respiration considerably influences the intensity and character of the rub, which, in extreme examples, may disappear during inspiration. A related phenomenon is the pleuro-pericardial rub of pleuropericarditis. The patient should be auscultated during quiet breathing, and with respiration suspended in inspiration and expiration, and a thorough chest examination must be included.

Victor Collin, Laennec's chef de clinique, wrote that the rub *"resembles the squeak of leather of a new saddle under the rider, or grating in the knee joint on moving the patella over the femoral condoyles".*

The classic pericardial friction rub is triphasic, the components occurring with atrial systole, ventricular systole and ventricular diastole (Figure 1). These triphasic rubs are the easiest to identify, the triple cadence being as important as the quality of the sounds in making the diagnosis and distinguishing from other auscultatory phenomena, such as cardiac murmurs, mediastinal crunch and artefacts caused by motion of the skin over the stethoscopic diaphragm.

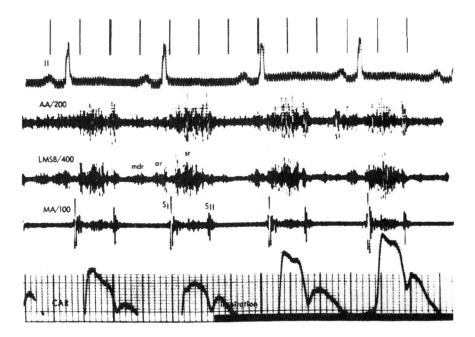

Figure 1. Triphasic pericardial friction rub. The rub is recorded in atrial systole (ar) ventricular systole (sr) and mid-diastole (mdr). (From *Spodick, 1971,* with permission)

The triple cadence is so characteristic of a pericardial friction rub, that there is little or no chance of mistaking it for anything else. Mistakes are more apt to be made when the rub is not triphasic, most commonly biphasic, in which case it may be taken as a to-and-fro cardiac murmur. The less common monophasic rub is easily confused with the murmur of mitral or tricuspid regurgitation. Pericardial friction rub thus has to be distinguished from cardiac murmurs, mediastinal crunch due to air in the mediastinum (Hammond's sign), sounds made by hydropneumopericardium, and various artefacts.

It is difficult to confuse the early diastolic blowing murmur of aortic regurgitation, or the low pitched rumbling mid-diastolic murmur of mitral stenosis, with or without presystolic accentuation, with a pericardial friction rub. Pericardial friction rubs fail to change, as expected, in response to physiological or pharmacological interventions designed to alter the duration, timing and intensity of cardiac murmurs. Patients with Hammond's sign usually have, in addition, palpable surgical emphysema of the chest wall. By far the most common causes of pneumopericardium are iatrogenic. It is almost inevitable that some air enters the pericardium during pericardiocentesis, and air or CO_2 may have been injected to image the pericardium. Much less common causes of pneumopericardium are infection by a gas-forming organism, or rupture of the oesophagus into the pericardium. allowing free communication between the pleura and pericardium. Advances in non-invasive imaging have greatly decreased the use of inducing pneumothorax to outline the pericardium in cases of congenital absence or partial absence of the pericardium. This change is just as well because, now that pneumothorax is no longer a therapy for pulmonary tuberculosis, few clinicians have experience in inducing artificial pneumothorax.

A scratching sound made by movement of the thoracic cage against the stethoscope can be a troublesome feature of the examination, particularly in very thin individuals, in whom it is difficult or impossible to seat the stethoscope evenly on the skin. Careful attention to technique, using a small chest piece, and avoiding areas of hyperdynamic precordial activity, serve to prevent this error which, in any case, is more common in individuals without experience and training in auscultation of the heart.

Acute pericarditis is somewhat unusual in that one symptom, pericardial pain, one physical finding, the friction rub, and one laboratory abnormality on the electrocardiogram, deviation of the ST or PR segment, suffice to make the diagnosis. Many additional symptoms and signs may be present, but they are not due to the acute pericarditis per se; rather, they are features of a complication such as pericardial effusion or tamponade, or are manifestations of the causative disease.

Uncommon but well-documented symptoms of acute pericarditis include dysphagia or else pain on swallowing, cough and hiccup.

6. THE ELECTROCARDIOGRAM

The electrocardiogram can be exceedingly helpful in making the diagnosis, but distinguishing normal variants, such as early repolarisation (*Wanner, Schaal, Bashore, 1983*) and myocardial pathology, can create difficulties. The electrocardiogram, and certainly serial electrocardiograms, can be pathognomonic of acute pericarditis. Four phases of the electrocardiographic progression have been recognised now for many years (*Spodick, 1977*). The original description goes back to the legendary pioneer of electrocardiography, Richard Langendorf (Figure 2).

Das Elektrokardiogramm der Perikarditis.

Von

Dr. MAX WINTERNITZ und Dr. RICHARD LANGENDORF.

I. Teil.

Bei der Redaktion am 26. Oktober 1937 eingegangen.

· —

Die moderne Elektrokardiographie ist zu einem unentbehrlichen Rüstzeug der internen Diagnostik geworden. Die Krankheitszustände, bei denen ihre Ergebnisse im Zentrum der Diagnostik stehen, sind allerdings eng umgrenzt. Es sind dies einerseits die Myokarditiden, anderseits die sklerotischen Myokardaffektionen, bei denen die Elektrokardiographie mitunter sogar ohne Hilfe der Klinik entscheidende Ergebnisse liefert. Wenn nun in den letzten Jahren eine dritte Krankheitsgruppe, die der Perikarditiden[1] elektrokardiographisch erforscht worden ist, so verdient die Frage eingehende Prüfung, ob das EKG auch hier imstande ist, die Diagnostik entscheidend zu fördern. Die vorliegende Arbeit ist diesem Problem gewidmet.

Die ersten Mitteilungen über Veränderungen des EKG bei Perikardaffektionen liegen weit zurück. Cybulski und Surzycki (1) beobachteten 1912 bei einem Patienten mit Perikarderguss niedrige Ausschläge des EKG mit starker Abflachung der T-Zacken, wobei diese Veränderungen mit Abklingen der Erscheinungen noch zunahmen. 1923 betonten Oppenheimer u. Mann (2)

---

[1] Im folgenden bedeutet P. Perikarditis, EKG Elektrokardiogramm, Zst Zwischenstück, IK Initialkomplex.

Figure 2. Title page of the first description of the electrocardiogram in acute pericarditis (From *Winternitz M, Langendorf R 1938, with permission*)

The first stage, which is now well recognised, is elevation of the ST segment in a distribution of leads incompatible with a local abnormality, such as acute ischemia or the onset of a myocardial infarction. Stage one usually begins soon after the onset of acute pericarditis, but may be delayed for a few days. The ST segment tends to retain its normal concavity and can be present in all leads except V1 and aVR. These features of the ST segment are different from those in ischemic heart disease. More specific, but less sensitive than ST segment deviation, is PR segment depression (*Spodick, 1973*), which is a less well-known feature of acute pericarditis (Figure 3). The second stage, which may be quite brief, is a return of the ST segments to the baseline. In the third stage, diffuse T wave inversion develops. The fourth stage, which does not occur in all the patients, is a return of the tracing to normal.

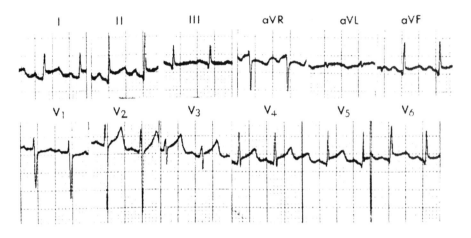

Figure 3. Electrocardiogram showing widespread ST segment elevation, and PR depression.

The vector of the ST segment points to the injury, which, in the case of pericarditis, is diffuse; therefore, it points downward, to the left and posteriorly (Figure 4). The injury current of acute pericarditis is weaker than that of myocardial infarction, and it covers a wider area of the heart's surface. In pericarditis, ST deviation seldom exceeds 5 mvolts and a monophasic pattern is not seen (*Surawicz and Lasseter 1970*). In a patient with severe precordial pain and ST segment elevation, the obvious first consideration is usually acute myocardial infarction. ST elevation in as many leads as is usual in acute pericarditis is distinctly unusual in acute myocardial infarction. One would not expect to see ST elevation in all three standard limb leads in a case of acute myocardial infarction and reciprocal depression in leads subtending uninvolved myocardium. In acute pericarditis, ST segment depression in leads V1 and aVR simply reflects the ST vector's direction. When an electrocardiogram is taken in the very early stage of acute myocardial infarction, the Q wave may be absent, only to appear on subsequent tracings.

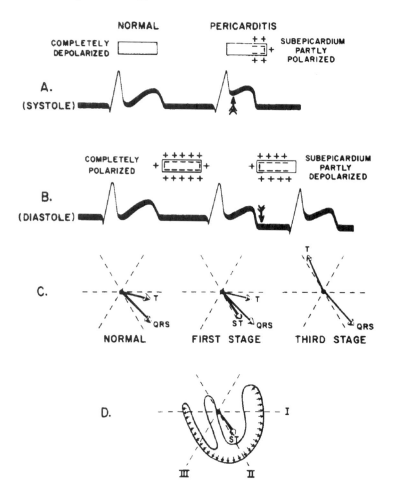

Figure 4. Genesis of the electrocardiographic changes in acute pericarditis. **A:** A systolic current of injury flows from the normally depolarised deep layers of the myocardium to the partly repolarised superficial layers and causes true ST segment elevation. **B:** The diastolic current of injury depresses the TQ segment, which, on the clinical ac coupled electrocardiograph, is manifest as apparent ST segment elevation. **C:** Transient development of an abnormal ST vector in the first stage, and rotation of the T vector in the third stage. **D:** Orientation of the mean ST vector in the first stage, accounting for the almost universal ST elevation. The small arrows represent the instantaneous ST vector due to the current of injury.
(From *Spodick 1959, with permission*)

6.1   Early repolarisation

Early repolarisation is a normal variant that changes the ST segment in a way very similar to acute pericarditis; indeed, without serial tracings it can be impossible to tell the difference (Figure 5). This variant has been said to be commoner in young black men (*Ashman 1941*). This topic has been revisited on many occasions, some reports being in agreement but others not, as reported in a review article (*Mehta, Jain, Mehta 1999*).

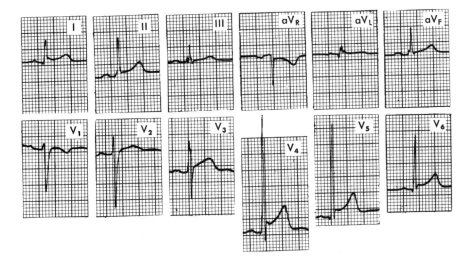

Figure 5. Early repolarisation in a normal subject .The resemblance to acute pericarditis is striking. (*From Goldberger and Goldberger 1981, with permission*)

The hallmark of the third stage is T-wave inversion, indistinguishable from T-wave inversion from other causes. This difficulty is obviated if one has seen tracings from earlier stages. The duration of T inversion is highly variable, lasting weeks, months or indefinitely. This pattern is called chronic pericarditis (Figure 6). T-wave abnormalities of chronic pericarditis cannot, like some non-specific T-wave changes, be reversed by isoproterenol infusion (*Daoud, Surawicz, Gettes, 1972*). Striking T-wave abnormalities seen in patients soon after cardiac surgery are often benign, reflecting only surgical irritation of the pericardium.

6.1.1   Mechanisms

The genesis of early repolarisation is not known, but several observations shed light on the possible mechanisms. Vagal stimulation accelerates repolarisation, which is often found in sinus bradycardia. Stimulation of the right stellate ganglion causes ST elevation with a concave contour through an electrical gradient between the antero-apical wall, which recovers earlier than the posterior wall. Early repolarisation of the anterior wall is thought to result from stimulation of the right sympathetic nerve. Sympathetic stimulation also can depress and shorten the PR segment, and this can be seen in early repolarisation as well as acute pericarditis. Increased dispersion of repolarisation from the subendocardium to the subepicardium may also contribute to early repolarisation. These features suggest a role of the autonomic nervous system in the genesis of early repolarisation.

6.2   Electrocardiographic morphology

Elevation of the ST segment 1 to 4 mv from the isoelectric line takes off from the J junction, the segment is concave upwards, the downstroke of the R wave is notched or slurred, and the T waves are often abnormally large and symmetrical. The ratio of ST elevation to the amplitude of the T wave is less than 0.25. These features help in distinguishing between early repolarisation, acute myocardial infarction and acute pericarditis, but the lack of change on serial tracings is the most reliable criterion for early repolarisation (*Surawicz and Knilans, 2001*). Only the clinical aspects of a case distinguish persistent T-wave inversion (chronic pericarditis) from other causes of T-wave abnormalities.

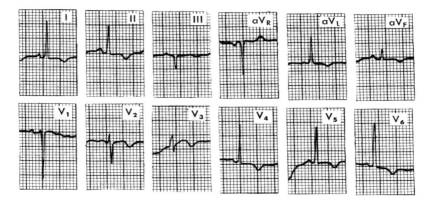

Figure 6. Chronic constrictive pericarditis

6.3   Atypical electrocardiogram

The electrocardiogram is not always typical; in one study this was true in 19 of 44 cases, likely a higher than average prevalence. ST elevation was altogether absent in some, and restricted in a way that simulates ischemic heart disease in others (*Bruce and Spodick, 1980*). In four of the patients, PR depression was the only evidence of pericarditis.

6.4   Atrial arrhythmia

Atrial arrhythmia, including atrial tachycardia and fibrillation or flutter, may complicate acute pericarditis, but in my experience, this is uncommon. Pathologists have ascribed the disturbed rhythm to inflammation in the vicinity of the sino-atrial node that occupies a subpericardial location near the superior vena caval right atrial junction (*James, 1962*).

7.   OTHER LABORATORY FINDINGS

In idiopathic or viral pericarditis, the erythrocyte sedimentation rate and C-reactive protein are almost invariably elevated and an increase in the white cell count is usual. Early in the course, leukocytosis is common, but later in the course gives way to lymphocytosis. The hematological picture in other causes of acute pericarditis often differs. The MB fraction of creatinine kinase is modestly elevated in severe cases, reflecting inflammation of the epicardium (*Karjalainen and Heikkila, 1986*). The troponin$_i$ level may, likewise, be slightly elevated. Higher elevations suggest myopericarditis. Scintigraphy has been used with gallium (*O'Connell, Robinson, Henkin, 1980*), or pyrophosphate (*Fleg, Siegel, Williamson, 1978*) to image pericardial inflammation. Alternatively, pericardial inflammation can be imaged using gadolinium-enhanced magnetic resonance imaging (*Matsouka, Hamada, Honda, 1994*).

8.   CLINICAL COURSE

The prodromal syndrome is often quite severe. Acute pericarditis is usually a short, sharp, self-limiting disease, often occurring in patients without discernible risk factors for ischemic heart disease, although, in an unlucky few, the syndrome recurs, sometimes frequently and over a prolonged period of time (*vide infra*). Other relatively infrequent complications are cardiac tamponade, clinically significant myocarditis, and the eventual development of constrictive pericarditis. The risk of cardiac tamponade is greatest early in the course, and may recur if acute pericarditis recurs. It is my practice, when seeing patients with acute pericarditis for the first time, to admit them to hospital for observation and, in appropriate circumstances, to exclude ischemic heart disease. The patients should be followed for several months to watch for recurrence or evidence of constriction or pericardial effusion. It should be recalled that, after acute pericarditis, constriction may be transient and disappears with pharmacological treatment.

Recognisable myocarditis is an early complication that fortunately is relatively uncommon. Clues are excessive dyspnoea or tachycardia, conduction disturbance and ventricular arrhythmias, greater elevation of cardiac enzymes or a third heart sound. If heart size increases, it is important to distinguish between pericardial effusion and the onset of heart failure, both of which are possible in the setting of recent acute pericarditis.

The adjective "benign" was used by Osler in his description of acute pericarditis, and the phrase, acute benign pericarditis, is still current, but should only be used after the illness has proven to be benign as, occasionally, serious complications, troublesome recurrences, or even death have followed.

9.   TREATMENT

The goals are relief of pain, resolution of effusion, when significant, and, in some cases, relief of tamponade. Aspirin, ibuprofen, indomethacin, or other non-steroidal antiinflammatory agents usually produce prompt relief in most patients. Ketorolac tromethamine, an NSAID for parenteral use, is effective, and can be a way around gastric intolerance to this class of drugs (*Arunasalam and Siegel, 1993*). Aspirin is the safest antiinflammatory drug with which to treat acute pericarditis complicating acute myocardial infarction, because the alternatives may impair healing with scar formation (*Berman, Haffajee.Alpert, 1981*).

10.   RECURRENT PERICARDITIS

In this vexing syndrome, the inciting agent is absent or no longer active (*Robinson and Brigden 1968*). Since that early description, recurrent pericarditis has been recognised as an auto-immune process. The exact recurrence rate after an acute attack is not known, but may be in the range of 15 to 32 percent (*Fowler, 1990*). One cannot predict in which cases recurrence will be likely. The original episode may have been typical "dry" pericarditis, a pericardial effusion of any size, or possibly with cardiac tamponade.

Since recurrent pericarditis is considered to be an autoimmune phenomenon, one would anticipate a good therapeutic response to immunosuppressive and antiinflammatory drugs. The syndrome shares many of the features of pericarditis of various aetiologies that are considered due to autoimmunity. These include the postpericardiotomy syndrome, Dressler's syndrome and posttraumatic pericarditis, all of which may be associated with recurrence. There is no feature of the original episode of acute pericarditis that predicts the likelihood of recurrence.

Treatment with a corticosteroid should be considered only for patients who have clearly failed a thorough trial of nonsteroidal therapy. When corticosteroid therapy is inevitable, the drug must be given in high dose for a month and then tapered slowly, to lessen the risk of relapse.

10.1   Diagnosis

The diagnosis is usually apparent on clinical grounds, but investigators working in a laboratory devoted to inflammatory diseases of the pericardium and myocardium perform extensive studies in patients suspected of having recurrent pericarditis or, as they term it, autoreactive pericarditis *(Maisch, Ristic, Pankuweit 2002)*. These studies include pericardioscopy and multiple epicardial biopsies. It should be noted, however, that these techniques are not available in most cardiology services and clinics. Endomyocardial biopsy is not helpful. Pericardial fluid shows an increase in the number of monocytes and lymphocytes. The fluid is sterile to culture and polymerase chain reaction; malignant cells, likewise, are absent.

10.2   Clinical course

The patient is asymptomatic between episodes. The recurrence may be a single event, or may return after days, weeks, months, or even years, in some cases even 15 years *(Fowler 1990)*. Earlier, Fowler had reported on 31 patients, followed up to 19 years. Relapses occurred over periods ranging from five or more years in 19 patients to eight or more years in seven patients. *(Fowler and Harbin 1986)*.

The most important symptom is disabling pain; less commonly, the patients' symptoms related to cardiac tamponade. Constrictive pericarditis is a very rare complication.

While a typical first attack of acute pericarditis can be relied on to respond promptly to the administration of antiinflammatory drugs, recurrences are often much more recalcitrant. The episodes can recur over a long time during which the patient usually is miserable, anxious, and often unable to carry on an occupation, or with schooling. It is therefore essential to communicate well and early with the patient who needs to know that it is not the infection that recurred, and made to understand the broad concept of an autoimmune disease and the rationale of treatment. The patient needs frequent reassurance that permanent sequelae are rare and that eventually the process will die down and disappear. The patient also needs to be informed about the side effects and dangers of steroids and non-steroidal medication. Discussion of immunosupression and its possible consequences is also in order. All this requires much time and patience on the part of both patient and physician. For patients who do not tolerate any of these drugs, a formulation for parenteral administration is available and effective (*Arunasalam and Siegel, 1993*).

10.3   Treatment of recurrent pericarditis

The majority of patients respond promptly and completely to a course of prednisone or prednisolone, given initially at high dose and then tapered while monitoring the response. The use of steroidal agents, however, is a source of controversy and can create many problems, some of them serious. The use of prednisone should therefore be strictly limited. The ideal is to avoid the use of steroids altogether, but this is not always possible, as some patients do not respond to any other medication.

10.3.1   Non-steroidal antiinflammatory agents

Some physicians treat an initial episode of acute pericarditis with prednisone or another steroid without first trying alternatives. That is unfortunate, because it may well increase the difficulty of avoiding or restricting their use in the event of recurrence. Ibuprofen is effective, but its use may be prevented by gastro-intestinal intolerance. The dose usually needs to be high, 400 to 800 mg or more, four times daily. Prophylaxis with an H_2 blocker or antispasmodic should be offered, and treatment is essential if the drug causes abdominal pain or related symptoms. COX-2 non-steroidal antiinflammatory agents, such as Cerebrex and Vioxx, are less apt to irritate the stomach. When symptoms have been absent for two or three weeks, the dose should be slowly and progressively decreased. If symptoms return, the dose should be increased to at least the last dose that suppressed all symptoms, and be maintained there for two or three weeks before attempting to taper the dose again. In some cases it is necessary to return to the initial high dose. Common errors are to use too low a dose, or to taper it too rapidly.

A large number of these agents is available, and the number continues to grow. Many patients claim that only one is effective for them, and, in general, I have no reservations about complying with their wishes. Indomethacin is often effective but, since it is a coronary vasoconstrictor, it is probably best avoided, when possible, in patients with coronary disease. The COX-2 inhibitors, such as Vioxx and Cerebrex, have somewhat less gastrointestinal effects, and may be less nephrotoxic, but whether they are better at suppressing pericardial inflammation remains to be seen.

10.3.2   Steroid therapy.

When a thorough trial of alternative treatment fails to relieve the patient, one may have to resort to therapy with a steroid, usually prednisone, and sometimes, especially in Europe, prednisolone. For many years now, some investigators have suspected that steroids may perpetuate rather than suppress pericardial inflammation. This paradoxical response may be related to the use of doses that are too low (*Marcolongo, Russo, Laveder, 1995*). Marcolongo et al. reviewed the cases of 12 patients admitted to the clinical immunology service of the University of Padova for persistence of recurrent pericarditis. All had been treated previously for 7 to 45 days with prednisone or deflazacort; but the doses were low, and the duration of treatment short, the highest ranging from 0.07 to 0.9 mg/k/day. Before this treatment, 11 had been treated with nonsteroidal agents, without success. Believing that the cause of the poor response to corticosteroid treatment may have been inadequate dosage and duration of treatment, the investigators treated the patents again, this time with prednisone 1.0 to 1.5 mg/k/day for at least four weeks and tapered slowly over the next three months. During the period when the dose of prednisone was being lowered, the patients received 1.6g of aspirin daily. The dose of aspirin was cut in half when prednisone was finally discontinued, and this dose was maintained for a further three months.

Thirty-nine relapses were documented (two to six in each patient) after the shorter, lower-dose regimens. In treatment with high-dose prednisone, supplemented in some cases with other immunosuppressing drugs, only one recurrence was observed in a period of four to fifty months. The favourable results of using a high dose of immunosupressant drugs are illustrated in Figure 7. Most physicians who often treat recurrent pericarditis, and did so before the publication cited here, adhere to the basic principles of Marcolongo's protocol, namely prescribing a high dose when initiating therapy and maintaining that dose for a month, taking a matter of months to taper the dose to zero, and adding a nonsteroidal antiinflammatory agent, and, in severe cases, a more potent immunosuppressor.

Using corticosteroids to treat recurrent pericarditis is thus more hazardous than using them for a single attack of acute pericarditis. The high doses needed and the longer duration of treatment that may need to be repeated several times poses a real risk of osteopenia. Patients who appear to be headed for a protracted regimen of prednisone treatments should have bone density measured, and, if treatment is in fact prolonged, bone densitometry should be repeated. Prophylaxis or treatment should be decided on an individual basis, after discussion with the patient. Some patients find acne, gain in appetite and weight, or severe Cushing's syndrome intolerable. Euphoria and other mental changes can be problematic. Gastric side effects require prophylaxis. In pre-diabetes, the induced hyperglycaemia may need treatment; usually an oral agent suffices. The general precautions in patients receiving immunosuppressive drugs are appropriate, but need not be applied as rigorously as in patients who have undergone solid organ transplantation. In older patients or those with renal insufficiency or diabetes, renal function should be monitored serially for the duration of treatment with nonsteroidal antiinflammatory drugs.

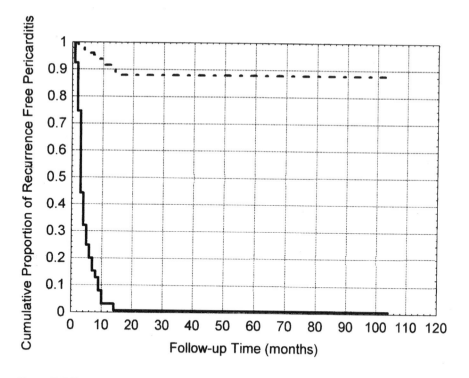

Figure 7. Effect of high dose immunosuppressive therapy (dashed line) versus ineffective low dose antiinflammatory treatment (solid curve) to prevent recurrence of acute pericarditis. (From *Marcolongo, Russo, Laveder, 1995*)

10.3.2.1 **Colchicine**

Whenever possible, colchicine should be included in the treatment regimen, as it may reduce, or even obviate the need for corticosteroid treatment (*Rodriguez de la Serna, Guindo Soldevila, Marti Claramunt 1987*; *Guindo, Rodriguez de la Serna, Ramio 1990*). Colchicine is an old and remarkable drug used to treat gout (*Porter and Rousseau 1998*) with many actions, including inhibition of mitosis, and binding to tubulin. It blocks some leukocyte functions (*Dinarello, Chusid, Fauci 1976*) and interferes with transcellular movement of collagen (*Kershenobich, Vargas, Garcia-Tsao 1988*). Colchicine is highly concentrated in white blood cells. On this basis, it may reduce or prevent immunopathic reactions. Colchicine is an effective drug for treating familial Mediterranean fever (*Gedalia, Adar, Gorodischer, 1992*) and a relationship between this familial disorder and recurrent pericarditis is known to exist (*DeLine and Cable 2002*). Furthermore, the best results from treating recurrent pericarditis with colchicine have been reported from countries in which familial Mediterranean fever is common (*Adler, Finkelstein, Guindo 1998*). This finding may partially explain the variable success rates found by different investigators who have used colchicine in the treatment regimen for recurrent pericarditis (*Adolph 1990*). Thus, it is likely that genetic factors influence the response to colchicine in recurrent, autoreactive pericarditis.

10.3.2.2 **Topical therapy**

Triamcinolone, a nonabsorbable corticosteroid instilled into the pericardium, was a therapy frequently employed in the past for pericarditis complicating dialysis for renal failure. Recently, this mode of treatment has been tried in 84 patients with recurrent pericarditis (*Maisch, Ristic, Pankuweit 2002*). Three (3) to 500 mg/m^2 were injected in 100 ml of normal saline into the pericardium and the fluid was removed after 24 hours. The patients then received 0.5 mg of colchicine thrice daily for six months. Recurrence was prevented in 90 percent at three months and 84 percent at one year. This method of treatment deserves further evaluation.

10.4 **Pericardiectomy**

Pericardiectomy would seem to be a rational treatment but, as mentioned previously, cure is not guaranteed and criteria that predict who will or will not respond have not been published. Most cardiologists therefore are reluctant to advise pericardiectomy unless driven to it (*Fowler 1990*). Not surprisingly, more enthusiasm for the operation is found in surgical circles

(Tuna and Danielson 1990). Success depends on performing as complete a pericardiectomy as possible; it is therefore necessary to refer the patient to those with experience in performing the operation for this indication.

10.5   New and prospective treatment strategies

Given the difficulties and frustrations of treating this difficult syndrome, it is not surprising that new methods are under active investigation. These include administration of agents such as triamcinolone, a non-absorbable steroid drug, or colchicine. The presence of a pericardial effusion deemed large enough to tap safely is no longer a prerequisite, in view of techniques that have been developed to catheterise the pericardium safely even when there is little or no effusion. These methods include percutaneous insertion of a needle and blunt cannula *(Sosa, Scanavacca, d'Avila 2000),* percutaneous puncture of the right atrial appendage *(Verrier, Waxman, Lovett 1998),* and the "perducer," an instrument designed to achieve this object from the subxiphoid approach (see also Chapter 6) *(Macris and Igo 1999).* Clinical trials, sponsored by the task force on pericardial disease of the World Heart Federation, are now underway *(Maisch, Ristic, Seferovic 2000).*

References

Adler Y, Finkelstein Y, Guindo J, Rodriguez de la Serna A, Shoenfeld Y, et al. Colchicine treatment for recurrent pericarditis. A decade of experience. Circulation 1998; 97:2183-2185.

Adolph RJ. Old drugs with new uses. Colchicine for treatment of recurrent pericarditis. Circulation. 1990; 82:1505-1506

Arunasalam S, Siegel RJ. Rapid resolution of symptomatic acute pericarditis with ketorolac tromethamine: a parenteral nonsteroidal antiinflammatory agent. Am Heart J. 1993 May;125(5 Pt 1):1455-1458.

Ashman R. An electrocardiographic study of caucasians and negroes. Tri-State Med J 1941; 13:2686.

Berman J, Haffajee CI, Alpert JS. Therapy of symptomatic pericarditis after myocardial infarction: retrospective and prospective studies of aspirin, indomethacin, prednisone, and spontaneous resolution. Am Heart J 1981; 101:750-753.

Bruce MA, Spodick DH. Atypical electrocardiogram in acute pericarditis: characteristics and prevalence. J Electrocardiol 1980; 13:61-66.

Daoud FS, Surawicz B, Gettes LS. Effect of isoproterenol on the abnormal T wave. Am J Cardiol 1972; 30:810-819.

DeLine, Cable. Clustering of recurrent pericarditis with effusion and constriction in a family. Mayo Clin Proc 2002; 7:39-43

Dinarello CA, Chusid MJ, Fauci AS, Gallin JI, Dale DC, et al. Effect of prophylactic colchicine therapy on leukocyte function in patients with familial Mediterranean fever. Arthritis Rheum 1976; 19:618-622.

Fleg JL, Siegel BA, Williamson JR, Roberts R. 99mTc-pyrophosphate imaging in acute pericarditis: a clinical and experimental study. Radiology 1978; 126:727-731.

Fowler NO, Harbin AD III. Recurrent acute pericarditis: Follow-up study of 31 patients. J Am Coll Cardiol 1986; 7:300.

Fowler NO, Manitsas GT. Infectious pericarditis. Prog Cardiovasc Dis 1973; 16:323-336.

Fowler NO. Recurrent pericarditis. Cardiol Clin 1990; 8:621-626.

Gedalia A, Adar A, Gorodischer R. Familial Mediterranean fever in children. J Rheumatol Suppl 1992; 35:1-359

Goldberger Al, Goldberger E. Clinical electrocardiography (ed 2) St Louis, CV Mosby 1981, p126.

Guindo J, Rodriguez de la Serna A, Ramio J, de Miguel Diaz MA, Subirana MT, et al. Recurrent pericarditis. Relief with colchicine. Circulation 1990; 82:1117-1120.

James TN. Pericarditis and the sinus node. Arch Intern Med 1962; 110:305-311.

Karjalainen J, Heikkila J. "Acute pericarditis": myocardial enzyme release as evidence for myocarditis. Am Heart J 1986; 111:546-552

Kershenobich D, Vargas F, Garcia-Tsao G, Perez Tamayo R, Gent M, et al. Colchicine in the treatment of cirrhosis of the liver. N Engl J Med 1988; 318:1709-1713.

Laennec RTH. A Treatise On The Diseases of the Chest. Translated by John Forbes.. T&G Underwood, London, 1821.

Macris MP, Igo SR. Minimally invasive access of the normal pericardium: initial clinical experience with a novel device. Clin Cardiol 1999; 22(Suppl I):I36-I39.

Maisch B, Ristic A, Pankuweit S. Intrapericardial treatment of autoreactive pericardial effusion with triamcinolone; the way to avoid side effects of systemic corticosteroid therapy. Eur Heart J. 2002; 23:1503.

Maisch B, Ristic AD, Seferovic PM. New directions in diagnosis and treatment of pericardial disease. A project of the Taskforce on Pericardial Disease of the World Heart Federation. Herz 2000; 25:769-780.

Marcolongo R, Russo R, Laveder F, Noventa F, Agostini C. Immunosuppressive therapy prevents recurrent pericarditis. J Am Coll Cardiol 1995; 26:1276-1279.

Matsouka H, Hamada M, Honda T, Kawakami H, Abe M, et al. Evaluation of acute myocarditis and pericarditis by Gd-DTPA enhanced magnetic resonance imaging. Eur Heart J 1994; 15:283-284.

Mehta M, Jain AC, Mehta A. Early repolarization. Clin Cardiol. 1999; 22:59-65.

O'Connell JB, Robinson JA, Henkin RE, Gunnar RM. Gallium-67 citrate scanning for noninvasive detection of inflammation in pericardial diseases. Am J Cardiol 1980; 46:879-884.

Osler W: The Principles and Practice of Medicine. New York, D Appleton, 1892, p 582.

Permanyer-Miralda G, Sagrista-Sauleda J, Soler-Soler J. Primary acute pericardial disease: a prospective series of 231 consecutive patients. Am J Cardiol 1985; 56:623-630.

Porter R, Rousseau GS. Gout, the Patrician Malady. London, Yale University Press, 1998.

Robinson J, Brigden W. Recurrent pericarditis. Br Med J 1968; 2:272.

Rodriguez de la Serna A, Guindo Soldevila J, Marti Claramunt V, Bayes de Luna A. Colchicine for recurrent pericarditis. Lancet 1987; 2:1517

Sosa E, Scanavacca M, d'Avila A, Oliveira F, Ramires JA. Nonsurgical transthoracic epicardial catheter ablation to treat recurrent ventricular tachycardia occurring late after myocardial infarction. J Am Coll Cardiol 2000; 35:1442-1449.

Spodick DH. Acoustic phenomena in pericardial disease. Am Heart J 1971; 81:114-124.

Spodick DH. Diagnostic electrocardiographic sequences in acute pericarditis. Significance of PR segment and PR vector changes. Circulation 1973;48:575-80

Spodick DH. Pathogenesis and clinical correlations of the electrocardiographic abnormalities of pericardial disease. Cardiovasc Clin 1977;8:201-213.

Spodick DH: Acute Pericarditis. New York, Grune and Stratton, 1959, p22.

Surawicz B and Knilans TK. Chou's Electrocardiography in Clinical Practice Philadelphia, WB Saunders, 2001, pp 239-255

Surawicz B, Lasseter KC. Electrocardiogram in pericarditis. Am J Cardiol 1970; 26:471-474

Tuna IC, Danielson GK. Surgical management of pericardial diseases. Cardiol Clin 1990; 8:683-696.

Verrier RL, Waxman S, Lovett EG, Moreno R. Transatrial access to the normal pericardial space: a novel approach for diagnostic sampling, pericardiocentesis, and therapeutic interventions. Circulation 1998; 98:2331-2333.

Wanner WR, Schaal SF, Bashore TM, Norton VJ, Lewis RP, et al. Repolarization variant vs acute pericarditis. A prospective electrocardiographic and echocardiographic evaluation. Chest 1983;83:180-184.

Winternitz M, Langendorf R. Das Elektrokardiogramm der Perikarditis. Acta Med Scand 1938; 94:141-188.

Zayas R, Anguita M, Torres F, Gimenez D, Bergillos F, et al. Incidence of specific etiology and role of methods for specific etiologic diagnosis of primary acute pericarditis. Am J Cardiol 1995; 75:378-382

Chapter 9

SPECIFIC PERICARDIAL DISORDERS
Congenital malformations and acquired diseases

1. CONGENITAL MALFORMATIONS

1.1 Partial and complete absence of the pericardium

1.1.1 Historical Background

The first description of this entity has been ascribed to Realdo Columbus, a contemporary of William Harvey, whose theory of circulation of the blood Columbus did not accept. Nasser, who studied this malformation quite intensively over thirty years ago (Nasser 1970), is more confident that the first unquestionable description was that of Baille, "On the want of a pericardium in the human body"(Baille 1793).

1.1.2 Embryology

Defects in the pericardium are thought to result from premature atrophy of the left duct of Couvier, which compromises the pleuropericardial membrane destined to form the left pericardium (Southworth and Stevenson 1938). In normal development, the left duct of Couvier atrophies to form part of the left superior intercostal vein. The right duct of Couvier becomes the superior vena cava that ensures closure of the right pericardial membrane, which explains why absence of pericardium is far more common of the left than the right (Morgan, Rogers, Forker 1971). A case was reported, however, of a defect in the right pericardium through which parts of the right atrium and ventricle had herniated. The patient was treated by resection of the right side of the pericardium (Minocha, Falicov, Nijensohn, 1979). In a detailed discussion of the embryology (Kaneko, Okabe, Nagata, 1998), it was emphasised that, in the vast majority of cases, the phrenic nerve passes ventral to the defect. This information is important to thoracic surgeons seeking to avoid injuring the nerve; but a propos the embryology, Kaneko et al. reported an unusual case in which the phrenic nerve was split, passing both ventral and posterior to the defect. The posterior course of part of the nerve is inconsistent with the hypothesis that failure of the pericardial-pleural membrane to close underlies the embryology of absence of the pericardium. Kaneko et al. proposed that some pericardial defects result from a tear in the pericardio-pleural membrane secondary to the stretch it incurs during embryogenesis.

1.1.3   Associated congenital malformations

Congenital absence of the pericardium is an isolated malformation in about 60 percent of cases, but may be found with patency of the arterial duct, atrial septal defect, congenital mitral stenosis, tetralogy of Fallot, tricuspid regurgitation (van Son, Danielson, Callahan 1993), and the Eisenmenger complex. An association of billowing mitral valve and congenitally absent left pericardium has been noted (Pocock, Lakier, Benjamin 1977). In other instances, pericardial absence is associated with congenital malformations of the lung, including sequestration and bronchogenic cysts. Reporting on their experience with absence of the pericardium among over 1,400 necropsies, Southworth and Stevenson emphasised the frequent occurrence of pleuro-pericarditis, secondary to pulmonary infection, in these patients and concluded that the chief danger of deficient pericardium is that it allows pulmonary infection via the resultant communication between the pleural and pericardial cavities (Southworth and Stevenson 1938). It is now widely accepted, however, that strangulated herniation of part of the heart, usually the left atrium or its appendage, is by far the most important complication of critically sized pericardial deficiencies, although recent literature on this subject is surprisingly scant. This complication, when it strangulates the appendage, is life threatening and requires emergency surgical operation.

Absent left pericardium was found in two members of the same family. Other members had hypoplastic left heart and tetralogy of Fallot (Taysi, Hartmann, Shackelford, 1985). Absence of the anterior pericardium may be found in a complex that includes severe congenital heart disease, and deficiencies in the sternum and abnormal facies (Cottrill, Tamaren, Hall, 1998). A case discovered during investigation for sick sinus syndrome displayed marked changes in the electrocardiogram, heart rate and sinus node recovery time with changes in posture, suggesting that the sick sinus syndrome was induced by stretching the vagus when the patient assumed the right decubitus position (Hano, Baba, Hayano, 1996).

1.1.4 Clinical Features

1.1.4.1 Radiological and bedside examination

Most individuals with absence of the pericardium do not have symptoms directly related to the lesion, and the physical findings when present (and often they are not) are non-specific and therefore tend to be elicited after the diagnosis is known; they seldom lead to the diagnosis. Probably the lesion is first suspected from a compatible abnormality on imaging performed for a different purpose. Sometimes surgeons come across the abnormal pericardium accidentally while performing thoracotomy or sternotomy. Spontaneous pneumothorax permits some of the air to enter the pericardial space via the defect, another instance in which the lesion is found by sheer chance.

Excessive mobility of the heart when the patient changes posture can be appreciated on clinical examination when the left side of the pericardium is totally missing (the commonest variant) and when the whole pericardium is absent, but not when the defect on one side is partial and most of the heart remains intrapericardial.

1.1.4.2 Plain chest radiogram

Both partial (Figure 1A) and the less common total absence of the pericardium (Figure 1B) are readily recognised by chest radiography. When the left side of the pericardium is altogether missing, or when there is substantial deficiency, several abnormalities combine to produce a virtually diagnostic appearance (Figure 1B). These findings are: (1) a leftward shift of the heart's position, (2) elongation of the left heart border, prominent aortic knob and a long well-demarcated pulmonary arterial segment, (3) a radiolucent band between the aortic knob and the main pulmonary arterial segment, and (4) another radiolucent band separating the left hemidiaphragm from the heart. These lucencies are caused by interposition of lung between the aorta and the pulmonary artery, and between the heart and diaphragm; they are seen best on overexposed films. In some cases of partial absence, the findings are less specific, consisting only of prominence of the pulmonary artery or left atrial appendage, or both (Nasser, Helmen, Tavel, 1970)

Lateral displacement of the entire heart causes the right heart to appear enlarged but, by echocardiography and computer-assisted tomography, the right atrium and ventricle are normal in size. When the patient is lying on the left side, the heart shifts to the left more than it normally does.

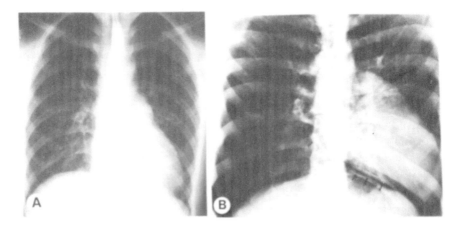

Figure 1. **A:** Partial absence of the left side of the pericardium. **B:** Complete absence of the left side of the pericardium.

The abnormal chest radiogram triggers bedside examination, but it is much less helpful. Chest pain resembling angina or less typical pain is reported by a significant number of the patients and may lead to further evaluation and establishing the diagnosis. Pain is more common in patients who experience intermittent herniation of the left atrium, without strangulation; accordingly, the pain may be worse when lying on the left side. An alternative suggestion is that torsion of the great vessels due to the increased mobility of the heart with changing posture causes chest pain *(Ellis, Leeds, Himmelstein 1959)*. Other findings are not specific; for example, a conspicuous left ventricular heave palpable in the anterior, mid or even posterior axillary line, not accompanied by a third or fourth heart sound or evidence of other disease that would cause left ventricular hypertrophy. A soft ejection murmur may be audible, but the mechanism has not been explained. The electrocardiogram shows a vertical orientation in the frontal plane and clockwise rotation in the horizontal plane. Right bundle branch block is common, and non-specific T-wave changes may be present *(Di Pasquale, Ruffini, Piolanti, 1992)*. A syndrome comprising abnormal facies, mental retardation and growth hormone deficiency with complete absence of the left pericardium has been described (*Boscherini, Galasso. Bitti, 1994)*, as has familial incidence *(Taysi, Hartmann, Shackelford, 1985)*. The jugular pulse may show V instead of the normal A dominance (*Matsuhisa, Shimomura, Beppu, 1986)*, and Doppler interrogation of the superior vena caval blood flow demonstrates diminished systolic and increased diastolic flow and velocity (*Fukuda, Oki, Iuchi, 1995*).

1.1.4.3 Other imaging

Absence of the pericardium can be identified after pneumothorax, be it spontaneous (*Krishnan, Babu, Govindan, 1996; Pickhardt 1998*) or therapeutic for pulmonary tuberculosis (*Nasser, Feigenbaum, Helmen 1966*), or else it may be discovered by chance when performing intrathoracic surgery. At the time of Nasser's first publication in 1966, the acceptable standard for making the diagnosis was to induce artificial pneumothorax (Figure 2). At that time, chest physicians were experienced in, and successful in, safely performing artificial pneumothorax, because it was a common intervention for the treatment of pulmonary tuberculosis with cavitation. At present, few physicians are competent with this technique.

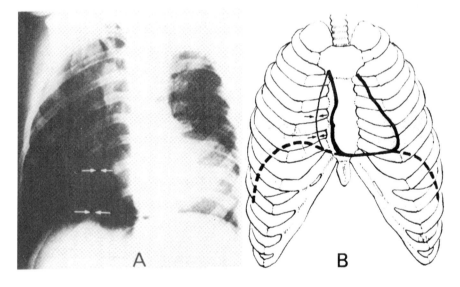

Figure 2. **A:** Left lateral decubitus chest radiogram following left artificial pneumothorax. **B:** Line drawing of air outlines the left pericardium and the right pleuropericardium is outlined against air in the right lung. (From Nasser, Feigenbaum, Helmen, 1966, by permission of the American Heart Association)

The diagnosis can often be established by echocardiography *(Connolly, Click, Shattenberg 1995)* which obviates the need for pneumothorax. The echocardiographic abnormalities are unusual imaging windows, hypermobility of the heart, swinging of the heart, and abnormal septal motion by M mode (Figure 3).

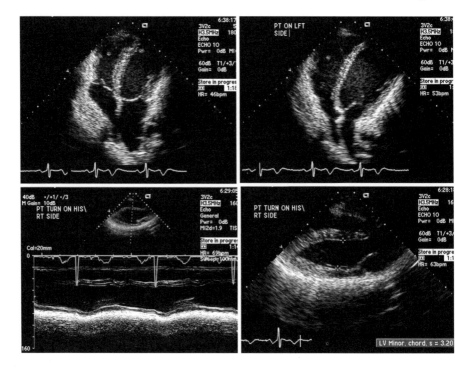

Figure 3. Congenital absence of the pericardium demonstrated echocardiographically. **Top Left**: Four chamber view with the patient in the standard left decubitus position. **Top Right**: The patient has been repositioned to right decubitus. Note how the position of the heart has shifted. **Bottom Left**: M-Mode. Note abnormal septal motion due to excessive motion of the heart as a whole. **Bottom Right:** The long axis view is unusual in that the apex is easily seen. (Images kindly supplied by Wm Keen, M.D., Kaiser Permanente Hospital, San Diego CA.)

Both magnetic resonance imaging and computer-assisted tomography (Figure 4) (*Jacob, Souza, Parro 1995*) are now the standard means of making the diagnosis in cases in which it is not obvious from the plain chest radiogram. These tomographic images provide superior and more detailed information concerning the location and extent of the pericardial deficiency. These additional data are useful for assessing the risk of herniation or strangulation and the need for surgical intervention (*Gassner, Judmaier, Fink 1995*). In a review of ten patients seen at the Mayo Clinic between 1982 and 1992, the electrocardiographic and the features of three imaging modalities were compared. The echocardiographic windows were abnormal in all ten, there was excessive mobility of the heart in nine, abnormal motion of the ventricular septum in eight, and abnormal swinging motion of the heart in seven (*Connolly, Click, Schattenberg, 1995*). Abnormal septal motion may be observed in systole, diastole or both (*Oki, Tabata, Yamada, 1997*).

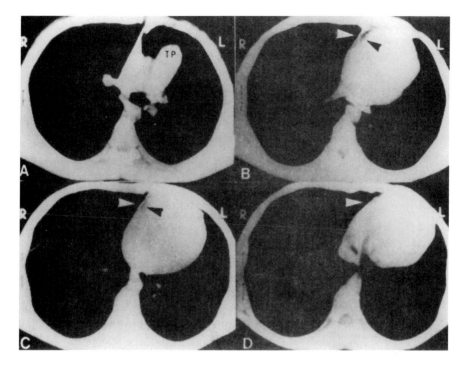

Figure 4. Computer assisted tomogram of absent left pericardium. **A:** left and lateral displacement of the pulmonary trunk (TP). **B**: at the level of the left atrium; the heart is displaced to the left, the left pericardium is absent, the right pericardium is visible (white arrowhead) contrasting with the fat (black arrowhead). **C**: at the level of the ventricles, showing leftward displacement of the heart and absent left pericardium. The white arrowhead indicates the right pericardium. **D**. ventricular level showing leftward displacement of the heart. (From Jacob, Souza, Parro 1995, with permission)

1.1.4.4   Clinical course and treatment

Total absence of the whole or of the left pericardium does not cause significant clinical events. Minor deficiencies, likewise, do not create symptoms, signs, or abnormal radiological or other images. It is the medium-sized defects that can cause chest pain and may allow herniation of part of the heart, usually the left atrial appendage. Strangulation of the hernia demands prompt relief of incarceration, most commonly at open operation, but sometimes via thoracoscopy. The threat of strangulation of cardiac tissue through a critically-sized defect should be obviated, either by enlarging it, by performing partial pericardiectomy (with or without excision of the appendage), or closing it at open operation or thoracoscopically (*Yamagishi., Ishikawa, Yoshida, 1997; Risher, Rees, Ochsner 1993*). Not all pericardial defects are congenital, as a pericardial incision may be made during thoracic or cardiac surgery, and not closed, allowing cardiac herniation. This event may be suspected on clinical grounds and be corrected with thoracoscopic surgery (*Rodgers, Moulder, DeLaney, 1979*).

2.   PERICARDIAL CYST

Pericardial cysts are not common (Figure 5). The overwhelming majority are located in the right cardio-phrenic angle, and the typical appearance is that of a circular smooth edged opacity with a density close to that of water; hence their designation as "spring water" cysts. Much less commonly, the cyst is located at the left cardio-phrenic angle. Other locations are rare. They are usually only 3 to 4 cm in diameter, but can be considerably larger, and occasionally are so massive. that their appearance on the chest radiogram simulates a large pleural effusion (*Satur, Hsin, Dussek, 1996*). Very large pericardial cysts occasionally mimic a pericardial effusion and, even more rarely, actually cause tamponade (*Bandeira, de Sa, Moriguti, 1996*). Some of these patients report dyspnea due to compression of the lung by the huge cyst. Spontaneous disappearance of a pericardial cyst has been reported, trauma being the assumed cause. Rarely, the wall of the cyst calcifies. Pericardial cysts do not cause symptoms unless they compress a vital structure. Pericardial diverticula are cysts that communicate with the pericardial cavity.

Some pericardial cysts form when a pericardial diverticulum closes and leaves behind a cyst, that usually is intrapericardial, but may migrate to an extrapericardial position. The contained "spring water" is acellular, sterile to culture and polymerase chain reaction, does not contain immune reactants and is lined with methothelial cells. Pericardial cysts may be confused with a rare pericardial tumour, the cystic teratoma.

The typical asymptomatic cyst is usually discovered after chest radiography for an unrelated reason. The typical lesion is almost unmistakable, but an opacity on the chest radiogram is always a matter for concern. Fortunately, both computer assisted tomography and magnetic resonance imaging can usually clarify the diagnosis. Echocardiography is perhaps less reliable for this purpose.

The differential diagnosis may be difficult when the location is atypical. Several decades ago, one of our patients had undergone myectomy for hypertrophic cardiomyopathy. Postoperatively, a bulge on the left heart border raised the possibility of a pseudo-aneurysm, but at exploration turned out to be a pericardial cyst. In the present era, thoracotomy would have been obviated by diagnostic imaging.

Congenital partial eventration of the diaphragm is the result of deficient muscularisation of the membranous diaphragm that divides the coelomic cavity into the peritoneal, pericardial and pleural cavities in the 8th to 10th week of embryologic development. The eventration permits migration of liver or other abdominal contents to herniate into the mediastinum in infants. The radiologic appearance of this abnormality simulates a large pericardial cyst. Recognition of eventration is important, since the treatment differs from that of pericardial cyst (*Hesselink, Chung, Peters, 1978*). Pericardio-diaphragmatic hernia in adults is due to injury of the diaphragm (*Larrieu, Wiener, Alexander, 1980*}.

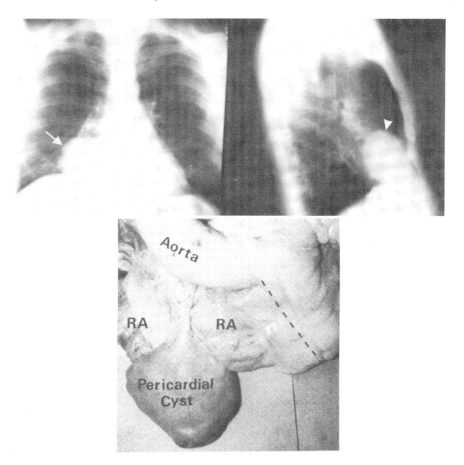

Figure 5. **Top::** The typical pericardial cyst appears as a large opacity in the right cardiophrenic angle (arrow) and lies anteriorly in the lateral projection (arrow head). **Bottom:** Photograph of a pathological specimen of a pericardial cyst. (From Roberts WC and Spray TL, in Spodick DH (ed). Pericardial Diseases. Philadelphia, FA Davis, 1976, with permission)

2.1   Treatment

Although pericardial cysts are benign and usually asymptomatic, patients may be sufficiently concerned that they request treatment. Typical cysts can be removed via a thoracoscope, or absolute alcohol can be injected into the cyst, which then disappears. Large or atypical cysts are usually treated by open chest surgical operation.

3.   MULIBREY NANISM

This is a rare autosomal recessive disease for which the abnormal genes have been mapped. Most of the patients are Finnish. The patients have low body weight and height (Nanism or dwarfism) and abnormalities of muscle, brain, and liver, but what makes the disease of interest to cardiologists is that a considerable proportion of them have diastolic dysfunction and many, but not all of that subset, have constrictive pericarditis. Pericardiectomy helps some of the patients but, in others, effects no improvement. When many of these patients were investigated, modern means to separate myocardial from pericardial aetiology of diastolic dysfunction had not been developed; therefore, clinicians lacked the means to predict the outcome of pericardiectomy, performing the operation empirically when diastolic dysfunction was severe. It may be that, in future, evaluation of respiratory variation of peak ventricular filling rates, colour Doppler, and tissue Doppler will enable physicians to predict the outcome of pericardiectomy.

4.   NONVIRAL INFECTIOUS PERICARDITIS

4.1   Tuberculous pericarditis

Tuberculosis remains an important cause of pericarditis but, unfortunately, diagnosis is not always straightforward and the mortality rate remains appreciable. This is not a trivial problem, because failure to recognise and treat a tuberculous pericardial effusion may lead to effusive constrictive pericarditis and eventually to severe chronic constriction. Since the publication of the first edition of this book, this situation has been eased somewhat by tests based on microbiology and enzymology. The diagnosis of tuberculous pericarditis is too often presumed on the basis of tuberculin skin testing, or contact with known cases of tuberculosis. Thus patients may be exposed to unnecessary chemotherapy and be wrongly labelled as having tuberculosis. A major cause of the difficulty in diagnosis is the low yield of tubercle bacillus in pericardial fluid from affected patients, because tens of millions of bacilli need to be present if they are to be reliably detected on stained smears, and because pericardial effusion in some cases is a reaction to tuberculin. The organisms grow faster on the newer liquid culture media, such as BACTEC radiometric broth, than they did on the time-honoured Lowenstein-Jensen solid culture medium used in the past for growing tubercle bacillus. The solid Middlebrook medium is now more commonly used than the Lowenstein-Jensen and tubercle bacilli grow on it. The *M tuberculosis* can thus now be grown in 8 days and drug sensitivity testing requires only two more days (*Roberts, Goodman, Heifets, 1983*). Culture of pericardial tissue can pick up some of the few cases missed by culturing pericardial fluid.

In developed countries, tuberculosis is an uncommon cause of pericarditis, although in the landmark study from a municipal hospital in Barcelona (*Permanyer-Miralda, Sagrista Sauleda, Soler-Soler, 1985*), tuberculosis accounted for 4 percent of 231 consecutive new cases of pericarditis and for 7 percent of 65 cases with tamponade. The epidemiology of pericardial effusion depends on the population studied, which means that one must be aware that the data from published studies cannot necessarily be extrapolated to the patients in one's own practice. For example, in contrast to the study from Barcelona, an American veterans hospital study of pericardial tissue and fluid, obtained by biopsy from 57 of 75 patients with a new large pericardial effusion, showed that tuberculosis was not the cause in a single case (*Corey, Campbell, Van Trigt, 1993*).

The most common mode of pericardial infection is spread from an adjacent infected lymph node, which usually is asymptomatic.

4.1.1   Diagnosis

It is important to enquire whether a patient newly diagnosed with pericarditis has had tuberculosis or contact with cases of pulmonary tuberculosis, especially sputum-positive cases. Most of the patients, however, do not have active parenchymal pulmonary tuberculosis. Otherwise, the history, clinical examination and image studies are not specific for tuberculosis, but depend on whether the manifestation is a haemodynamically insignificant effusion, cardiac tamponade, constrictive pericarditis, or acute pericarditis. Discussion of these entities in other chapters is not repeated here. Patients with acute tuberculous pericarditis usually have the general systemic symptoms of this infection, such as malaise and excessive sweating and often have fever. A negative skin test, particularly in patients with a positive reaction to mumps or candida, would mean that tubercular infection of the pericardium is highly unlikely. Although pericardial disease complicates only 1 or 2 percent of patients with pulmonary tuberculosis, 70 percent of patients with AIDS-related pericardial disease may have extrapulmonary tuberculosis, including tuberculous pericarditis as well (*Barnes, Bloch, Davidson, 1991*). Acid-fast bacilli should be sought in the pericardial fluid when present, otherwise in the sputum and gastric washings where their presence does not necessarily implicate the pericardium. Any pericardial fluid obtainable should be cultured in a liquid medium that yields rapid results. Pericardial and pleural fluid should be analysed for adenosine deaminase concentration. A level higher than 40 units/l indicates the diagnosis of tuberculosis with a sensitivity of 93 percent and specificity of 97 percent (*Koh, Kim, Cho, 1994*), although some false positives in cases of malignant pericardial effusion have been reported, but in these, the content of carcino-embryonic antigen is usually elevated. It is my practice to determine the adenosine deaminase concentration in all patients with a pericardial effusion of uncertain aetiology.

4.1.1.1   Role of polymerase chain reaction

Early recognition of tuberculous pericarditis is of the essence, because we have ample evidence that the sooner the treatment begins the better the outcome. In spite of the recent advances in diagnostic tools, certain diagnosis is often delayed by the shortcomings that persist. When acid-fast bacilli are demonstrated on a smear or section, the organisms may not be M *tuberculosis* but a related species, such as *M avium,* that can also cause pericardial disease (*Choo and McCormack 1995*). This infection must be considered, especially in immuno-incompetent patients with pericardial effusion, after excluding other infectious and non-infectious causes to which these patients are prone. It should be recalled, however, that the pericardial effusion may be of other aetiology. *M avium* pericarditis has been reported in several patients with AIDS. The application of nucleic acid amplification to prove the presence of DNA of *M tuberculosis* is therefore a welcome addition to the diagnostic armamentarium, because it is much faster, usually requiring only two days (*Cegielski, Devlin, Morris, 1997*). False positive results occasionally occur, however, but research continues and PCR should be done on pericardial fluid when the diagnosis of tuberculous pericarditis is under serious consideration.

4.1.2   Tuberculous pericardial effusion

The effusive phase follows an acute phase characterised by fibrinous pericarditis. In this phase, histological examination may disclose tubercles and acid-fast bacilli. The acute phase may pass unrecognised. Tuberculous pericardial effusion is usually more indolent than viral pericarditis, but can develop rapidly and become very large (Figure 6), and is an important cause of cardiac tamponade. In other cases, massive pericardial effusion accumulates slowly, in which case tamponade is mild or subclinical. The fluid is usually bloody, but occasionally is not. The predominating cell is the lymphocyte. When the effusion is infectious rather than reactive, the protein content is high, indicating its exudative nature. In the absorptive phase, the effusion lessens and pericardial thickening occurs, leading to effusive constrictive pericarditis with disease of the visceral pericardium and eventually to chronic constrictive pericarditis, often calcific. Tuberculosis of the pericardium may be discovered late and unexpectedly in the course of chronic effusive pericarditis, previously considered idiopathic (*Sagrista-Sauleda, Merce, Permanyer- Miralda, 2000*). See also Chapter 3.

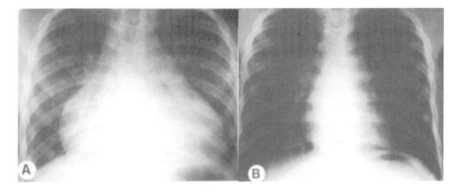

Figure 6. Primary tuberculous pericardial effusion **A:** on admission; **B:** after two weeks treatment with prednisone

Pericardial effusion in patients with tuberculosis does not necessarily imply tubercular infection of the pericardium. These non-infectious "primary" effusions are a reaction to tuberculin. Fifty percent of pericardial effusions associated with tuberculosis resorb spontaneously (*Permanyer–Miralda, Sagrista Sauleda, Soler-Soler, 1985*); presumably, these are of the reactive variety. How many of these patients later acquire tuberculosis of the pericardium is not known. This tendency of primary pericardial effusion in tuberculosis to disappear without treatment complicates interpretation of the effect of prednisone, as illustrated in Figure 6.

4.1.3   Treatment

The medical treatment of tuberculous pericarditis does not differ from that of other kinds of extrapulmonary tuberculosis. No effort should be spared before commencing antituberculous chemotherapy. All too often, patients are treated for a presumptive diagnosis of tuberculous pericarditis, based on findings such as conversion to positive of the tuberculin skin test, or contact with infected individuals. In general, this approach should not be taken but, in the case of immuno-incompetent patients with a large pericardial effusion, is sometimes acceptable. Many patients require, in addition, invasive intervention or surgical operation. The standard initial regimen comprises four antituberculous drugs given for 8 weeks, as follows:

Isoniazide 300 mg by mouth, once daily,

Rifampin 600 mg by mouth, daily,

Pyrazinamide 15 to 30 mg/k but not exceeding 2g/day,

Ethambutal, 15 to 25 mg by mouth, once daily, **OR** streptomycin 20 to 40 mg/k intramuscularly to a maximum of one gram daily.

Upon completion of this phase of treatment, most patients need to continue only with the isoniazide and rifampin for a total duration of treatment of six months *(Li, Corey, Sexton 2002)*.

The emergence of drug resistant strains of *M tuberculosis* is a major and growing concern *(Drobniewski, Eltringham, Graham, 2002)*, especially in underprivileged populations, and is due in part to poor compliance with the pharmacological regimen. In these circumstances, it is highly desirable to supervise the taking of every dose *(Dye, Garnett, Sleeman, 1998)*.

The above regimen applies to acute fibrinous pericarditis due to tuberculosis, tuberculous pericardial effusion and tamponade. Additional treatment required for specific syndromes is discussed below.

4.1.3.1   Pericardial effusion

If the effusion is not hemodynamically significant, the patient should be treated medically without pericardial invasion beyond the initial pericardiocentesis that established the diagnosis. Cardiac tamponade must be managed in the standard manner and be accompanied by the medical treatment outlined above. Large chronic pericardial effusion of unknown cause should be followed long term for the development of late tamponade and evidence of tuberculosis. Cardiac tamponade is still a significant contributor to death in tuberculous pericarditis, even though the decline in mortality is attributable in part to proper management of cardiac tamponade.

Effusive-constrictive pericarditis is a serious development in the natural history of pericarditis because it is a precursor of chronic constriction with its high morbidity and mortality. It therefore demands aggressive pharmacological treatment. Serious consideration of pre-emptive pericardiectomy is certainly warranted (*DeValeria, Baumgartner, Casale* 1991). Before embarking on this course, it is worthwhile to observe the effects of medical treatment, because the constrictive element of constrictive pericarditis may disappear after such treatment (*Gupta and Lokhandwala, 1996*).

One of the major aims of therapy is to prevent chronic constrictive pericarditis. Nevertheless, constriction eventually ensues in 40 to 50 percent of cases in spite of clinically effective chemotherapy. A study of the predictors of constriction showed that tamponade in the effusive phase was the leading predictor, in spite of complete resolution by pericardiocentesis (*Suwan and Potjalongsilp 1995*). A likely explanation is that tamponade presents earlier when the pericardium already is thickened, and that this thickening almost invariably proceeds to severe constriction.

4.1.3.2   Role of adrenal corticosteroid therapy

We now have data that support the addition of prednisone. Earlier, it had been suggested from clinical experience, but without the benefit of a placebo control trial, that inclusion of prednisone in the treatment regimen improved outcome. In Trankei, South Africa, tuberculous pericarditis is the commonest cause of right heart failure. This otherwise sad situation provided investigators with a database of tuberculosis of the pericardium that can never be matched in Europe or North America. The first of two large, randomised, placebo control trials examined the addition of 5 mg. of prednisolone for the first 11 weeks of treatment to directly supervised pharmacological therapy in 143 patients who had acute tuberculous constrictive pericarditis, proven by rigorous investigation (*Strang, Kakaza, Gibson 1987*). Four percent of the patients who received prednisolone died, versus 11 percent taking placebo. Likewise, the clinical status of those who received prednisolone improved more than those who did not. Prednisolone also lessened the severity of raised jugular pressure and reduced the requirement for eventual pericardiectomy from 30 to 21 percent.

The authors subsequently reported the effects of adding prednisolone to the standard treatment of 234 patients with effusive or effusive-constrictive pericarditis. Prednisolone reduced the mortality of patients treated by draining the fluid, from 14 to 3 percent. *(Strang, Kakaza, Gibson 1988).* A meta-analysis that included the data from Strang et al. and two smaller trials found the relative risk for the superiority of prednisone in 411 patients was only 0.36 to 1.16. Nevertheless, I and others (*Trautner and Darouiche, 2001; Mayosi, Volmink, Commerford 2000*) recommend adjuvant corticosteroid treatment for these patients. One mg/k/day for one month, and then tapered, is a suitable regimen.

Radical pericardiectomy is indicated for constrictive pericarditis with fluid retention and cardiac filling pressures exceeding 10 mmHg after four months of medical treatment including prednisolone. Best results are obtained, and with substantially less mortality, when the operation is performed early, and certainly before the advent of atrial fibrillation, wasting and ascites.

4.1.4   Pathology

Caseating necrosis found on examination of the pericardium excised at pericardiectomy or seen on biopsy or at necropsy (Figure 7) confirms the aetiology was pericarditis. In cases where tuberculosis was strongly suspected, but was unproven preoperatively, these lesions may or may not be found. In long-standing inactive cases, it is likely that the lesions had been replaced by fibrosis and calcification, but it is also possible that the aetiology was not tuberculosis. Postoperative antituberculous medical therapy is mandated when active lesions are found on operative specimens of pericardium.

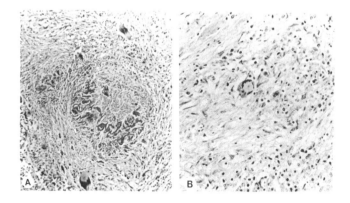

Figure 7: Tuberculous pericarditis. **Left:** Photomicrograph X40 of a typical granuloma of the pericardium. Central necrosis with aggregates of epithelioid cells at the periphery and several giant cells can be seen. **Right:** Photomicrograph X100 of a granuloma with Langerhans giant cells in the centre. (From Bloor CM. Cardiac Pathology. Philadelphia, Lippincott, 1978, with permission)

4.2   Fungal pericarditis

The more common fungal infections and inflammatory reactions of the pericardium are histoplasmosis, coccidiomycosis and candidiasis.

4.2.1   Histoplasmosis

In patients who live in areas where histoplasmosis is endemic, pericarditis or pericardial effusion that elsewhere would first be considered viral, tuberculous, or idiopathic, infection by H *capsulatum* deserves serious consideration (*Wheat, Stein, Corya 1983*). Pericardial histoplasmosis may be a true infection of the pericardium or be a sensitivity reaction to the antigen. Endemic areas are the Ohio and Mississippi valleys, and the Western Appalachians. Young, otherwise healthy persons, often male, are usually affected. As with tuberculosis, however, immunoincompetence, for any reason, increases susceptibility to the infection. Like tuberculosis, histoplasmosis of the pericardium is usually caused by spread from an infected hilar node and, less commonly, by haematogenous dissemination from infection anywhere in the body. Construction demolition and related activities release the organisms from their habitat in the ground to the air, and thus can trigger an outbreak of the disease. Again, as with tuberculosis, histoplasmosis sometimes progresses to severe constrictive pericarditis that requires pericardiectomy (*Wooley and Hosier 1961*). Physicians who see patients with pericardial effusion who live in or have recently been in endemic areas need to be aware that histoplasmosis is yet another cause of large recurrent pericardial effusion. When evaluating massive recurrent pericardial effusion, they should ascertain whether the patient has been in an endemic area (*Kilburn and McKinsey 1991*). In the spectrum of histoplasmosis, however, pericardial involvement is uncommon; only one of 61 patients seen in a thoracic surgical unit had pericardial disease, but that was tamponade (*Prager, Burney, Waterhouse 1980*).

4.2.1.1   Diagnosis

Distinguishing histoplasmosis from tuberculosis can be difficult. Pericardial effusion is more often the presenting feature. In both infections, hilar adenopathy is common, distinguishing them from viral pericarditis.

When the pericardium is tapped, the dominant cell found is the lymphocyte; histoplasmosis has been proven by biopsy, even when the organism was not seen or cultured from the fluid (*Zakowski and Ianuale-Shanerman 1993*). The pericardial fluid is usually an exudate, but only rarely are the organisms seen on smear, or by biopsy. More often, the diagnosis depends on serological testing. A single titre of 1:32 or more is strong evidence in favour of active or recent infection. Latex agglutination tests become positive in two or three weeks. The complement fixation test is positive in only half of the cases. It is most important not to perform skin testing until serological studies have been completed, because intradermal injection of histoplasmin interferes with the result. In some cases, *H capsulatum* can be isolated from peripheral blood or bone marrow. DNA of *H capsulatum* can now be identified by polymerase chain reaction with 100 percent specificity from biopsy specimens (*Bialek, Feucht, Aepinus, 2002*).

4.2.1.2   Treatment

In severe cases, the regimen should include ketoconozole, usually 200 mg daily by mouth suffices. Patients allergic to the conozoles may have to be treated with the much more toxic amphotericin B, which used to be the standard treatment and is effective. The dose is 35 to 40 mg/k daily, but because of renal and other toxicity, the initial dosing is sometimes less. In many cases, probably the majority, pericarditis and pericardial effusion are self-limiting and require no pharmacological treatment.

4.2.2   Coccidioidomycosis and blastomycosis

The responsible fungus, Coccidioides, is endemic in the South-West of the United states, causing "San Joaquin fever," and in Argentina it is often a component of disseminated infection (*Oudiz, Mahaisavariya, Peng 1995*). The infection spreads from pulmonary or mediastinal nodes; haematogenous spread, equivalent to miliary tuberculosis, also occurs, and then may lead to tamponade and constrictive pericarditis (Figure 8). Pericardiectomy, when required, should be done early in the course of effusive constrictive or frank constrictive pericarditis (*Faul, Hoang, Schmoker 1999*). An antifungal agent, such as fluconozole, should be administered preoperatively.

Other fungal infections of the pericardium include aspergillosis and candidiasis. The patients we see have AIDS, or are receiving immunosuppressive drugs after placement of a cardiac allograft.

4.3   Bacterial and purulent pericarditis

4.3.1   Historical note

Galen recognised purulent infection of the pericardium while removing the "putrefied" sternum of a patient with traumatic pericarditis (*Sexton and Corey 2002*). He also trephined the sternum of another young man with septic mediastinitis, removing a small piece of the pericardium (*Spodick 1970*).

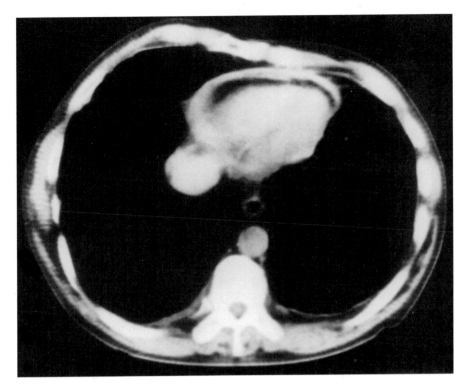

Figure 8. Computer assisted tomogram of the thorax of a patient who lived in the San Joaquin valley and developed constrictive pericarditis secondary to blastomycosis with widespread pulmonary and mediastinal involvement.

4.3.2   Epidemiology

The incidence of bacterial pericarditis and its aetiology have changed since the pre-antibiotic era, but it remains a serious disease with a high mortality. The diagnosis is elusive and too often missed or seriously delayed. The highest mortality occurs at the extremes of age. The miracles of modern medicine have not been wrought without a price. The easily handled pneumococcus as a cause of purulent infection of the pericardium has been displaced by the less tractable coagulase-positive *Staphylococcus aureus*, which is increasingly resistant to antibiotic treatment. The changes in the spectrum of infectious pericarditis were noted over 25 years ago (*Klacsmann, Bulkley, Hutchins, 1977*). They still apply and the trend continues. Pneumococcal pneumonia has ceased to be a common source of pericardial infection. In its place, we now see pericardial infection by direct spread from a variety of thoracic foci of infection, such as extension from a diaphragmatic or myocardial abscess, and a greater proportion of cases with haematological dissemination. Pre-existing pericardial disease, for instance, congenital absence, trauma, dialysis-associated pericardiopathy, or collagen vascular disease increase the susceptibility of the pericardium to infection. Pericarditis is a known complication of meningitis; often, it is a sensitivity reaction, but sometimes the pericardium is infected by *C Neisseria meningitidis* (*Blaser, Reingold, Alsever 1984*). A recent reclassification divides meningeal pericarditis into three syndromes: (1) disseminated meningococcal disease; (2) isolated meningococcal meningitis in which cerebral meningitis is absent; and (3) reactive, which occurs late in the course of meningitis and in which the effusion is sterile (*Finkelstein, Adler, Nussinovitch 1997*). A large variety of pyogenic organisms, including fungi, may be responsible. Fungal infection is a feature of the postoperative course of a patient with an infected valvular prosthesis or when immunosuppressed after cardiac transplantation (Figure 9). Candidiasis causes an aggressive purulent pericarditis that requires equally aggressive treatment. Anti-fungal drugs, complete evacuation of the pus, and pericardiectomy may all be needed (*Canver, Patel, Kosolcharoen, 1998*).

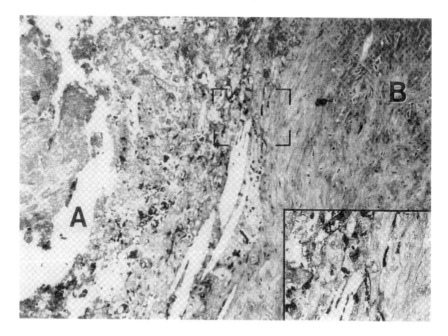

Figure 9. Photomicrograph of the pericardium of a patient with purulent pericarditis due to *C albicans*. The patient was a cardiac allograft recipient receiving immunosuppressive treatment. It shows the characteristic tangled mass of fungal hyphae, inflammatory debris (**A**), and organizing fibroblastic reaction (**B**). (Reproduced from Canver, Patel, Kosolcharoen 1998, with permission.)

Most of the patients we now see being treated in an intensive care unit have multi-system disease, and many have received antibiotics in doses that would be insufficient for purulent infection of a body cavity. Extensive investigation by intensivists and pulmonologists quite frequently has not included echocardiography. Most of the patients have a number of alternative reasons for oedema, such as raised venous pressure, fever and leukocytosis. Some are recovering from thoracic or cardiac surgical operation. Education to make physicians more aware of the possibility of purulent pericarditis would be helpful.

Any reasonable suspicion that a pericardial effusion may be purulent should lead to pericardial drainage. Patients admitted for cardiac tamponade may have pus in the pericardium and thus have two indications for draining the pericardium.

4.3.3   Diagnosis

In view of the elusive nature of the diagnosis, we need to maintain a high level of awareness of its existence. Patients with conditions and under the circumstances described above should heighten our index of suspicion. When suspicion has been aroused, the next step after the history and examination is to image the pericardium. Echocardiography will reveal the presence of pericardial effusion, and may show fibrin or other evidence that the effusion is organising but, to determine whether the effusion is a transudate or an exudate, its density should be measured by computer assisted tomography or magnetic resonance imaging. Unless imaging has definitively excluded purulent pericardial fluid, pericardiocentesis or pericardiotomy, followed by detailed analysis of the fluid, should be carried out promptly. If the common causative bacteria are not found, the clinician needs to seek less common ones, for example, E *coli,* Proteus, N *gonorrhoea,* B *melitensis,* T *tulerensis,* lseudomonas, Klebsiella and various salmonella species, to name some cited in the literature. The prudent cardiologist will turn this aspect of managing the case to an infectious disease specialist who has some control over the bacteriology laboratory.

4.3.3.1   The fluid

When the fluid is an exudate, the protein content is high. Glucose is less than 35 ml/dl (2 mmol/l). Leukocytosis is intense. Gram staining and culture usually furnish the aetiological diagnosis, but when these tests fail, the laboratory must conduct a systematic search for other pathogens.

4.3.4   Treatment

All agree that the pericardium must be evacuated as completely as possible. When the exudate is still liquid, this aim can be satisfied by pericardiocentesis followed by catheter drainage for several days. If the effusion is fibrinous, a fibrinolytic agent can be instilled into the pericardium (*Ustunsoy, Celkan,* Si;vri;koz *2002),* but this manoeuvre does not always succeed in making it possible to empty the pericardial space of purulent fluid (*Bridgman 2001*). When the exudate is thick and sticky, the pericardium should be drained surgically. This approach requires pericardiotomy using a subxiphoid incision, or thoracotomy with more extensive pericardiectomy. It is wise to consult an infectious disease specialist who will participate in selecting and managing the antibiotic regimen. High pericardial concentration of antibiotics is achieved with systemic administration; thus intrapericardial administration has no place in the treatment. Many of these patients are severely debilitated, calling for maximal measures to preserve their overall status.

4.3.5   Other infective agents

A number of other agents may infect the pericardium, including, *amoeba histolytica,* (*Singh, Singh, Didwania 1987*), *nocardia asteroides* (*Chavez, Causey, Conn 1972*), E *coli*, and C psittaci. I followed a patient with rheumatoid arthritis and a small pericardial effusion. Subsequently, he developed severe tamponade and was treated by pericardiocentesis. He then travelled to Mexico where he acquired E *coli* septicemia. Upon return, he again had severe cardiac tamponade, but this time the effusion was purulent and grew E *coli*. He underwent pericardiectomy. I mention this case because the aetiology of pericardial effusion in a patient may change.

4.4   Purulent pericarditis in children

Purulent pericarditis is an uncommon disease in early childhood, but carries a high mortality and may lead to the extraordinarily rapid development of constrictive pericarditis (*Caird, Conway, McMillan 1973*). The children are desperately ill. Until severe tamponade or constriction appears, the clinical picture, as in adults, is dominated by the extrapericardial source of infection, and by systemic findings, such as high fever and heart rate. The two most common infecting organisms are S *aureus* and H *influenzae* followed by N *meningitis*. Children acquire bacterial pericarditis from a variety of illnesses that are common in the young. These include streptococcal tonsillitis, otitis media, pharyngitis, and meningitis (*Lorrell and Braunwald 1992*).

5. METABOLIC CAUSES OF PERICARDIAL DISEASE

5.1 Renal disease and dialysis-related

Pericarditis, usually with effusion, may complicate the course of patients receiving chronic haemodialysis. The effusion causes tamponade in a significant proportion of the cases. Tamponade associated with dialysis has now displaced end-stage as the commonest cause of pericarditis due to renal disease. Dialysis-related pericardial disease presents the problem that its diagnosis, and certainly the treatment, is made difficult by dialysis-induced hypovolemia in a substantial proportion of the patients. Fortunately, this problem, while still an important threat to these patients, has become much less frequent following the use of new membranes on the machines. This change suggests that some as yet unidentified molecules, that were able to cross the membranes on older machines, are filtered by the newer membranes. Pericarditis is less frequent when peritoneal dialysis rather than haemodialysis or ultra-filtration is used to treat end-stage renal disease. It is possible that peritoneal dialysis blocks the absorption of middle molecules formed during nitrogen metabolism.

There were eight cases of pericarditis in the series of 100 autopsied patients who died from renal failure, reported by Richard Bright *(Bright 1836)*. Renal disease, because of the advent of dialysis, has increased the prevalence of 8 percent, noted by Bright, to about 20 percent (*Colombo, Olson, Egan 1988*). In end-stage renal disease, pericardial disease manifests when the blood urea nitrogen is above 60 mg/dl, and often considerably higher than that, whereas much lower levels may affect the pericardium in the case of dialysis (*Rostand and Rutsky 1990*).

5.1.1 Aetiology

The reasons why patients with uraemia, or undergoing chronic dialysis, are susceptible to pericarditis and pericardial effusion are not known. Furthermore, the cause may be different in the two patient groups. The immune system in uraemia is depressed, leaving the patients more likely to catch infection. Clustering of cases supports possible viral infection.

Alternatively, the pericardial disease may be an immune response, as suggested by the observation that more than half a series of 25 uremic patients had complement-fixing antimyolemmal antibodies with cytolytic myocardial properties. This immunopathy was not seen in acute pericarditis of other aetiology (*Maisch and Kochsiek 1983*).

5.1.2   Clinical features

Patients with acute uremic pericarditis, but no effusion, have pain characteristic of pericarditis and a coarse friction rub that may be palpable. The electrocardiographic findings that would be expected, however, are absent because pericarditis of uremic aetiology spares the epicardium (*Black, 2002*). When complications are absent, the physical exam is unremarkable, but the patient should be observed for signs of tamponade. Rarely, uremic pericarditis leads to constrictive pericarditis. The pericardial fluid is almost always bloody, and the presence of retained blood may give rise to fever. Patients with uraemia are notorious for hemorrhagic diathesis that likely leads to blood in the pericardium. Certainly, the pericardial granulation tissue is highly vascular. Patients with late stage chronic renal disease often have platelet dysfunction and increased capillary permeability. Systemic heparinisation aggravates bleeding; therefore, regional heparinisation is preferred.

5.1.3   Pathology

Uremic pericarditis is a dense fibrinous reaction (Figure 10) with very few cells visible; it may be dry, or there may be a sanguineous pericardial effusion. Viewed in the operating suite, the pericardium is red and the underlying heart muscle is often friable. In more chronic cases, the effusion is organised, the pericardium thickens and becomes densely fibrotic, giving rise to its "onion-peel" appearance.

5.1.4   Treatment

Acute dry uremic pericarditis is treated in the same way as acute pericarditis of other aetiology, except that it is wise not to use aspirin, because it may increase the liability to bleeding. If pericardiocentesis is required, the operator needs to know the clotting profile and to be aware of the increased risk for a poor outcome should the myocardium be injured.

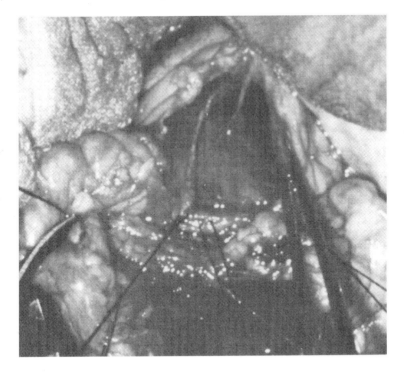

Figure 10. Uremic pericarditis. Photograph taken during pericardiectomy for uremic pericarditis.

For dialysed patients, the standard treatment of pericardial effusion is to increase the intensity of dialysis, although it is effective in only about half of the patients with a large symptomless pericardial effusion (*Frommer, Young, Ayus 1985*). In euvolemic patients, the response is usually gratifying, but patients undergoing rigorous dialysis may be hypovolemic in consequence. Increasing dialysis in such patients can precipitate low-pressure cardiac tamponade that can be hard to detect on clinical examination. The pericardial effusion must be monitored by a cardiologist, trained in echocardiography, for signs of cardiac compression. This situation calls for high quality decision-making because, depending on their volume status, some of the patients respond to increased dialysis, but others to volume loading, and the presentation of tamponade is often atypical. In the past, non-absorbable corticosteroid was instilled into the pericardium to dampen the inflammatory response (*Buselmeier, Davin, Simmons 1978*). This mode of treatment is now less popular, but still advocated by some (*Quigg, Idelson, Yoburn 1985*).

Recurrence of pericardial effusion, persistence beyond three weeks, or cardiac tamponade should be treated by pericardiotomy. The easiest approach is a subxiphoid incision with removal of the xiphoid process. Local anaesthesia usually suffices, and when necessary, the procedure can be performed at the bedside (*Prager, Wilson, Bender 1982*; *Rostand and Rutsky, 1990*).

5.2   Hypothyroidism: Myxoedema

Pericardial effusion occurs in some hypothyroid states but, except for cases with myxoedema, is seldom clinically significant. Pericardial effusion is found in a third of frankly myxoedematous patients and may be very large. The presence of pericardial effusion does not correlate with the level of thyroxine or thyroid stimulating hormone, although the heart rate is slower in those with pericardial effusion than in those without (*Kerber and Sherman, 1975)*. Pericardial effusion is a result of the pathophysiology of myxoedema; namely, slowed lymphatic drainage, sodium and water retention, and increased capillary permeability with extravasation of protein.

Radiological cardiomegaly is mostly due to the pericardial effusion, which can be of enormous volume, but sometimes it is due to myxoedematous cardiomyopathy, or independent heart disease. These effusions may be asymptomatic. When the effusion is symptomatic, the symptoms could just as easily be attributed to myxoedema itself. Myxoedema effusions seldom cause tamponade, although cases have been reported (*Smolar, Rubin, Avramides,1976)*.

The pericardial fluid is generally clear and straw-coloured, with a high content of protein and cholesterol. Myxoedema is thus a cause of cholesterol pericarditis. For discussion of cholesterol pericarditis, see Chapter 3.

Electrocardiographic features are sinus bradycardia, low QRS and P voltage, and decreased amplitude or inversion of the T wave. The severity of the ECG and radiological changes correlate quite well. QT is prolonged; the precise measurement of the interval is prevented by inability to locate the end of the T wave because of its low amplitude. Disturbance of atrioventricular and intraventricular conduction are present more often than in the general population. Torsade de pointes, causing syncope, most likely is explained by the prolonged repolarisation time (*Surawicz 2001)*.

5.3   Chylopericardium

This topic is covered in Chapter 3. Briefly, the chylopericardium is an effusion of chyle from the thoracic duct into the pericardium. It may be caused by a congenital anomaly or by injury of the duct.

6. THE PERICARDIUM AND MYOCARDIAL INFARCTION

6.1 Infarction pericarditis and pericardial effusion

The pericardium may be affected in two principal ways by a myocardial infarction. Firstly, within two or three days, pericarditis with or without effusion may supervene (infarction pericarditis). Secondly, in a smaller proportion of patients, an immune response causes delayed pericardial effusion (post cardiac injury syndrome).

A report from the GISSI study stated that introduction of fibrinolysis for the early management of acute myocardial infarction has reduced the incidence of infarction pericarditis (*Correale, Maggioni, Romano 1993*). The true incidence of pericarditis can be arrived at only by frequently repeated auscultation for a pericardial rub in a large number of consecutive patients who have sustained an acute myocardial infarction not more than three days earlier. The rub has to be relied upon, because pericardial pain may be absent and, in any case, can be very hard to tell from myocardial ischemia. Comparable problems confound interpretation of the electrocardiogram. A clue, however, is that the evolution of T-wave abnormalities is atypical. This T-wave evolution, atypical for myocardial infarction, is present in most cases with clinical pericarditis, but also in half the cases with a pericardial effusion, without other evidence of pericarditis (*Oliva, Hammill, Talano 1994*). Even the rub is not without its problems; it may be there one hour or one day and not another. Pericarditis occurs more frequently after a large anterior infarction. The effusion worsens the prognosis, not directly, but because it indicates that the infarction was substantial (*Wall, Califf, Harrelson-Woodlief 1990*). The proportion of cases with pericarditis discovered at autopsy far exceeds the best clinical estimates (*Dubois, Smeets, Demoulin 1985*).

Treatment is seldom indicated and, in fact, may be deleterious, because steroidal and nonsteroidal antiinflammatory drugs impair healing of the infarction and may thus lead to myocardial rupture and death, or ventricular aneurysm. An observational retrospective analysis of 41 cases so treated reported that half of them had sustained rupture of the infarction (*Hammerman, Alker, Schoen 1984*). Pericardial effusion frequently occurs early in the course, but almost always makes no clinical impact. The true incidence can therefore only be determined by serially performed echocardiograms. These studies have shown that effusion appears early in the course of acute infarction, is present in about a third of the patients, and persists for a surprisingly long time (*Galve, Garcia-del-Castillo, Evangelista*

1986). The majority are small and asymptomatic, but sometimes they are large, and can complicate the course with severe tamponade (*Fuchs, Weiss, Elami, 1997*). Rupture of the infarcted myocardium creates a haemorrhagic effusion that can easily progress to tamponade. It may well be a fatal error to attribute greatly depressed blood pressure and cardiac output to cardiogenic shock, when the real cause is decompensated cardiac tamponade.

6.1.1   Pericardial injury (Dressler's syndrome)

A second pericardial complication of acute myocardial infarction is the post-pericardial injury syndrome, a delayed reaction of the pericardium to any kind of injury to the heart or pericardium. That pericardial pain, fever, leukocytosis and pericardial effusion may occur weeks, months or years after a myocardial infarction was first reported by Dressler as the "post-myocardial infarction syndrome" (*Dressler 1959*). In the early days of cardiac surgery, a similar syndrome was noted to follow cardiac operation and was called the post-cardiotomy syndrome, until it was appreciated that when the pericardium was opened, but no cardiac incision had been made, the syndrome occurred nevertheless, so its name was changed to the post-pericardiotomy syndrome. Chest trauma is yet another cause of this syndrome, so now all these syndromes are considered as one, namely, the post-pericardial injury syndrome. Eponymous titles for diseases are attractive because the intent is to memorialise those who were the first to describe them, but too often the attribution is erroneous, and such terminology conveys nothing concerning pathophysiology or clinical aspects.

6.1.1.1   Pathogenesis

Myocardial injury stimulates the formation of antigens that in turn form complexes with the antigens and deposit them on the pericardium, pleura and lung parenchyma. Consistent with this explanation are the latency between the insult and the beginning manifestations of the syndrome, its response to corticosteroid treatment, and its tendency to relapse.

6.1.1.2   Clinical features

Typically, the onset is weeks or months after the heart attack, but occurrences after only a few days or, alternatively, years afterwards have been reported. Pericardial and pleural pain, fever, leukocytosis, an elevated erythrocyte sedimentation rate and other markers of acute inflammation are common. If the effusion progresses to tamponade, the associated symptoms appear and may dominate.

On examination, the patient appears ill and distressed. Pericardial and pleural friction rubs may be auscultated, and signs of pleural effusion elicited. If the repolarisation changes of myocardial infarction have resolved, evidence of acute pericarditis may well be seen on the electrocardiogram; otherwise, electrocardiographic changes are subtle. The chest radiogram often shows pleural effusion and, less often, lung infiltrates. Administration of nonsteroidal antiinflammatory drugs or, failing that, a corticosteroid brings about rapid resolution. When the syndrome is very severe, 1 mg/k of prednisone can be given for a few days, and then tapered. If tamponade is severe, pericardiocentesis should not be delayed while awaiting a response to pharmacological treatment. The syndrome may end as constrictive pericarditis (*Cheung, Myers, Arnold, 1991*) but fortunately, only rarely.

7. TRAUMATIC PERICARDIAL DISEASE

7.1 Historical note

The first successful closure of a pericardial laceration was performed in Chicago in 1893, a time when surgeons were taught, "Any surgeon who would attempt to suture a wound of the heart is not worthy of the serious consideration of his colleagues," an admonition attributed to Theodore Billroth *(Dupre and O'Leary, 1997)*.

7.2 Syndromes of pericardial injury

As discussed elsewhere in this volume, trauma may play an important role in the aetiology of pericardial effusion, cardiac tamponade and constrictive pericarditis, the latter being a late sequel. The injury may be sharp, including iatrogenic, or blunt. Major causes of blunt injury of the pericardium include vehicle accident, motorcycle crash, a serious fall, and crushing. Major causes of sharp pericardial injury include gunshot, stabbing, impalement and interventional cardiac procedures. All are manifestations of the pericardial injury syndrome discussed in the preceding paragraphs. Most of the cases are seen in trauma centres. Emergency or urgent operative treatment is frequently needed. Mortality is high, but prompt treatment lowers it *(Fulda, Rodriguez, Turney 1990)*.

Contusion of the heart may be associated with blunt chest trauma, thereby simulating myocardial infarction. Non-haemorrhagic effusions may develop slowly after blunt trauma, or rapidly, with consequent tamponade. Thus trauma is another cause of the pericardial injury syndrome. Gunshot wounds of the heart can be expected to produce early tamponade, but exceptions occur. A 12 year old girl who sustained multiple pellets in the heart was treated initially with a pericardial drain, but one month later she had a large pericardial effusion, without evidence of tamponade (*Tutar, Atalay, Uysalel, 1999).* Between these extremes are cases in which tamponade is delayed only a matter of hours (*Narins, Cunningham, Delehanty, 1996).* Severe blunt chest trauma calls for careful follow-up for tamponade or rhythm disturbance, and electrocardiographic changes resulting from contusion of the heart. Blunt chest injuries can rupture the diaphragmatic or pleural aspect of the pericardium, with early or delayed herniation of abdominal contents into the pericardium, or of the heart into a pleural cavity, usually the left (*Roebuck and Minford, 1983).* An intrapericardial haematoma may form when pericardial haemorrhage fails to resorb completely. These haematomata may calcify, and may be mistaken for granulomata or neoplasm. They may cause regional constriction of the heart, or even constrictive pericarditis (*Meleca and Hoit, 1995). They* may compress a saphenous venous graft and cause ischemia (*Shehata and Gillam, 1996)* or obstruct the right ventricular outflow tract (*Phillips, Rodriguez, Cowley 1983).* Clearly, these pericardial haematomata can be responsible for diagnostic dilemmas and create interesting anomalies of physiology. Pericardial trauma from puncture by another animal's horn is common in cattle (*Simeonov 1978).* To end this account of unusual pericardial injuries, I mention the case of a fur seal that swallowed the barbed spine of a ray, which punctured the right ventricle (*Obendorf and Presidente 1978).*

8.   HYPERSENSITIVITY, AUTOIMMUNITY, AND THE COLLAGEN VASCULAR DISEASES

8.1   Acute rheumatic fever

From Osler we learned that rheumatic carditis is generally a pancarditis. Rheumatic pericarditis, however, is sometimes present without carditis, may be fibrinous, effusive or, in children, purulent. We know that the pericarditis resolves spontaneously, because we seldom see autopsy evidence of it in patients who die of rheumatic heart disease. Clinically apparent pericarditis denotes severe carditis. Pain, pericardial friction rub and the characteristic abnormalities of cardiac repolarisation are found. The patient may develop pericardial effusion. Pericarditis is distinctly uncommon in children, except in the case of acute rheumatic carditis, in which it is sometimes the first clue to myocardial involvement.

The diagnosis is often straightforward but, depending on the findings and clinical circumstances, it is sometimes necessary to consider other diseases in this category, including juvenile rheumatoid arthritis and lupus erythematosus. Other considerations include purpura and infective endocarditis.

Evidence of carditis demands bed rest. Although bed rest for many other conditions so treated is now deprecated, it remains important when carditis is active. Penicillin should be given to eradicate the causative streptococcal infection, and any later pharyngitis should lead to culture for this organism or, failing that, prophylactic administration of penicillin. High dose aspirin is standard treatment, but corticosteroid treatment is needed for refractory cases. Pericardial effusion usually responds to this therapy. Tamponade is not common but, if present, is treated in the standard manner.

8.2   Lupus erythematosus

More than half the patients develop pericarditis somewhere along the course of lupus erythematosus *(Ansari, Larson, Bates 1986)*. Echocardiographic abnormalities are more frequent than clinical findings. In some cases, pericardial effusion is the first finding. Lupus is sometimes discovered after an echocardiogram has been performed for a different purpose. Other patients have the classic signs of acute fibrinous pericarditis. Pericarditis often accompanies a flare-up of lupus activity. Both pericardial and myocardial involvement are seen by necropsy in a high proportion of the cases *(Doherty, Feldman, Maurer. 1988)*. Constrictive pericarditis and cardiac tamponade are rare complications.

Tamponade can appear at any stage, and may even be the first manifestation of lupus *(Kahl 1992)*. Valvular disease or cardiac conduction disturbances, as well as extra-cardiac manifestations of the disease and lupus antibodies furnish evidence of lupus pericarditis.

The correct diagnosis can be assured by endomyocardial biopsy. At necropsy, verrucous vegetations of non-infectious endocarditis (Liebman Sach disease) may be superimposed on lupus lesions, but are seldom detected by echocardiography.

Lupus erythematosus is not confined to the naturally occurring disease, but also occurs in that form of the disease induced by drugs such as hydralazine, mexilitine and procainamide. It can be difficult to decide if pericarditis is caused by the uraemia of lupus nephritis or lupus immune complexes.

8.3   Rheumatoid arthritis

The nature of pericardial involvement in rheumatoid arthritis is incompletely understood. The pathology in most cases is obliterative pericarditis. Acute fibrinous pericarditis and pericardial effusion make up the remainder. Specific granulomatous infiltration is not common; when present, it takes the form of small rheumatoid nodules located superficially in the myocardium. The pericardium is infiltrated with CD8+ and T lymphocytes. The number of these cell types in the peripheral blood is increased (*Travaglio-Encinoza, Anaya, Dupuy D'Angeac 1994*). Cholesterol crystals and IgE immune complexes may be found in the pericardial fluid (*Van Offel, De Clerck, Kersschot, 1991*). The onset of pericarditis is not related to the duration of the disease and is more common in middle-aged men. Serological tests for rheumatoid arthritis are almost invariably positive. Many of the patients have extra-articular lesions, particularly rheumatoid lung and pleural nodules, with or without effusion. Pericardial fluid is high in protein, but low in glucose, typically 20 to 45 mg./dl. Rheumatoid arthritis is an important cause of constrictive pericarditis (*Thould, 1986*) in which it may develop with surprising rapidity. This syndrome has been observed in children. Pericardial disease complicates variants such as Still's disease (systemic juvenile rheumatoid arthritis) (*Alukal, Costello, Green 1984*), adult Still's disease in which, rarely, it may be a cause of cardiac tamponade (*Jamieson, 1983)* and ankylosing spondylitis *(Shah and Askari 1987*).

8.4   Mixed connective tissue disease

An excellent, beautifully illustrated description of this complex entity has been published recently (*Bennett, 2002*). Raynaud's phenomenon is common; renal and central nervous system disease tends to be mild. Arthritis is severe. Pulmonary hypertension comes on insidiously and is not related to pulmonary fibrosis, as it is in scleroderma. Skin involvement is common.

Pericardial disease is the commonest cardiac abnormality. Although a large pericardial effusion is sometimes found, the most common clinical manifestations of cardiac involvement are those due to right ventricular hypertrophy or failure.

8.5   Progressive systemic sclerosis – scleroderma

Limited cutaneous scleroderma (CREST) is confined to the skin of the hands, face, feet, and forearms. Raynaud's phenomenon is a late manifestation. Diffuse cutaneous scleroderma eventually becomes a multi-system disease, the skin thickening is severe and limits mobility of the affected parts. Dysphagia, secondary to involvement of the oesophagus, is common. Pulmonary fibrosis leads slowly to pulmonary hypertension. As in lupus and rheumatoid disease, pericardial disease is a frequent finding at autopsy (*Byers, Marshall, Freemont, 1997*).

The pericardiopathy is usually associated with cardiomyopathy, accounting for the ominous prognosis of pericarditis in scleroderma. Both pericardium and myocardium are fibrotic. A number of autoimmune antibodies are present in the blood of a significant number of the patients.

8.6 Drug-induced pericarditis

Pericardial disease may develop after exposure to a variety of drugs, including hydralazine, psicofuranine, procainamide, isonicotinic acid, warfarin, penicillin, phenylbutazone, methysergide, and daunorubicin. Procainamide, hydralazine and isoniazid produce a pericardial lesion that shares many of the characteristics of lupus erythematosus, and may occasionally lead to constrictive pericarditis or, even less commonly, cardiac tamponade. Methysergide, when it causes constrictive pericarditis, does so as part of a generalised mediastinal fibrosis. Pericarditis, induced by penicillin, is presumed to be a hypersensitivity reaction. Pericardial effusion may follow the use of minoxidil. Pericardial effusion and eosinophilia have been reported following the use of cromolyn sodium to treat bronchial asthma. Mesalamine, a drug used in the treatment of inflammatory bowel disease, has been cited as a cause of recurrent pericarditis (*Sentongo and Piccoli 1998*).

The list of possible culprits is too long to memorize, and new drugs may well be added. The mechanisms and, consequently, the manifestations and pathology differ. The pharmacists have made the data on drug interactions readily available; the wise course, when faced with a new case of pericardial disease, is to obtain a complete list of the patient's medications, and then consult a pharmacist, or access the database.

9. NEOPLASTIC PERICARDIAL DISEASE

Neoplasm is a leading cause of pericardial disease. This topic is covered in earlier chapters. I will not repeat most of that material in this section, the resulting brevity of which by no means reflects the importance of neoplasm in pericardial disease. Malignant tumours metastasise to the myocardium and pericardium with equal ease; but it is only in the latter that they commonly cause significant clinical findings. The highest involvement of the pericardium in malignancy is with carcinomas of the lung and breast in which about 35 percent have a significant pericardial effusion. Leukaemia, lymphoma and melanoma also often metastasise to the heart and pericardium, although less commonly. Many other malignant tumours may cause pericardial disease. These include carcinomas of the gastrointestinal tract, kidney, ovary *(Winter, Seidman, Krivak 2002)* and prostate *(Hayes-Lattin, Kovach, Henner, 2002)*. AIDS has brought about an increase in Kaposi's sarcoma and other tumours of the pericardium *(Barbaro and Klatt, 2002)*.

The number of primary pericardial neoplasms of the pericardium is surprisingly high, but they are infinitely less common than secondary pericardial neoplasm. Primary pericardial neoplasms include stromal tumours, the most common of which is the mesothelioma. Magnetic resonance imaging is helpful in identifying these tumours *(Gossinger, Siostrzonek, Zangeneh 1988)*. This tumour can cause a remarkable increase in the thickness of the pericardium with severe constriction of the heart. *(Llewellyn, Atkinson, Fabri, 1987)*: Mesothelioma may be disclosed by magnetic resonance imaging of patients with pericardial effusion of unknown cause that are refractory to treatment. Among the rarer pericardial tumours are various nonmyxomatous neoplasms. A non-diagnostic lesion is detectable by echocardiography, but certain diagnosis requires cross-sectional magnetic resonance imaging *(Smith, Shaffer, Patz 1998)*. Vascular tumours such as lymphangioma and haemangioma may invade the pericardium *(Burke, Johns, Virmani 1990)*. Developmental rests, for instance, teratoma *(Arciniegas, Hakimi, Farooki, 1980)*, and a miscellaneous group of neoplasms, such as neuro-fibroma, may also invade the pericardium.

The pericardial involvement may be via direct extension, as in cancer of the lung or breast, by retrograde lymphatic spread, which also may be the mechanism of dissemination of bronchogenic and mammary carcinoma, or by haematogenous spread, of which a common example is melanoma. Pericardial pheochromocytoma *(Saad, Frazier, Hickey 1983)* is difficult to localise and treat, but fortunately is very rare.

9.1   Syndromes of malignant pericardial disease

A number of different pericardial syndromes may be encountered. One is fibrinous pericarditis that does not differ from acute fibrinous pericarditis of other aetiology, except that pericardial effusion is more common and often is larger. Both the pathogenesis and the pathophysiology of malignant pericardial effusion are variable. Some are manifestations of advanced disease and are owing to invasion of the pericardium by the neoplasm; these effusions are often bloody and constitute an important aetiology of cardiac tamponade, especially on a hospital medical service. In other patients who have neoplastic disease and a pericardial effusion, the effusion is not malignant in the sense of containing "malignant" cells, but is "sympathetic"; which is to say that it is most likely an immune response. These effusions also may cause cardiac tamponade.

Another important syndrome is constrictive pericarditis, in which there may be, in addition, "superior vena caval syndrome" due to encasement of this great vein by tumour. This venous obstruction complicates bedside evaluation of central venous pressure. The jugular pressure is greatly elevated *(Wang, Yang, Chao, 2000)* in contradistinction to tamponade, and venous pulsations are absent on the side of obstruction, commonly the right side. The typical contour of venous pressure in tamponade can be obtained from the inferior vena cava and often the right atrium. Instead of classical constrictive pericarditis, some patients have effusive-constrictive pericarditis.

9.2   Treatment.

A number of options are open to the physician whose lot it is to treat patients with malignant pericardial disease ((*Shepherd 1997*). These options include pericardiocentesis, pericardiotomy, pericardiectomy, and balloon pericardiotomy (*Wang, Hsu, Chiang, 2002*). Intrapericardial instillation of a sclerosing agent, OK-432, interferon (*Maher, Shepherd, Todd 1996; Wilkins, Cacioppo, Connolly, 1998*), ^{32}P-colloid and a variety of cytostatic drugs (*Dempke and Firusian 1999*), and radiation, especially for highly radiosensitive neoplasm, such as leukaemia, must be strongly influenced by the age and general condition of the patient, and the wishes of the patient and family. Other factors that enter the recommendations are the prognosis of the malignancy itself and of any co-morbidity that may be present. Symptoms such as dyspnea may demand treatment. When the prognosis is poor, therapeutic efforts should be directed at relief of symptoms and the patient's comfort and peace of mind. While removal of pericardial fluid is usually the correct treatment for patients with moderate or severe tamponade, some patients with end-stage disease and severe pain and depression may prefer to be allowed to die with only sedation to relieve the dyspnea and other symptoms; their wishes should be respected. Thus for some patients with malignant pericardial disease, hospice care, not pericardiectomy or pericardiocentesis, is appropriate. It is vitally important for cardiologists and emergency room physicians to spare no effort to contact the patient's primary care physician before proceeding with invasive treatment. All too often, emergency room physicians or cardiologists, confronted with patients they have never set eyes on before, rush instinctively to pericardiocentesis, only to be greeted by an angry patient, family member and primary caregiver, instead of their anticipated gratitude.

When the prognosis is not so grim, a more vigorous and more conventional approach is proper. Patients with malignancy of the pericardium may survive with relative well-being for a year or more. Even those patients with tamponade of malignant aetiology are not necessarily doomed to imminent death; many of them require evacuation of the pericardial fluid, and perhaps partial or total pericardiectomy. Ethically, when encountering a patient with neoplastic pericardial disease with whom one is not thoroughly familiar, and knowing little or nothing of the social and family situation, the physician should give the patient the "benefit of the doubt" and treat aggressively; all well and good if the patient's doctor and family cannot be reached in reasonable time.

Where possible, pericardiocentesis is preferable to pericardiotomy or pericardiectomy for a first episode of tamponade. Subxiphoid pericardiotomy, using local anaesthesia for patients whose general health has greatly deteriorated, is appropriate for recurrence of tamponade. Some physicians favour this approach for first episodes of tamponade; it is well within the standard of care. Pericardiotomy is preferred when a physician skilled at pericardiocentesis is not available. Pericardiotomy allows biopsy if indicated, and recurrences are less likely than after pericardiocentesis without subsequent prolonged catheter drainage. In unlucky individuals, the pericardial injury syndrome may cause additional distress postoperatively.

A bewildering number of sclerosing agents have been instilled into the pericardium in an attempt to prevent recurrence of malignant pericardial effusion. The procedure often evokes considerable pericardial pain. Recently, it has been shown that if pericardiocentesis is followed by catheter drainage until the drain collects only 50 ml/24 hours or less, the resulting prevention of recurrent pericardial effusions equals that obtained after instillation of a sclerosing agent *(Gibbs, Watson, Singh, 2000)* (see also Chapter 6). My own practice is to avoid sclerosing agents whenever I can, which is almost always.

9.3   Cytology

Exfoliative cytological examination of pericardial fluid is useful for the diagnosis of malignancy, but also for excluding this diagnosis. A definite reading of malignancy is 100 percent specific, but sensitivity is less, according to most published accounts *(Wiener, Kristensen, Haubek, 1991)*. A difficulty in interpretation arises from cells described as atypical, usually secondary to inflammation. Cells of this type are, in turn, classified as definite, atypia, or suspicious for malignancy. Cytological examination may also provide prognostic information, as in the case of small cell carcinoma of the lung (*Wang, Yang, Chao 2000).*

10. IONISING RADIATION

Radiation injury of the pericardium usually is a consequence of therapeutic radiation. Much less commonly, the cause is accidental exposure, as in laboratory accidents, a breakdown of, or leak from a nuclear power generator, as in the case of Chernoble and Three Mile Island. Massive exposure to radiation followed the detonation of atomic bombs in Japan at the end of World War II, and a number of military personnel who participated in, or witnessed, tests of atomic bombs before effective shielding was in routine use were similarly exposed.

Much of our knowledge derives from the experience at Stanford University accumulated after an otherwise dramatically successful program of radiotherapy for Hodgkin's disease during which radiation-induced heart disease was a frequent serious complication (*Schultz-Hector, 1992*). The commonest form of radiation-induced heart disease is pericardial injury. Pericardiopathy induced by radiation falls into several categories, although these may overlap. (*Stewart, Fajardo, Gillette,1995).*

Acute pericarditis, with or without pericardial effusion, may arise during treatment or, less commonly, soon afterwards. Cardiac tamponade complicates some of these cases. Quite frequently, however, early acute pericarditis is a benign illness, self-limiting and responsive to antiinflammatory treatment. Delayed acute pericarditis develops weeks, months or years after the initiating radiotherapy. It too, may be dry or effusive and can be associated with cardiac tamponade. Constrictive pericarditis is a late phenomenon and may be delayed several decades. Radiotherapy is a major cause of effusive-constrictive pericarditis (see Chapter 6). Mediastinal radiation induces myocardial as well as pericardial fibrosis; therefore, many patients have a component of cardiomyopathy as well as constrictive pericarditis, accounting for the well known less satisfactory outcome after pericardiectomy compared with constrictive pericarditis of other aetiology (see Chapter 6).

10.1 Pathology

Fourteen (14) of 20 patients autopsied at Mayo Clinic, in whom pericardial tissue was available, had pericardiopathy. The mean radiation dose was 4,400 rads. Six of these had presented with pericardial effusion, three with constrictive pericarditis and two with effusive constrictive pericarditis. Constriction developed considerably later than effusion.

The parietal pericardium is predominantly affected, but the visceral pericardium is not always spared. The histology includes replacement of pericardial fat by collagen, and large bizarre fibroblasts (*Arsenian 1991*). Involvement of the visceral layer explains effusive-constrictive pericarditis. It should be noted that the visceral pericardium in effusive-constrictive pericarditis, although the source of severe constriction, need not be greatly thickened. In the myocardium, thick bundles of Type 1 collagen replace the thinner, more elastic Type 2 collagen, contributing to reduction of ventricular compliance (*Chello, Mastroroberto, Romano 1996*). It is tempting to speculate that the same alteration of the ratio of Type 1 to Type 2 collagen also occurs in the pericardium but, to my knowledge, this has not been demonstrated.

10.2   Dose response

Many patients treated had at least 60 percent of the cardiac silhouette irradiated. The incidence of cardiac or pericardial injury varied from 6.6 to 29 percent of various series, reviewed for a consensus conference. When a small volume of the heart was irradiated, tolerance was greater and incidence less (*Stewart, Fajardo, Gilllette 1995*). These investigators reported that when a large volume of the heart was exposed to irradiation, a dose 40 Gy in 20 fractions over a four-week period was well tolerated, but with higher doses, the incidence increased. When a small heart volume was irradiated,, the tolerated dose increased to 60 Gy in fractions of 30 in six weeks. Again, the incidence of cardio-pericardial injury increased sharply when the dose was increased above that. The thickness of the pericardium increases in proportion to the radiation dose. Anti-neoplastic agents, especially adriamycin, induce cardiomyopathy and, not surprisingly, decrease tolerance to cardiovascular radiation exposure. Most likely, this synergism applies to the pericardium as well.

10.3   Associated lesions of the heart

Mediastinal radiation damages the heart as well as the pericardium, as mentioned above and in earlier chapters of this volume. Ionising radiation causes premature coronary occlusions, valvular stenoses, and endocardial fibrosis, and thus is often an element of pancardiopathy. The severity of these cardiac lesions, in relation to that of the pericardium, has a lot to do with the clinical course and response to treatment. They deserve serious consideration when planning management.

For the last several years, I have been following a patient who, while in the Navy, witnessed an atomic explosion while on the deck of a warship. He was not wearing any protective clothing. The first sequel to be recognised was severe hypothyroidism, soon followed by a pericardial effusion requiring pericardiocentesis. When I saw him first, many years later, he had severe diastolic dysfunction, moderately severe aortic stenosis and mild stenosis of the pulmonary valve. The aortic stenosis progressed over the years to the point that the valve needed to be replaced. The findings at extensive preoperative evaluation suggested constriction of the right ventricle and left ventricular diastolic dysfunction of myocardial origin. At operation, the pericardium over the right heart was greatly thickened and constricted the right ventricle. Constriction of the left ventricle was mild. He improved considerably after aortic valve replacement and removal of pericardium from the right heart.

Improved dosimetry, and increased awareness by radiotherapists of the risk and consequences of inadvertent heavy exposure of large volumes of the heart are responsible for a decreasing incidence of this complication; and this trend will likely continue. Surgeons are increasingly appreciative of the risk for a poor outcome of pericardiectomy for constriction in patients who have had mediastinal radiation. These patients will be evaluated for evidence of myocardial damage so that more patients at high risk for mortality or inadequate relief will be excluded from selection for pericardiectomy.

References

Alukal MK, Costello PB, Green FA. Cardiac tamponade in systemic juvenile rheumatoid arthritis requiring emergency pericardiectomy. J Rheumatol 1984; 11:222-225.

Ansari A, Larson PH, Bates HD. Vascular manifestations of systemic lupus erythematosus. Angiology. 1986; 37:423-432

Arciniegas E, Hakimi M, Farooki ZQ, Green EW. Intrapericardial teratoma in infancy. J Thorac Cardiovasc Surg 1980; 79:306-311.

Arsenian MA. Cardiovascular sequelae of therapeutic thoracic radiation. Prog Cardiovasc Dis 1991; 33:299-311.

Baille M. On the want of a pericardium in the human body. Trans Soc Improve Med Chir Knowl 1793; 1:91-102.

Bandeira FC, de Sa VP, Moriguti JC, Rodrigues AJ, Jurca MC, et al. Cardiac tamponade: an unusual complication of pericardial cyst. J Am Soc Echocardiogr 1996; 9:108-112.

Barbaro G, Klatt EC. HIV infection and the cardiovascular system. AIDS Rev. 2002; 4:93-103.

Barnes PF, Bloch AB, Davidson PT, Snider DE Jr. Tuberculosis in patients with human immunodeficiency virus infection. N Engl J Med 1991; 324:1644-1650

Bennett RM. Clinical manifestations of mixed connective tissue disease. UpToDate,2002,10.3.

Bialek R, Feucht A, Aepinus C, Just-Nubling G, Robertson VJ, et al. Evaluation of two nested PCR assays for detection of Histoplasma capsulatum DNA in human tissue. J Clin Microbiol. 2002; 40:1644-1647.

Black, RM. Pericarditis in renal failure. UpToDate 2002, 10.2

Blaser MJ, Reingold AL, Alsever RN, Hightower A. Primary meningococcal pericarditis: a disease of adults associated with serogroup C Neisseria meningitidis. Rev Infect Dis 1984; 6:625-632

Boscherini B, Galasso C, Bitti ML. Abnormal face, congenital absence of the left pericardium, mental retardation, and growth hormone deficiency. Am J Med Genet 1994; 49:111-113.

Bridgman PG. Failure of intrapericardial streptokinase in purulent pericarditis. Intensive Care Med. 2001; 27:942

Bright R. Tabular view of the morbid appearances in 100 cases connected with albuminous urine. Guy's Hospital Rep 1836; 1:380-400

Burke A, Johns JP, Virmani R. Hemangiomas of the heart. A clinicopathologic study of ten cases. Am J Cardiovasc Pathol 1990; 3:283-290. Review.

Buselmeier TJ, Davin TD, Simmons RL, Najarian JS, Kjellstrand CM. Treatment of intractable uremic pericardial effusion. Avoidance of pericardiectomy with local steroid instillation. JAMA 1978; 240:1358-1359.

Byers RJ, Marshall DA, Freemont AJ. Pericardial involvement in systemic sclerosis. Ann Rheum Dis 1997; 56:393-394.

Caird R, Conway N, McMillan IK. Purulent pericarditis followed by early constriction in young children. Br Heart J 1973; 35:201-203

Canver CC, Patel AK, Kosolcharoen P, Voytovich MC. Fungal purulent constrictive pericarditis in a heart transplant patient. Ann Thorac Surg 1998; 65:1792-1794

Cegielski JP, Devlin BH, Morris AJ, Kitinya JN, Pulipaka UP et al. Comparison of PCR, culture, and histopathology for diagnosis of tuberculous pericarditis. J Clin Microbiol 1997; 35:3254-3257.

Chavez CM, Causey WA, Conn JH. Constrictive pericarditis due to infection with Nocardia asteroides. Chest 1972; 61:79-81

Chello M, Mastroroberto P, Romano R, Zofrea S, Bevacqua I, Marchese AR. Changes in the proportion of types I and III collagen in the left ventricular wall of patients with post-irradiative pericarditis. Cardiovasc Surg. 1996; 4:222-226.

Cheung PK, Myers ML, Arnold JM. Early constrictive pericarditis and anemia after Dressler's syndrome and inferior wall myocardial infarction. Br Heart J 1991; 65:360-362.

Choo PS, McCormack JG. Mycobacterium avium: a potentially treatable cause of pericardial effusions. J Infect 1995; 30:55-58.

Colombo A, Olson HG, Egan J, Gardin JM. Etiology and prognostic implications of a large pericardial effusion in men. Clin Cardiol 1988; 11:389-394.

Connolly HM, Click RL, Schattenberg TT, Seward JB, Tajik AJ. Congenital absence of the pericardium: echocardiography as a diagnostic tool. J Am Soc Echocardiogr 1995; 8:87-92.

Corey GR, Campbell PT, Van Trigt P, Kenney RT, O'Connor CM, et al. Etiology of large pericardial effusions. Am J Med 1993; 95:209-213.

Correale E, Maggioni AP, Romano S, Ricciardiello V, Battista R, et al. Comparison of frequency, diagnostic and prognostic significance of pericardial involvement in acute myocardial infarction treated with and without thrombolytics. Gruppo Italiano per lo Studio della Sopravvivenza nell'Infarto Miocardico (GISSI). Am J Cardiol 1993; 71:1377-1381

Cottrill CM, Tamaren J, Hall B. Sternal defects associated with congenital pericardial and cardiac defects. Cardiol Young 1998; 8:100-104.

Dempke W, Firusian N. Treatment of malignant pericardial effusion with 32P-colloid. Br J Cancer 1999; 80:1955-1957.

DeValeria PA, Baumgartner WA, Casale AS, Greene PS, Cameron DE, et al. Current indications, risks, and outcome after pericardiectomy. Ann Thorac Surg. 1991; 52:219-224.

Di Pasquale G, Ruffini M, Piolanti S, Gambari PI, Roversi R, et al. Congenital absence of pericardium as unusual cause of T wave abnormalities in a young athlete. Clin Cardiol 1992; 15:859-861.

Doherty NE 3rd, Feldman G, Maurer G, Siegel RJ. Echocardiographic findings in systemic lupus erythematosus. Am J Cardiol 1988; 61:1144

Dressler W. The post-myocardial infarction syndrome. Arch Intern Med 1959; 103:28-42.

Drobniewski F, Eltringham I, Graham C, Magee JG, Smith EG, et al. A national study of clinical and laboratory factors affecting the survival of patients with multiple drug resistant tuberculosis in the UK. Thorax 2002; 57:810-816.

Dubois C, Smeets JP, Demoulin JC, Pierard L, Henrard L, Frequency and clinical significance of pericardial friction rubs in the acute phase of myocardial infarction. Eur Heart J 1985; 6:766-768.

Dupre M, O'Leary JP. The first successful closure of a laceration of the pericardium. Am Surg 1997; 63:372-374.

Dye C, Garnett GP, Sleeman K, Williams BG. Prospects for worldwide tuberculosis control under the WHO DOTS strategy. Directly observed short-course therapy. Lancet 1998; 12; 352:1886-1891.

Ellis K, Leeds NE, Himmelstein A. Congenital deficiencies in the parietal pericardium. A review with two new cases including successful diagnosis by plain roentgenography. Am J Roentgenol 1959; 82:125-137.

Faul JL, Hoang K, Schmoker J, Vagelos RH, Berry GJ. Constrictive pericarditis due to coccidiomycosis. Ann Thorac Surg 1999; 68:1407-1409.

Finkelstein Y, Adler Y, Nussinovitch M, Varsano I, Amir J. A new classification for pericarditis associated with meningococcal infection. Eur J Pediatr. 1997;;156:585-588

Frommer JP, Young JB, Ayus JC. Asymptomatic pericardial effusion in uremic patients: effect of long-term dialysis. Nephron 1985; 39:296-301.

Fuchs S, Weiss AT, Elami A, Zahger D. Sudden hemorrhagic tamponade simulating subacute ventricular rupture after acute myocardial infarction. Int J Cardiol 1997; 60:219-220.

Fukuda N, Oki T, Iuchi A, Tabata T, Manabe K, et al. Pulmonary and systemic venous flow patterns assessed by transesophageal Doppler echocardiography in congenital absence of the pericardium. Am J Cardiol 1995; 75:1286-1288.

Fulda G, Rodriguez A, Turney SZ, Cowley RA. Blunt traumatic pericardial rupture. A ten-year experience 1979 to 1989. J Cardiovasc Surg (Torino) 1990; 31:525-530

Galve E, Garcia-del-Castillo H, Evangelista A, Batlle J, Permanyer-Miralda G, et al. Pericardial effusion in the course of myocardial infarction: Incidence, natural history, and clinical relevance. Circulation 1986; 73:294-299

Gassner I, Judmaier W, Fink C, Lener M, Waldenberger F, et al. Diagnosis of congenital pericardial defects, including a pathognomic sign for dangerous apical ventricular herniation, on magnetic resonance imaging. Br Heart J 1995; 74:60-66.

Gibbs CR, Watson RD, Singh SP, Lip GY. Management of pericardial effusion by drainage: a survey of 10 years' experience in a city centre general hospital serving a multiracial population. Postgrad Med J 2000; 76:809-813.

Gossinger HD, Siostrzonek P, Zangeneh M, Neuhold A, Herold C, et al. Magnetic resonance imaging findings in a patient with pericardial mesothelioma. Am Heart J 1988; 115:1321-1322.

Gupta S, Lokhandwala YY. Transient tuberculous constrictive pericarditis. Indian Heart J 1996; 48:65-67.

Hammerman H, Alker KJ, Schoen FJ, Kloner RA. Morphologic and functional effects of piroxicam on myocardial scar formation after coronary occlusion in dogs. Am J Cardiol 1984; 53:604-607

Hano O, Baba T, Hayano M, Yano K. Congenital defect of the left pericardium with sick sinus syndrome. Am Heart J 1996; 132:1293-1295.

Hayes-Lattin BM, Kovach PA, Henner WD, Beer TM. Successful treatment of metastatic hormone-refractory prostate cancer with malignant pericardial tamponade using docetaxel. Urology. 2002; 59:137.

Hesselink JR, Chung KJ, Peters ME, Crummy AB. Congenital partial eventration of the left diaphragm. AJR Am J Roentgenol 1978; 131:417-419.

Jacob JL, Souza Junior AS, Parro Junior A. Absence of the left pericardium diagnosed by computed tomography. Int J Cardiol 1995; 47:293-296.

Jamieson TW. Adult Still's disease complicated by cardiac tamponade. JAMA. 1983; 249:2065-2066.

Kahl LE. The spectrum of pericardial tamponade in systemic lupus erythematosus. Report of ten patients. Arthritis Rheum 1992; 35:1343-1349.

Kaneko Y, Okabe H, Nagata N. Complete left pericardial defect with dual passage of the phrenic nerve: a challenge to the widely accepted embryogenic theory. Pediatr Cardiol 1998; 19:414-417.

Kerber RE, Sherman B. Echocardiographic evaluation of pericardial effusion in myxedema. Incidence and biochemical and clinical correlations. Circulation 1975; 52:823-827.

Kilburn CD, McKinsey DS. Recurrent massive pleural effusion due to pleural, pericardial, and epicardial fibrosis in histoplasmosis. Chest. 1991; 100:1715-1717.

Klacsmann PG, Bulkley BH, Hutchins GM. The changed spectrum of purulent pericarditis: an 86 year autopsy experience in 200 patients. Am J Med. 1977; 63:666-673

Koh KK, Kim EJ, Cho CH, Choi MJ, Cho SK, et al. Adenosine deaminase and carcinoembryonic antigen in pericardial effusion diagnosis, especially in suspected tuberculous pericarditis. Circulation 1994; 89:2728-2735.

Krishnan MN, Babu KM, Govindan KP. Congenital partial absence of left pericardium: demonstration by computed tomography after artificial pneumothorax. Indian Heart J 1996; 48:63-64.

Larrieu AJ, Wiener I, Alexander R, Wolma FJ. Pericardiodiaphragmatic hernia. Am J Surg 1980; 139:436-440.

Li JS. Corey RG, Sexton DJ. Tuberculous pericarditis. UpTo Date. Online 10.2. 2002

Llewellyn MJ, Atkinson MW, Fabri B: Pericardial constriction caused by primary mesothelioma. Br Heart J 1987; 57:54-57.

Lorrell BH, Braunwald E. Pericardial Disease. In Heart Disease: A Textbook of Cardiovascular Medicine (Ed 4). E Braunwald (Editor) Philadelphia, W. B. Saunders Company, 1992.

Maher EA, Shepherd FA, Todd TJR. Pericardial sclerosis as the primary management of malignant pericardial effusion and cardiac tamponade. J Thorac Cardiovasc Surg 1996; 112:637-643.

Maisch B, Kochsiek K. Humoral immune reactions in uremic pericarditis. Am J Nephrol 1983; 3:264-271.

Matsuhisa M, Shimomura K, Beppu S, Nakajima K. Jugular phlebogram in congenital absence of the pericardium. Am Heart J 1986; 112:1004-1010.

Mayosi BM, Volmink JA, Commerford PJ. Interventions for treating tuberculous pericarditis. Cochrane Database Syst Rev. 2000;(2):CD000526. Review.

Meleca MJ, Hoit BD. Previously unrecognized intrapericardial hematoma leading to refractory abdominal ascites. Chest. 1995; 108:1747-1748.

Minocha GK, Falicov RE, Nijensohn E. Partial right-sided congenital pericardial defect with herniation of right atrium and right ventricle. Chest 1979; 76:484-486.

Morgan JR, Rogers AK, Forker AD. Congenital absence of the left pericardium. Clinical findings. Ann Intern Med 1971; 74:370-376.

Narins CR, Cunningham MJ, Delehanty JM, Risher WH, Singh DV. Nonhemorrhagic cardiac tamponade after penetrating chest trauma. Am Heart J 1996; 132:197-198

Nasser WK. Congenital absence of the left pericardium. Am J Cardiol 1970; 26:466-470.

Nasser W, Feigenbaum H, Helmen C. Congenital absence of the left pericardium. Circulation 1966; 34:100-104.

Nasser WK, Helmen C, Tavel ME, Feigenbaum H, Fisch C. Congenital absence of the left pericardium. Clinical, electrocardiographic, radiographic, hemodynamic, and angiographic findings in six cases. Circulation 1970; 41:469-478.

Obendorf DL, Presidente PJA. Foreign body perforation of the esophagus mitiating traumatic pericarditis in an Australian fur seal. J Wildl Dis 1978; 14:451-454.

Oki T, Tabata T, Yamada H, Manabe K, Fukuda K, et al. Cross sectional echocardiographic demonstration of the mechanisms of abnormal interventricular septal motion in congenital total absence of the left pericardium. Heart 1997; 77:247-251.

Oliva PB, Hammill SC, Talano JV. T wave changes consistent with epicardial involvement in acute myocardial infarction. Observations in patients with a postinfarction pericardial effusion without clinically recognized postinfarction pericarditis. J Am Coll Cardiol 1994; 24:1073-1077.

Oudiz R, Mahaisavariya P, Peng SK, Shane-Yospur L, Smith C, et al. Disseminated coccidioidomycosis with rapid progression to effusive-constrictive pericarditis. J Am Soc Echocardiogr 1995; 8:947-952.

Permanyer-Miralda G, Sagrista-Sauleda J, Soler-Soler J. Primary acute pericardial disease: a prospective series of 231 consecutive patients. Am J Cardiol 1985; 56:623-630

Phillips TF, Rodriguez A, Cowley RA. Right ventricular outflow obstruction secondary to right-sided tamponade following myocardial trauma. Ann Thorac Surg 1983; 36:353-358.

Pickhardt PJ. Congenital absence of the pericardium confirmed by spontaneous pneumothorax. Clin Imaging 1998; 22:404-407.

Pocock WA, Lakier JB, Benjamin JD. Billowing mitral valve syndrome in association with absent left pericardium. A case report. SA Med J 1977; 52:813-816.

Prager RL, Burney DP, Waterhouse G, Bender HW Jr. Pulmonary, mediastinal, and cardiac presentations of histoplasmosis. Ann Thorac Surg 1980; 30:385-390.

Prager RL, Wilson CH, Bender HW Jr. The subxiphoid approach to pericardial disease. Ann Thorac Surg 1982; 34:6-9

Quigg RJ Jr, Idelson BA, Yoburn DC, Hymes JL, Schick EC, et al. Local steroids in dialysis-associated pericardial effusion. A single intrapericardial administration of triamcinolone. Arch Intern Med 1985; 145:2249-2250.

Risher WH, Rees AP, Ochsner JL, McFadden PM. Thoracoscopic resection of pericardium for symptomatic congenital pericardial defect. Ann Thorac Surg 1993; 56:1390-1391.

Roberts GD, Goodman NL, Heifets L, Larsh HW, Lindner TH, et al. Evaluation of the BACTEC radiometric method for recovery of mycobacteria and drug susceptibility testing of Mycobacterium tuberculosis from acid-fast smear-positive specimens. J Clin Microbiol 1983; 18:689-696.

Rodgers BM, Moulder PV, DeLaney A. Thoracoscopy: new method of early diagnosis of cardiac herniation. J Thorac Cardiovasc Surg. 1979; 78:623-625.

Roebuck EJ, Minford J. Traumatic rupture of the pericardium with herniation of the heart. Br J Radiol 1983; 56:585-588.

Rostand SG, Rutsky EA. Pericarditis in end-stage renal disease. Cardiol Clin 1990; 8:701-707.

Saad MF, Frazier OH, Hickey RC, Samaan NA. Intrapericardial pheochromocytoma. Am J Med 1983; 75:371-376.

Sagrista-Sauleda J, Merce J, Permanyer-Miralda G, Soler-Soler J. Clinical clues to the causes of large pericardial effusions. Am J Med 2000; 109:95-101.

Satur CM, Hsin MK, Dussek JE. Giant pericardial cysts. Ann Thorac Surg 1996; 61:208-210.

Schultz-Hector S. Radiation-induced heart disease: review of experimental data on dose response and pathogenesis. Int J Radiat Biol 1992; 61:149-160.

Sentongo TAS, Piccoli DA. Recurrent pericarditis due to mesalamine hypersensitivity: a pediatric case report and review of the literature. J Pediatr Gastroenterol Nutr 1998; 27:344-347.

Sexton DJ, Corey GR. Purulent pericarditis UpTodate 10.2: 2002.

Shah A, Askari AD. Pericardial changes and left ventricular function in ankylosing spondylitis. Am Heart J 1987; 113:1529-1531.

Shehata AR, Gillam LD, Weisburst MR, Chen C. Pericardial hematoma causing saphenous vein graft compression. Am Heart J 1996; 131:598-599.

Shepherd FA. Malignant pericardial effusion. Current Opinion Oncol 1997; 9:170-174

Simeonov SP. Clinical and paraclinical changes in cattle with traumatic pericarditis before and after pericardial puncture. Vet Med Nauki 1978; 15:114-119.

Singh S, Singh AB, Didwania SK, Singh RJ. Amoebic pericardial effusion. J Indian Med Assoc. 1987; 85:271-273

Smith DN, Shaffer K, Patz EF: Imaging features of nonmyxomatous primary neoplasms of the heart and pericardium. Clinical Imaging 1998; 22:15-22

Smolar EN, Rubin JE, Avramides A, Carter AC. Cardiac tamponade in primary myxedema and review of the literature. Am J Med Sci 1976; 272: 345-352.

Southworth H, Stevenson CS. Congenital defects of the pericardium. Arch Intern Med 1938; 61:223-240.

Spodick DH. Medical history of the pericardium. Am J Cardiol 1970; 26:447-454.

Stewart JR, Fajardo LF, Gillette SM, Constine LS. Radiation injury to the heart. Int J Radiat Oncol Biol Phys 1995; 31:1205-1211.

Strang JI, Kakaza HH, Gibson DG, Allen BW, Mitchison DA, et al. Controlled clinical trial of complete open surgical drainage and of prednisolone in treatment of tuberculous pericardial effusion in Transkei. Lancet 1988; 2:759-764.

Strang JI, Kakaza HH, Gibson DG, Girling DJ, Nunn AJ, et al. Controlled trial of prednisolone as adjuvant in treatment of tuberculous constrictive pericarditis in Transkei. Lancet. 1987; 2:1418-1422.

Surawicz B. Diseases of the Heart and Lungs. In Chow's Electrocardiography in Clinical Practice. B Surawicz and TK Knilands (eds). Philadelphia, W.B. Saunders Company, 2001.

Suwan PK, Potjalongsilp S. Predictors of constrictive pericarditis after tuberculous pericarditis. Br Heart J 1995; 73:187-189.

Taysi K, Hartmann AF, Shackelford GD, Sundaram V. Congenital absence of left pericardium in a family. Am J Med Genet 1985; 21:77-85.

Thould AK. Constrictive pericarditis in rheumatoid arthritis. Ann Rheum Dis 1986; 45:89-94.

Trautner BW, Darouiche RO. Tuberculous pericarditis: optimal diagnosis and management. Clin Infect Dis. 2001; 33:954-961.

Travaglio-Encinoza A, Anaya JM, Dupuy D'Angeac AD, Reme T, Sany J. Rheumatoid pericarditis: new immunopathological aspects. Clin Exp Rheumatol 1994; 12:313-316.

Tutar HE, Atalay S, Uysalel A, Ozberrak H, Kocak G. Recurrent pericardial effusion due to gunshot wound of the heart in a hemodynamically stable child--a case report. Angiology. 1999; 50:337-340.

Ustunsoy H, Celkan M, Si;vri;koz M, Kazaz H, Kilinc M. Intrapericardial fibrynolytic therapy in purulent pericarditis. Eur J Cardiothorac Surg. 2002; 22:373

Van Offel JF, De Clerck LS, Kersschot IE. Cholesterol crystals and IgE-containing immune complexes in rheumatoid pericarditis. Clin Rheumatol. 1991; 10:78-80.

van Son JA, Danielson GK, Callahan JA. Congenital absence of the pericardium: displacement of the heart associated with tricuspid insufficiency. Ann Thorac Surg 1993; 56:1405-1406.

Wall TC, Califf RM, Harrelson-Woodlief L, Mark DB, Honan M, et al. Usefulness of a pericardial friction rub after thrombolytic therapy during acute myocardial infarction in predicting amount of myocardial damage. The TAMI Study Group. Am J Cardiol 1990; 66:1418-1421.

Wang HJ, Hsu KL, Chiang FT, Tseng CD, Tseng YZ, et al. Technical and prognostic outcomes of double-balloon pericardiotomy for large malignancy-related pericardial effusions. Chest 2002; 122:893-899.

Wang PC, Yang KY, Chao JY, Liu JM, Perng RP, et al. Prognostic role of pericardial fluid cytology in cardiac tamponade associated with non-small cell lung cancer. Chest 2000; 118:744-749.

Wheat LJ, Stein L, Corya BC, Wass JL, Norton JA, et al. Pericarditis as a manifestation of histoplasmosis during two large urban outbreaks. Medicine (Baltimore). 1983; 62:110-119.

Wiener HG, Kristensen IB, Haubek A, Kristensen B, Baandrup U. The diagnostic value of pericardial cytology: An analysis of 95 cases. Acta Cytol 1991; 35:149-153

Wilkins HE 3rd, Cacioppo J, Connolly MM, Marquez G, Grays P. Intrapericardial interferon in the management of malignant pericardial effusion. Chest 1998; 114:330-331.

Winter WE 3rd, Seidman J, Krivak TC, Pujari SG, Boice CR, et al. Papillary serous adenocarcinoma of the ovary diagnosed after malignant pericardial tamponade and embolic stroke. Gynecol Oncol. 2002; 84:453-455.

Wooley CF, Hosier DM. Constrictive pericarditis due to Histoplasma capsulatum. N Engl J Med 1961; 264:1230-1232

Yamagishi T, Ishikawa S, Yoshida I, Ohtaki A, Takahashi T, et al. Thoracoscopic closure of a congenital partial pericardial defect. Surg Today 1997; 27:874-875

Zakowski MF, Ianuale-Shanerman A. Cytology of pericardial effusions in AIDS patients. Diagn Cytopathol. 1993; 9:266-269

Index